PATHOLOGY
ANNUAL
1969

SERIES EDITOR

SHELDON C. SOMMERS, M. D.

Director of Laboratories, Lenox Hill Hospital, New York, New York;
Clinical Professor of Pathology, Columbia University College of
Physicians and Surgeons, New York, New York; Clinical Professor
of Pathology, University of Southern California School of Medicine,
Los Angeles, California

PATHOLOGY
ANNUAL

VOLUME 4

1969

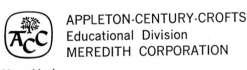
APPLETON-CENTURY-CROFTS
Educational Division
MEREDITH CORPORATION

New York

CONTRIBUTORS

Ralph Alley, M.D.

Subdepartment of Thoracic Surgery, Albany Medical Center Hospital, Albany, New York

Roland E. Berry, M.D.

Chief of Laboratory, Department of Clinical and Anatomic Pathology, St. Francis Hospital, Escabana, Michigan

Maurice M. Black, M.D.

Professor of Pathology and Attending Pathologist, New York Medical College-Flower and Fifth Avenue Hospitals, New York, New York

Drummond H. Bowden, M.D.

Professor, Department of Pathology, Faculty of Medicine, University of Manitoba, Winnipeg, Manitoba, Canada

Ada B. Chabon, M.D.

Assistant Professor of Pathology and Assistant Attending Pathologist, New York Medical College-Flower and Fifth Avenue Hospitals, New York, New York

Diane W. Crocker, M.D.

Associate Pathologist, Peter Bent Brigham Hospital; Assistant Clinical Professor of Pathology, Harvard Medical School, Boston, Massachusetts

G. A. Fattal, M.D.

Associate Professor, Department of Pathology, Faculty of Medicine, University of Manitoba; Pathologist, Winnipeg General Hospital, Winnipeg, Manitoba, Canada

Gerald Fine, M.D.

Department of Pathology, Henry Ford Hospital, Detroit, Michigan

Edwin R. Fisher, M.D.

Professor of Pathology, University of Pittsburgh; Chief of Laboratory Service, Veterans Administration Hospital, Pittsburgh, Pennsylvania

George F. Gray, Jr., M.D.

Assistant Professor of Pathology, Cornell University Medical College; Assistant Attending Pathologist, The New York Hospital, New York, New York

Robert C. Horn, Jr., M.D.

Department of Pathology, Henry Ford Hospital, Detroit, Michigan

Aubrey Kagan, M.R.C.P., M.B., B.S., D.P.H.

Chief, Epidemiology of Non-Communicable Diseases Unit, Division of Research in Epidemiology and Communications Science, World Health Organization, Geneva, Switzerland

Jacqueline Mauro, M.D., F.A.C.P.

Department of Pathology, Albany Medical Center Hospital, Albany, New York

Robert W. McDivitt, M.D.

Associate Professor of Pathology, Cornell University Medical College; Associate Attending Pathologist, The New York Hospital, New York, New York

Vincent J. McGovern, M.D.

Director, Fairfax Institute of Pathology, Royal Prince Alfred Hospital, Camperdown, New South Wales, Australia.

Donald G. McKay, M.D.

Professor of Pathology, University of California School of Medicine; Pathologist, San Francisco General Hospital, San Francisco, California

Pamela Morgan, B.A. (Econ.)

Research Associate, Department of Pathology, Faculty of Medicine and Institute of Computer Studies, University of Manitoba, Winnipeg, Manitoba, Canada

Holde Puchtler, M.D.

Department of Pathology, Medical College of Georgia; Eugene Talmadge Memorial Hospital, Augusta, Georgia

Sidney L Saltzstein, M.D.

Associate Professor of Pathology, University of California, San Diego School of Medicine; Chief of Surgical Pathology, University Hospital of San Diego County, San Diego, California

Arthur A. Stein, M.D.

Professor of Pathology, Albany Medical Center Hospital, Albany, New York

Leland D. Stoddard, M.D.

Professor and Chairman, Department of Pathology, Medical College of Georgia; Eugene Talmadge Memorial Hospital, Augusta, Georgia

Lloyd Thibodeau

Electron Microscopy Senior Technician, Albany Medical Center Hospital, Albany, New York

Draga Vesselinovitch, M.D.

Department of Pathology, The University of Chicago School of Medicine, Chicago, Illinois

John P. Wyatt, M.D.

Professor and Head, Department of Pathology, Faculty of Medicine, University of Manitoba, Winnipeg, Manitoba, Canada

Robert W. Wissler, Ph.D., M.D.

Professor and Chairman, Department of Pathology, The University of Chicago School of Medicine, Chicago, Illinois

CONTENTS

PATHOLOGY
ANNUAL
1969

BREAKING THE BARRIER BETWEEN PATHOLOGIST AND EPIDEMIOLOGIST

AUBREY KAGAN

As an epidemiologist, I have been working closely with pathologists from several countries for nine years. Our relationship has been friendly and, we think, productive. I had long forgotten that there was a time when we could not understand one another. A reminder of those far off days came recently in reply to something slightly iconoclastic said at a multidisciplinary meeting. A pathologist rose and, with much emotion and little science, showed that his understanding of what had been said was far from complete. My quandary was whether to explain things clearly and at some length, or whether to say the minimum, make a joke, and tell him afterwards. I was still undecided when, as I was about to speak, I realized he had given me the subject and several of the headings for this paper. In gratitude I chose the second course.

Difficulties in understanding between epidemiologist and pathologist are not due to lack of intelligence; rather, the reverse is true. What is acceptable to a fool is not at all reasonable to an intelligent man without prior test.

Different Approaches

There are basic differences in the way in which pathologists and epidemiologists are trained to work. The former studies in detail, and with great care, many aspects of a particular problem at the molecular, cell, tissue, organ, or organism levels. The epidemiologist considers, usually with little detail, a few aspects of a particular problem in large numbers of subjects—groups, communities, populations.

1

Judgement is made in different ways. The epidemiologist tends to be more objective and to test his judgement by the application of rigid mathematical rules. The pathologist tends to be more subjective and to have less rigid rules and a fine disregard for mathematics. The epidemiologist, often unable to be deterministic, accepts with relief the idea of probability and happily makes decisions on this basis that can be applied to groups. The pathologist, wishing to make a decision on an individual case, shuns the idea of probability and seeks determinism.

There is no implication that one method of forming a judgement or decision will be right and the other wrong. They only represent trends. The epidemiologist is not always objective, and the pathologist is not always subjective. While it is desirable to use mathematical rules to test judgement, this needs to be tempered with common sense. Many people have good judgement without any knowledge of mathematics; they apply logical rules intuitively. There are times when the epidemiologist should be more deterministic, and there are times when the pathologist must accept the idea of probability. The differences in approach are due to training and they help to create a barrier of mutual suspicion between those who practice the two disciplines.

Breaking the Barrier

At first my pathologist colleagues often could not agree with each other on subjects in the domain of pathology. They were united in their disagreement with me on subjects concerning epidemiology. It is to their merit that they accepted the idea of submitting all procedures and hypotheses to scientific tests. From that moment we were able to work together, and our mutual understanding arose out of this.

The extraordinary thing is that scientifically minded people often neglect to apply scientific tests. These are particularly needed in developing methods and study design and in assessing results. However, the initial stages of an investigation involve stating hypotheses and defining terms. The former does not, in my experience, give rise to difficulties in communication; the latter does.

Working Definitions

Nicholas Kagan has drawn in symbolic terms the difficulty of agreement on definitions (see p. 3). The scientists stand at the frontier of a particular branch of pathology and are looking out to the future in different directions. Because of this, they all have a different viewpoint, and none can agree with the other on the basis of what he sees. The clouds prevent them from seeing that each is looking in a different direction. If they are given a chance to listen to each other, the clouds will blow away and they will see that they are all standing on the same bit of solid land. This area of common agreement will serve as a "working definition" and as a stepping stone to the next piece of firm ground.

Disagreement among scientists is usually on what is not known. Often the proponents of different theories disagree bitterly with each other on these unestablished areas without bothering to listen to each other. However, there is much they for normal and 6.5 to 11.5 μ for pernicious anemia. If we measured only one corpuscle from a patient with pernicious anemia, it might be small. By chance, a single corpuscle from a normal individual might be large (up to 9 μ). The more corpuscles we examine from normal blood, the more likely is the average value to be low, and vice-versa. The chance that a particular average value indicates abnormality can be estimated, depending on how many corpuscles have been counted and the known variation in size of corpuscles in the normal and abnormal case.

For example,* the chance of finding an average diameter of red corpuscles of 8 μ in a normal person would be: 1 in 4 if it is based on a count of 2 corpuscles; 1 in 7 if it is based on a count of 4 corpuscles; less than 1 in 100 if it is based on a count of 16 corpuscles. I have mentioned this at some length because epidemiologists often worry pathologists by asking for larger numbers of cases, and most people believe that you cannot make a "silk purse out of a sow's ear."

If observations are independent and variation is as likely to be too high as too low, discrimination can be improved by increasing the number of observations. This permits a decisive answer to be made when methods are too imprecise for single observations, or when natural variation makes group comparison necessary. The epidemiologist recommends larger numbers of observations for this reason.

Errors of bias can also be reduced by improving definitions, training observers, excluding unsatisfactory observers and apparatus, improving apparatus, and by standardizing techniques, reagents and apparatus. When standards are available, bias may be calculated and the combined observer-apparatus procedure calibrated. This is commonplace in the exact sciences but neglected in medicine.

Bias does not decrease with increased number of observations and thus, unless it is so small that it is not relevant, it must be allowed for or it will obscure differences or similarities. It is therefore essential to assess bias to see if it is large compared with differences found, and if so, to make allowances. Even if a method is not calibratable, it is still possible under some circumstances to reduce bias. The procedure is to convert it to imprecision and to reduce it by increasing the number of observations as necessary. Bias can be turned into imprecision when all objects can be examined independently by one or all observers, or when all objects from all sources to be compared can be shared equally between all observers. Again, the observations must be independent in all cases.

EXAMPLE. Suppose one observer uses a meter rule that is really 120 cm long (i.e., biased to read *low*) and another has a meter rule that is really 80 cm long (i.e., biased to read *high*). If they wish to compare the size of buildings in their own villages, even if they are the same size, the first observer will find his houses approximately 40 percent smaller than the second observer finds his. If each observer had examined houses in his own and the other village he would have found no difference between them. The same would be true if both observers had examined each house

---

*For the mathematician: $\sigma = 0.8$ $\quad \Delta = 0.8$ $\quad$

n = 2	t = 1.4	p = 0.3
n = 4	t = 2	p = 0.15
n = 16	t = 4	p < 0.01

For the near mathematician: I have assumed that 95 percent of the readings fall between 6.4 and 9.6 μ and 99 percent fall between 5.6 and 10.4 μ.

and taken the average value. In each of the ways described so far, the observer has to do twice as much work. The same effect could be obtained if each observer examined half the houses in each village. It would be necessary for the allocation to be made so that each would get an equal chance to examine every kind of house in each village. (It would be best for each observer not to know which village the house came from in case this knowledge biased his judgement. This would not be difficult to obscure in the case of aortas or coronary arteries.[3]) The comparison would now be between the average house in each village.

This method is applicable when there are large numbers of objects to be assessed, a large number of observers, and a means of allocating specimens from each source to be compared without disclosing the source (Professor A. L. Cochrane's "portable data")—for example, observations on preserved specimens or biopsies.

Quality Control

The concept of quality control, borrowed from industry and biochemistry, is designed to maintain high standards at reasonable cost. By examining a sample off the production line, the industrialist can determine if anything has gone wrong in the plant and avert disaster. In scientific investigations, by incorporating some standards or repeat objects in the observers' batches of material, quality control of each observer's "production" can be achieved. If the observer cannot tell which is the test object but knows some will appear, this helps to keep him alert. Abnormal readings will indicate at once that something wrong has happened to the observer or apparatus.

Differences between readings of the same object by the same observer, of the same object by different observers, or of the same object at two widely separated periods of time, will show up and quantify imprecision, inter-observer bias, and inter-sessional trends. These can be allowed for later in determining whether similarities or differences found are real.

Advice from Experts

Having considered the hypothesis one wishes to test and the methods available, one may find that the circumstances necessary for carrying out the study are difficult to attain. Advice from experts will probably be sought. This is quite likely to be false if it is not based on adequate tests.

For example, in a recent investigation, we thought it desirable to study autopsy material from *all* deaths occurring from ten years of age in several communities of about a quarter of a million people. The experts said that this was impossible.

After tests in eight areas, five were found where study was possible. In another area, the autopsy rate for all deaths was 33 percent. The pathologist felt that he saw nearly all coronary or cancer deaths because of special arrangements in the community. On testing, we found he saw very few. Surprisingly, and unknown before to him or to us, the test showed that he saw 84 percent of all deaths in the age group 50 to 54 without any special effort. A further test confirmed this. (Unfortunately we could not continue the study in this community because the pathologist accepted a post elsewhere, and the remaining pathologists in the community were not interested in our study.)

Representative Populations

My pathologist colleagues have, in the past, found the concept of representative population hard to understand. Judging from remarks at multidisciplinary meetings and from published papers, it must be obscure to many now.

Pathologists do not like the idea of studying populations. They cannot easily obtain material from random samples and therefore want to know why they cannot get all the information they want from studying a few selected cases—the material that comes to them easily—carefully. Why does the epidemiologist insist on obtaining a "representative sample," whatever that might mean?

Let me give an obvious example. It is not uncommon, so I am told by publishers of poems, for ladies who have just ceased to be maidens to rush pen in hand to write a serious sonnet on "Sex and the Universe," or something like that. It is absolutely no use, so the publishers say, telling those ladies at this stage that their experience is insufficient to extrapolate to the universe. So would it be too with the pathologist who had just written a dogmatic book on atherosclerosis or coronary thrombosis on the basis of the odd cases that end up at autopsy in his hospital.

An objective in a study is to be able to extrapolate findings beyond the material that has been examined. To do this, the material must be a representative sample of a larger body of material. In hospital studies in general, and in autopsy studies in particular, this is hard to arrange. Not all kinds of sickness are found in hospitals. People with certain diseases may die at home. If it is a speciality or teaching hospital, selection may be very one-sided. Trying to find out about a particular disease or frequency of disease from most hospital autopsy series is like trying to find out about a community by examining the people living in the best hotel.

There is much selection in autopsy, since in many hospitals, only a proportion (and not a representative sample) of people who die are autopsied. Thus, admission may be biased in one direction, death in another, and those who come to autopsy in a third. In such cases, unless the pathologist can show special cause otherwise, it should be assumed that the findings can refer only to the material examined and cannot be extrapolated. J. N. Morris, in searching the London Hospital Pathology Records, was surprised to find ruptured ventricle rarely mentioned, although myocardial infarction was common. Crawford and Morris[5] showed that this was because a large number of subjects with ruptured ventricle (sudden deaths and old people) did not die in the hospital. Many of them were seen in the Coroner's (Medical Examiner's) autopsy room.

Pathologists have claimed that, on the basis of hospital autopsy, thrombus is found in the extramural portion of a main coronary artery in 90 percent of patients dying from acute myocardial "infarction." In a recent series, all kinds of coronary heart disease death were studied and autopsy material examined in 86 percent of all deaths.[9] Of the 176 subjects aged 40 to 59 who died because of acute myocardial "infarction," 25 percent showed no occlusion or thrombus of the main extramural coronary artery. Sixty-three percent of these cases were "sudden deaths," i.e., occurring within six hours of the onset of symptoms. Usually few such cases reach a hospital. It is possible that the pathologist who bases his opinions on hospital autopsy has a false impression however carefully he may have examined such cases. Because he has not examined a *representative sample* of coronary heart disease deaths, he may have lacked the very cases in which thrombus does not occur. He should not extrapolate beyond his particular data because his data are not representative of anything except the material he has examined.

Nonrepresentative data cannot be used to give an indication of the frequency of events in a community. One could not say that, on the basis of hospital admissions or autopsies, disease X or condition Y never, always, seldom, or often occurs in a community. Of course, if it is seen in someone from the community, one can say it does occur, but information on frequency is confined to the data examined if the material is not representative of a wider group.

Association not Causation

Association does not imply causation. However, causation is often found through examination of associations, and the rule is forgotten because it is much easier to jump to a conclusion than to devise a test situation.

Strong associations can arise by chance and be meaningless; e.g., the increase in circulation of a well-known British Sunday newspaper with the increase in carcinoma of the bronchus in England and Wales. Sometimes, however, there is a subtly hidden malignant third factor.

A good example of the latter is the association of hepatitis with treatment of syphilis with arsenicals before penicillin was available. It was long thought that the hepatitis was due to the arsenical. The correct reason was, of course, the transmission of virus via the syringe. The practice was to withdraw the plunger of the syringe to see if blood entered a special viewing chamber between the syringe and the needle before injecting the arsenical. This was to ensure that the arsenical was not injected outside the vein. Unfortunately, although the viewing chamber and needle were changed between patients, it was common practice to use the same syringe, without intervening sterilization, on successive patients. The hepatitis was due to virus transmitted from one patient to another and not to the arsenical that went with it.

Although morphology often gives the clue to the nature of the causative agent, it is not always so. There are times when the same pathologic appearances may be caused by any of several possible agents. Irey[6] cites this as one of the difficulties in determining tissue reactions to drugs. Circumstantial evidence, such as the timing of events or experimental evidence of cause and effect, is needed before judgement can be made. Indeed, this seems to be essential for a rational jump from association to causation whatever the circumstances.

The dictum "association is not cause" is sometimes forgotten because classical teaching makes the issue seem clear. Thus, many, but not all, pathologists and clinicians believe that acute myocardial "infarction" is caused by leucocyte-platelet-fibrin thrombus occluding the large extramural branch of the coronary artery supplying the necrosed area of myocardium.[7] Much barren research and a whole branch of therapeutics and prophylaxis of dubious value has grown around this belief. (It has even been possible to sue a doctor for negligence for not using anticoagulants.) The firm belief is due to the sudden onset with ischemic pain; the frequent finding of an occluding leucocyte-platelet-fibrin thrombus in the artery supplying the area; classical teaching; and animal experimentation.

The first warning that all may not be well with the theory is the evident failure of anticoagulant therapy to prevent many acute attacks, although it does reduce thromboembolic events. Also, it is known that the morphology of the necrosed myocardium is not specific to infarction. Similar large areas of myocardial necrosis have been found in the absence of coronary occlusion. Marigo[8] has found extensive myocardial necrosis, indistinguishable from that found in acute coronary heart disease, in the absence of coronary artery lesions of any kind. Under these circumstances, an unconventional question that might have been asked from logical consideration must now be asked. Is coronary thrombosis the cause or effect of the myocardial lesion in acute myocardial "infarction"?

Circumstantial evidence of a combined epidemiologic-pathologic nature from material already mentioned[9] gives weight to this neglected question. Deaths that pathologists found were due to large acute myocardial "infarctions," but in which coronary occlusion and thrombosis were not found, were examined just as carefully as those in which this condition was found. The former differed from the latter in that sudden death occurred more often and, on the average, atherosclerosis of the coronary arteries was less. This would conform with the concept that myocardial necrosis occurred without the formation of thrombus. Death followed before the thrombus had time to form or because there was insufficient coronary intimal lesion to precipitate a leucocyte-fibrin thrombus. Further weight is given to the latter idea by the finding that the acute myocardial infarction deaths without coronary obstruction that were not sudden, had, on the average, even less coronary atherosclerosis than the sudden ones.[9] On the other hand, in the deaths with coronary occlusion or thrombus, there was no difference in amount of coronary atherosclerosis between those who died suddenly and those who did not.

I do not wish to imply that this proves that coronary thrombus of the type described is always the effect and never the cause of acute myocardial necrosis or vice-versa. The matter has been dealt with here at some length because it illustrates the obliteration of logical thought through classical teaching, and it shows how a combination of epidemiologic and pathologic thought and enquiry may focus attention on a change in direction of study. A great deal of attention is rightly being given by clinicians, pathologists, and epidemiologists to the initiating cause of the "acute coronary attack." Much of this should be deviated from the leucocyte-fibrin-thrombus, which may be innocent, to other possibilities such as embolus from platelet thrombus, arrhythmias, or metabolic disturbance.

Cooperation Between Pathologist and Epidemiologist

I have spent much time explaining some of the difficulties that pathologists have in understanding epidemiologists and have given some explanation of the latter's apparently peculiar behaviour. I hope it will be evident that sometimes the application of epidemiologic principles can be of use to pathologists. I have not dealt explicitly with the advantages to the epidemiologist of the disciplines of pathology. There is no doubt in my mind that these are enormous.

The pathologist's approach gives a chance of understanding the intimate details of vital processes. It permits a clearer diagnosis of disease, its precursors and mechanisms, than other methods, and it sometimes is the only way in which these factors may be assessed. This, coupled with the frequent possibility of quantitating these processes, makes it a valuable method of assessing frequency and extent of disease factors and their association. When pathologic endpoints of disease are frequent and clear-cut, and can be measured precisely on a quantitative scale, they are ideal for use as indicators of failure or success of intervention. This, plus the flexibility of the pathologic approach makes it ideal for testing hypotheses. The spirit of determinism of the pathologist is a salutary corrective to the epidemiologist, making him realize that some aspects of probability are unsatisfactory.

In the past, much of the cooperation between epidemiologist and pathologist has been the tossing of ideas, theories, techniques, from one to the other. Each has made use of this in his own discipline and has modified the theory; in successful cases, one or the other has ended up with a theory of causation or a method of control of diseases that works. The history of the gloriously successful approach to a large number of communicable diseases and some noncommunicable disease is a testimony to this method. It also shows that discoveries of behavior at molecular level can lead to application at the community level, and vice-versa.

For the future, I suspect that this type of cooperation will continue. But I hope a new type of cooperation will develop—the type I have been writing about in this essay, where the disciplines intermingle, give strength to each other, and grow together in unison. This combination of the precise, detailed knowledge in depth of pathology and the logic, analytical power, and breadth of epidemiology is needed to tackle the major problems of today and tomorrow. These are the problems of optimal control, when many factors are partly related to each other and, in combination, cause disease.

Cooperation between clinician and pathologist has led to great advances in clinical medicine and in pathology. The book of community pathology has yet to be written. I see it as a stepping stone to understanding disease in terms of biochemistry. I hope epidemiologists will cooperate with pathologists towards these goals. If my experience is anything to go on, those who do will not regret it.

References

1. Kagan, A. Information on thrombosis as a cause of death from studies promoted by the World Health Organization: Conference on Thrombosis. Washington, National Academy of Science, 1967.
2. Kagan, A., Katsuki, S., Sternby, N.H., and Vaneček, R. Reliability of death certificate data on vascular lesions affecting the central nervous system. Bull. W.H.O., 37:477, 1967.
3. Uemura, K., Sternby, N.H., Vaneček, R., Vihert, A.M., and Kagan, A. Grading atherosclerosis in aorta and coronary arteries obtained at autopsy. Bull. W.H.O., 31:297, 1964.

4. Dodgson, C.L. (alias Carroll, L.); 1876. "The Hunting of the Snark," (Fit the first, second verse) in "Complete Works of Lewis Carroll." Nonesuch Library, London, 1939. Page 680.
5. Crawford, M.D., and Morris, J.N. Ruptured ventricle: Incidence in the population of London, 1957-58. Brit. Med. J., 2:1624, 1960.
6. Irey, N.S. Diagnostic problems and methods in drug induced diseases. Washington, D.C., Registry of Tissue Reactions to Drugs, Armed Forces Institute of Pathology, 1967-8.
7. Mitchell, J.R.A., and Schwartz, C.J. Arterial Disease. Oxford, Blackwell Scientific Publications, 1965.
8. Marigo, C., and Livsic, A.M. Personal communication, 1967.
9. Kagan, A., Sternby, N.H., and Vihert, A.M. Lancet, in press, 1968.

COMPUTER-AIDED INSTRUCTION IN PATHOLOGY

DRUMMOND H. BOWDEN
PAMELA MORGAN

There is increasing concern among medical educators that the traditional methods of instruction are inadequate to meet the demands of modern medical science. The problems presented by the ever-increasing quantity of new knowledge that confronts the student and the rate at which this knowledge becomes obsolete are often compounded by an unfavorable ratio of faculty to students. It is not surprising, therefore, that we have seen, within the past few years, unprecedented activity directed towards the development of new and improved methods of instruction. These efforts usually have been directed to the design of instruments of programmed self-instruction.

Programmed instruction may be defined as the presentation of information by a logical series of steps in which the response of the student to a particular question determines the next question that will be presented. Many different instruments such as programmed texts, scrambled textbooks, and simple, mechanically operated teaching machines have been proven to be effective.[1, 2] Several advantages are usually cited in support of the use of these instruments. Students are thought to learn faster, they retain a larger proportion of the material, and they are enabled to progress at rates attuned to their individual abilities.[3]

There is an increasing awareness, however, that despite the proven merit of these methods in the areas of basic instruction and review, they offer to students of superior intellect few advantages over traditional teaching modes.[4] The programmed method of instruction, even when it is well constructed, may fail completely to motivate the superior student. The interest of this student is more likely to be stimulated when he is exposed to the process of active learning involved in solving problems. This situation is difficult to simulate with programmed texts or simple teaching machines.

The ideal instrument of programmed instruction would be designed with two objectives: first, the presentation of essential facts; second, a recapitulation that demands the use of these facts in the solution of problems. The first objective may be achieved in a number of ways; the second requires the replacement of the traditional interchange between student and instructor by a simulated dialogue in which the initiative is given directly to the student.

This paper recounts our experience with computer-aided instruction. It is presented in three sections: 1) an overall view of the problems encountered when the computer is used in this way; 2) an account of our program on thromboembolism; and 3) critique.

The Computer and Programmed Instruction

The development of teaching machines was already well advanced when it was suddenly overtaken by computer science. The introduction of the computer as a teaching device should, therefore, be regarded as a natural and logical sequence in the evolution of programmed instruction. The capacity of the computer to control the storage of information and access to that information appears to offer several advantages over mechanical teaching devices.

The computer may accept questions from a student and present him with relevant answers from its accumulated data. Thus, the student assumes an active role in his own instruction since the initiative in the computer dialogue rests with him. The computer maintains a continuous record of the dialogue and it uses this to decide whether the student has deficiencies in his knowledge and needs to be presented with a remedial program which he must study before proceeding to the next section of the course. On the other hand, the bright student who races through the exercise may be challenged by a branch of the program that presents a more detailed and penetrating analysis of the instructional material. The capacity of the computer to store a considerable amount of information also makes it possible to record the cumulative performance of the student over a prolonged period. This enables the instructor to observe the performance and assess the progress of the student at any time during the course.

These several attributes suggest that the computer may be, at least on theoretical grounds, the ideal instrument of programmed instruction. There is at present, however, a significant gap between this theoretical ideal and the practical application of the computer as an instructional instrument, although efforts are being made towards the solution of these problems.

The Problem of Language

The interpretation of oral or written responses occurring during an instructional dialogue between a student and a tutor involves a detailed knowledge of the formalities and inconsistencies of natural language. Complete replacement of the tutor demands a machine with a mastery of language equal to that of a man. It is clearly impossible, at present, to program a computer to understand language at this level.[5] Two reasons may be cited: first, and perhaps most important, not enough is known about the analysis of language and the theory of semantics; second, there is the technical problem involved in the construction of a computer large enough to hold the colossal quantity of information that would be necessary to operate such a free and adaptable system. Within these limits, we may now consider what adaptations of natural language are necessary for the development of an automated model of conversation. The interchange between the student and the teacher may be thought of as occurring in four stages: 1) the presentation of the question to the student; 2) the reception of the response from the student; 3) the evaluation of the response; 4) based on the evaluation, the choice of the next question.

The preparation of programmed material, whether for the computer or for conventional instruction, invariably follows this format. It is with the third stage— evaluation of the response—that the greatest difficulty is experienced. A teacher analyses the response of the student using his accumulated knowledge of the subject and, at a more fundamental level, of the language in which it is expressed. Thus, by a process of subconscious analysis, he may be able to understand an almost inarticulate response. When the interchange is automated, the method of analysis and the essential vocabulary of the subject matter must be precisely defined, programmed, and stored in the computer since, in order to evaluate an answer, the machine must be able to recognize or "understand" the correct answer.

Evaluation Techniques

Several techniques have been devised to meet the difficulties inherent in the evaluation of the student's response. Of these, the multiple choice machine devised by Crowder is perhaps the most simple.[6] It is evident, however, that its usefulness as a conversational instrument is limited, because it only tests recognition and does not allow the student to compose his own answers. This difficulty may be overcome by the use of a right-wrong machine. If it is provided with the correct answer, it will decide whether a response is correct or incorrect and, on this basis, present an appropriate new question or statement to the student. This offers a distinct advantage over the multiple choice device since the student is free to construct his own answers. Analysis of these answers, however, still presents a formidable problem.

Consider the length of the response; obviously, it is more difficult to analyze a long reply than a short one. But, there are problems even with the shortest of answers. The computer is able to recognize as correct only those answers that have been programmed and stored in the machine. Any response that has not been defined by the program is automatically stated to be incorrect. The question should, of course, be so worded as to limit the range of possible answers; nevertheless, it is essential that the instructor precisely define the correct response and the various deviations that may be totally or partially acceptable. All correct answers and all of their variations must be accepted. This means a clear declaration of all possible responses and all of the ways in which they may be expressed.

The subject of synonyms may be introduced here, e.g., platelets or thrombocytes, blood clotting or blood coagulation, thrombus or clot. Two approaches may be suggested: the acceptable synonyms may be written into the course material, or a synonym dictionary may be constructed and instructions given that all answers must be checked with this list. With regard to spelling, either the machine is programmed to accept alternative spellings, such as hemorrhage or haemorrhage, or rules must be established for converting words from one spelling to another. The easiest solution to the problem of vocabulary is to present the student with a lexicon containing words that are acceptable to the computer. This technique inevitably limits the freedom of the student to compose his answers.

Preparation of the Data

The various strategies for evaluation just discussed are necessary because the computer does not "understand" but must be presented with rules for comparing information it receives with that which is acceptable. Consequently, those who prepare programmed data for the computer must undertake for themselves most of the analysis that is implied in the term "understanding."

A number of computer "languages" such as Coursewriter (IBM),[7] PILOT (Starkweather),[8] LYRIC (Silvern and Silvern),[9] and our own, have been devised to facilitate the programming of instructional and other material.

There are two components to each of these computer "languages." The first and larger portion, allows the writing of data that already have been analysed under headings such as "information," "question," "acceptable answer," "alternative spelling," etc. This portion remains the same each time it is used, and it is not altered within the program. The second component is dynamic since it specifies how the progress of the student to date should determine his subsequent course. This means that the computer's assessment of each student's progress will be different each time he reaches a branching point.

In a typical system, when the analysis is complete, the coded data are punched on cards which are read into the computer and recorded on magnetic discs. Alternatively, the data may be directly typed into the system on one of the typewriter terminals of the computer. This "on-line" method, though more efficient from the viewpoint of the teacher, is less efficient from the computer-system point of view because it occupies an expensive terminal for a much longer period of time.

The format of the data is usually quite simple. It is not necessary for the instructor to spend many hours in its preparation; a secretary, with no knowledge of the subject matter, or of the computer, may easily be trained to prepare the data from written or tape-recorded source material.

Computer-Aided Instruction at the University of Manitoba

Pathology is at present taught in the second of the four years of medical education. Individual segments of the course are so integrated that the various modes of instruction, lectures, laboratory exercises, and small group tutorials are complementary and reinforce each other. Considerable emphasis is placed on techniques of self-instruction. One method in particular—the programmed clinicopathologic conference—has been shown to be very effective (Bowden, 1967).[10] The students discuss problems arising from their individual studies at weekly tutorial sessions. The system works well but, inevitably, it involves a delay of several days between formulation of a query by the student and discussion with the instructor. Many students have suggested that a more rapid feedback would be of considerable benefit since it would enable them to proceed at their own pace. Theoretical considerations suggested that programmed instruction controlled by the computer could provide this type of feedback to the student. Consequently, in September 1966, the Department of Pathology and the Institute for Computer Studies undertook, as a cooperative venture, the study of computer-aided instruction.

From the computer aspect, the objective was the production of a program that could control the presentation of teaching data and evaluate the response of the student. A secondary consideration was the development of a system which would allow the simultaneous and independent operation of a number of student terminals. From the educational aspect, it was necessary to determine whether the computer could usefully extend the repertoire of available teaching tools and to see if the material presented would be in any way restricted by the limitations of the computer. These two aspects of the project were investigated and developed in parallel.

The Computer Aspect

The requirements of the computer program were the ability to present data to the student in the form of a question or statement, to receive his response, and to provide immediate feedback. This pattern of communication was a basic requisite whatever the subject matter was. Therefore, a program was written which would handle material prepared in a format which indicated its purpose and use. In this way, the computer could manipulate data on any subject, regardless of its meaning. Figure 1 presents an overall plan of the organization of the computer program.

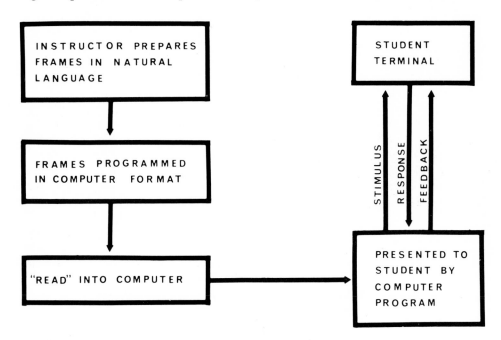

Fig. 1.   Organizational plan.

The preparation of the sequential frames that comprise the instructional program will be discussed in more detail when we consider the educational aspects of the project. At this point it is sufficient to state that the frames were written by the instructor in natural language and prepared for use in the computer.

EQUIPMENT.   The frames, programmed in computer format, were fed into an IBM 360/65 computer by a card reader which transliterates letters and numbers on punch cards into a form which the computer can use. In the early stages of the project, a typewriter was the sole means of communication to the student. Although the method was adequate for the initial testing of the program it was soon evident that the student, naturally anxious to read a whole sentence at a time, became impatient as the machine laboriously typed out a particularly long question or statement. The system was, therefore, adapted to use the IBM 2260 terminal which displays on a television-like screen up to twelve lines of information in less than a second. The terminal has a typewriter keyboard with which the student enters his answer on the screen (Fig. 2).

PROGRAM FORMAT.   The format of the program was such that the computer was used almost exclusively as a right-wrong machine. The student composed his own answers, though the questions were so formulated that only brief replies were necessary. The following example, taken from our instructional program on throm-

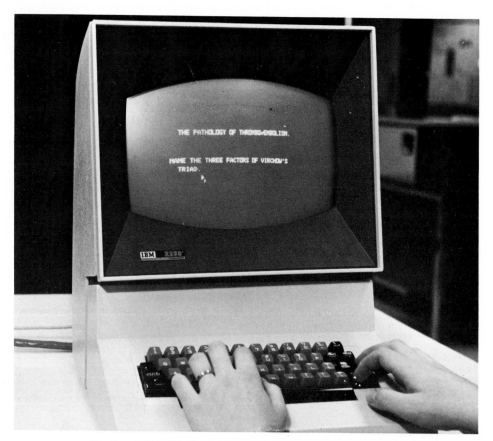

Fig. 2.   IBM 2260 display terminal with typewriter keyboard.

boembolism, illustrates the technique used to translate the frames into computer format.

Format Characters   *Data for Presentation*

D   RESOLUTION BY ENZYMATIC DIGESTION IS NOT ALWAYS ACCOMPLISHED. AS A RESULT OF ENDOTHELIAL AND FIBROBLASTIC PROLIFERATION THE THROMBUS MAY BECOME ORGANIZED.

Q   FUSION OF "INVADING" CAPILLARIES LEADS TO ....

AS   RE-ESTABLISHMENT OF LUMEN
RECANALISATION
RECANALIZATION
RECHANNELISATION
RECHANNELIZATION

The key to the format characters is as follows: D—information in the form of a statement or a display; Q—information in the form of a question, implying expectation of a response by the student; AS—acceptable answers (note that variations in form and spelling have to be written into the program).

The machine was also programmed for the use of multiple choice questions since situations arose in which there seemed to be some advantage to be gained by prompting the student with the display of several alternatives. The following example relates to the blood protein fibrinogen:

D   THE MOLECULAR WEIGHT OF THE CLOTTING PROTEIN ACTIVATED BY THIS ENZYME IS
          A.   69,000
          B.   400,000

AS   B

FEEDBACK AND BRANCHING. The feedback of information from the computer occurred at two levels. The student was provided with an immediate response as to whether his answer was correct or incorrect, and, at the end of the exercise, a cumulative record of his performance was available to the instructor as well as the student (Fig. 3).

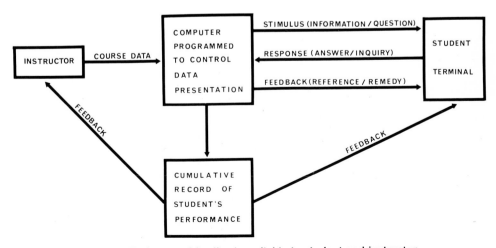

Fig. 3.   Pathways of feedback available to student and instructor.

The records of a group of students could be used by the instructor to evaluate his teaching program. For example, a high proportion of students having difficulty with one particular sector might indicate that this area had not been well taught. The record of the individual student's progress could also be used while the exercise was actually in progress. In our program, only three figures were recorded for each student: the number of questions answered correctly, the number answered incorrectly, and whether the previous answer was right or wrong. These figures could be tallied as integers or percentages so that the progress of the student could be checked at any point to determine whether he knew enough to proceed to the next section of the program.

In many instances, a wrong answer means a misunderstanding of an important fact. It was necessary, therefore, to include a branching mechanism that would automatically move the student forward if his answer were right or, if it were wrong, take him along another pathway which would teach him what was not understood before returning to the main line of the data. This side-stepping of the mainstream of the program is called a remedial loop. The branching technique was also used for clearing up obvious misconceptions. For example, it was found as a result of testing that certain wrong answers recurred more frequently than others. These answers were subsequently listed along with the correct responses that were stored in the computer. Each time a student gave one of these responses he was presented with a frame that explained his error (Fig. 4).

In the preparation of this type of program, the instructor must place the branching or decision points at strategic sites together with an indication, for each possible outcome, of the action that has to be taken. Thus, not only must he organize the presentation of the data by writing each frame with the acceptable answers, but he must also anticipate the student's errors and be prepared to re-explain an important point. The task also involves an assessment of the student's knowledge at specific stages of the exercise so that decisions may be made regarding his subsequent pathways through the course. The computer program allows these decisions to be made at predetermined points.

The Educational Aspect

PILOT STUDY. The first stage of the investigation was a pilot study in which a short and relatively simple exercise was constructed with the express purpose of delineating the major difficulties that may be encountered in a dialogue between a student and a machine. The computer was to be used as a combined teaching-testing machine and not as an instrument of primary instruction. The teaching of pathology would remain unchanged, but at the end of a particular segment of the course the students would, individually, test themselves with the computer.

The exercise was designed as a Socratic dialogue, based on the assumption that, although a student may know most of the basic facts about a particular topic, he may fail, through confusion of thought or lack of analysis, to make a logical use of this knowledge. The computer was programmed to question the student, receive his replies, and immediately correct his wrong answers. The cumulative record main-

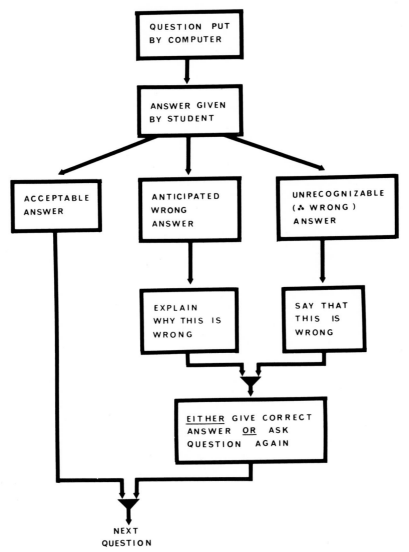

Fig. 4. Branching mechanisms in the computer program.

tained by the machine would enable the instructor to analyse the performance of each student and to extract more general information about the overall effectiveness of the course.

Thromboembolism was chosen as the subject of the computer dialogue because the type of information presented in this portion of the pathology course could easily be adapted to the logical, programmed sequences that are essential to this type of instruction. The program consisted of a series of questions and answers starting with basic clotting mechanisms and progressing to a consideration of the various factors that may be involved in normal flow, stasis, thrombosis, and embolism. A short portion of the program is shown in the following sequence of frames.

D	WE WILL FIRST CONSIDER VENOUS THROMBOSIS:
Q	CONSIDER BLOOD FLOW IN A VEIN. IF FOR ANY REASON THE RATE OF FLOW IS REDUCED, WHICH OF THE FORMED ELEMENTS OF THE BLOOD TEND(S) TO SETTLE OUT FIRST?
AS	PLATELETS THROMBOCYTES
Q	INTRAVASCULAR COAGULATION IS THEREFORE INITI-ATED BY THE ADHERENCE TO THE ENDOTHELIUM OF . . . . .
AS	PLATELETS THROMBOCYTES
Q	RELEASE OF THE PHOSPHOLIPID COMPONENT OF PLATE-LETS LEADS TO THE GENERATION OF . . . . .
AS	THROMBOPLASTIN

Testing of this program revealed a number of defects. Some were related to the limitations of the computer, others to the method in which the material was presented. The most serious problem may be expressed in one word—*language*. The program was designed on the premise that the basic language necessary to the presentation and understanding of thromboembolism was limited and readily defined. Consequently, it was assumed that anyone with an adequate knowledge of this subject would be so familiar with the language that he could readily communicate with the computer. In practice, however, we found that the student frequently used words that the machine did not recognize. This was true even for persons reputed to be expert in the field of thromboembolism.

The program was so constructed that the answers to the questions posed by the computer required the use of few words. But, in fact, they could be expressed in a number of different ways. As a result, correct alternative answers were scored as incorrect if they had not been listed in the computer. Theoretically, the machine should be able to handle all of the possible variations of correct answers, including the recognition of portions of phrases and incorrect spelling. The programming of all of the alternative synonyms, phrases, and spellings, although possible, proved to be an immense and laborious chore. One short example will suffice to illustrate this point.

Q	PHOSPHOLIPID "THROMBOPLASTINS" CAPABLE OF INI-TIATING COAGULATION MAY ALSO BE LIBERATED FROM . . . . .
AS	CELLS, INJURED CELLS, DAMAGED CELLS, ENDOTHE-LIUM, ENDOTHELIAL CELL(S), INJURED ENDOTHELIUM, TISSUE(S), INJURED TISSUE(S), DAMAGED TISSUE(S).

This list, though formidable, is by no means complete, yet any answer that did not match the given words was automatically recorded as wrong.

The difficulties of language resulted, therefore, in a very high rate of error. Since it was obvious that many of these errors were due not to deficiences of knowledge but to the failure of the computer program to recognize correct or partially correct answers, the student often became irritated and aggressive in his attitude to the machine and lost interest in the program.

At this time, the program was evaluated independently by two consultants (J. J. Pear and G. L. Martin) from the Department of Psychology, University of Manitoba. They agreed with our conclusion that it would be difficult to use the computer for the type of Socratic dialogue that we had originally planned.

Two possible solutions were open: either the machine should be programmed to recognize all possible variations of natural language—a prohibitive task, or the student should be taught the same language that was stored in the computer. We decided, therefore, to modify our approach to the investigation by designing a computer program that would instruct the student, simultaneously, in the language and the knowledge necessary to an understanding of the principles of thromboembolism. Subsequently, using the same language, the computer would present the student with a series of clinicopathologic problems related to this material.

The revision of the program was undertaken as a cooperative venture with our colleagues from the Department of Psychology, to whom we express our thanks.

REVISED PROGRAM.   The proposal fell naturally into two separate though interdependent segments: the first instructional; the second problem solving. The design of the instructional segment followed the basic principles of programmed instruction in which material is presented to the student in a series of small steps.[11, 12] At each step, the student was required to compose an answer to which he immediately received a response regarding its accuracy. Each step was built on the preceding ones so that, as the student acquired more knowledge and more words, the prompting that was necessary in the early steps to evoke appropriate responses was gradually eliminated. The following frames illustrate these points:

D	THE MAJOR STEPS IN INTRAVASCULAR BLOOD COAGULATION ARE AS FOLLOWS: A THROMBOPLASTIC SUBSTANCE IS RELEASED FROM AGGREGATED PLATELETS AND FROM INJURED ENDOTHELIUM. THE THROMBOPLASTIC SUBSTANCE(S) INITIATES A CHAIN OF EVENTS WHICH EVENTUALLY LEAD TO THE CONVERSION OF THE BLOOD PROTEIN, FIBRINOGEN, INTO FIBRIN THREADS. THESE FIBRIN THREADS ENTRAP MORE PLATELETS AND OTHER BLOOD ELEMENTS.
Q	THUS, A THROMBUS IS COMPOSED OF MASSED . . . . . AND BLOOD ELEMENTS ENTRAPPED IN A MESHWORK OF . . . . . THREADS.
AS	PLATELETS FIBRIN
Q	IN EXTRAVASCULAR—I.E., NORMAL—CLOTTING, THE . . . . . SUBSTANCE IS RELEASED INITIALLY BY DAMAGED TISSUE SURROUNDING OR WITHIN A SEVERED OR RUPTURED VESSEL. PLATELETS STICK TO THE DAMAGED ENDOTHELIAL WALL, AND THEY TOO RELEASE A . . . . . SUBSTANCE.
AS	THROMBOPLASTIC THROMBOPLASTIC

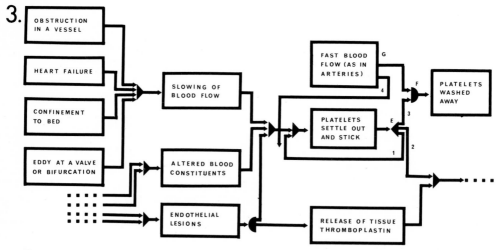

Fig. 5 (1,2,3).   Diagrams illustrating the logical construction of the flow charts on thromboembolism.

Q   A THROMBOPLASTIC SUBSTANCE MAY BE RELEASED BY
           . . . . . , OR BY . . . . . TISSUE.
AS   PLATELETS
           DAMAGED (INJURED)
Q   THROMBOPLASTIN IS THE GENERAL NAME FOR ANY
           THROMBOPLASTIC SUBSTANCE. A THROMBOPLASTIC SUB-
           STANCE IS ONE WHICH, WHEN RELEASED INTO THE

BLOOD, CAUSES . . . . . TO BE CONVERTED INTO . . . . .
THREADS.

AS   FIBRINOGEN
             FIBRIN

The preparation of the new program involved a detailed analysis of the principles of thromboembolism prior to the writing of the instructional frames. The organization of this task was facilitated by the construction of a series of flow charts. This diagrammatic scheme allowed a visual representation of simultaneous and recycling processes and the branching nature of the sequential events that occur in thromboembolism. The chart also presented a detailed description of the conditions that predispose to the formation and dissemination of thrombi.

Figure 5 demonstrates the logical construction of the flow charts. The chart represented in Figure 6 was presented to the student at the start of the exercise in order to provide him with an overall view of the program.

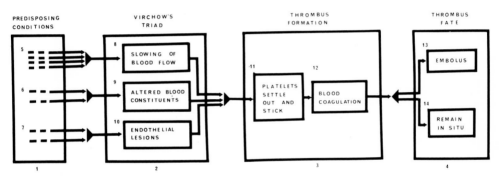

Fig. 6. Flow chart designed to give the student an overall view of the subject to be presented.

The flow charts were an important factor in the development of free communication between the pathologists and the psychologists with respect to addition, deletion, correction, and exact delineation of the subject matter. Furthermore, it provided an objective basis for constructing the instructional frames and for empirically comparing the relative merits of alternative sequences.

This type of program offered two advantages over the one developed for the pilot study. From the computer aspect, the problem of many alternative correct answers was eliminated through appropriate cueing of the desired response. From the educational aspect, this program was a teaching instrument.

Computer Approach to Problem Solving

In the introduction to this paper it was stated that an ideal instrument of programmed instruction should be able to present the basic principles of a topic to the student and, subsequently, to determine whether or not the student could use this knowledge to solve problems. In the specific context of medical education, the student must learn to use information that is available to him in the form of a case history and the results of a physical examination in order to determine what further investigations he should select to solve the problem and make a diagnosis.

With this objective in mind, the instructional program on thromboembolism is currently being extended to include a section which will test the ability of the student to apply his knowledge to problem solving. Briefly, the student is asked to reconstruct the clinical and pathologic findings in a patient who has died from thromboembolic disease. Bits of information from the clinical history and pathologic findings are presented on request. The student may, for example, request information concerning previous illnesses, age, sex, weight, hematologic examinations, blood pressure, state of the coronary arteries, and so on. Only one piece of information may be requested at a time, and the student may, at any time, elect to answer a series of questions regarding the site and nature of the thrombus or embolus, the elements of Virchow's triad that predispose to intravascular coagulation, and the significance of these findings in relation to the death of the patient.

The display of clinicopathologic data demands the free use of color slides, X-rays, and charts. This may be achieved by programming the computer to control the display of 35 mm slides stored in a projector such as the Kodak Carousel. With this simple device, the instructor retains the versatility necessary to the presentation of an interesting program (Fig. 7).

The attractive feature of this type of clinicopathologic reconstruction is that it places the initiative directly with the student and forces him to make judgements based on his knowledge. It is hoped that this approach may provide the instructor with objective evidence as to which students are likely to function best in applied situations.

It is not known whether the skills necessary to the solution of such problems

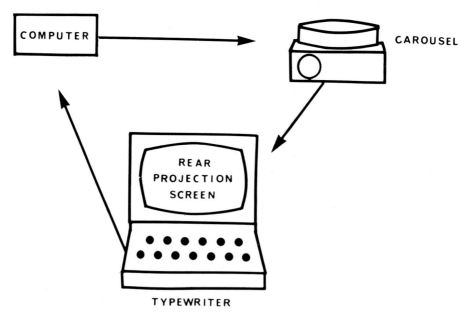

Fig. 7. Combined use of the computer and 35 mm slides add to the versatility of the program.

can be taught by the computer. In principle, however, this form of programmed instruction can be applied to the teaching of problem solving.

Critique

A complete analysis of our study is not possible at this time since the revised program on thromboembolism has only recently been completed and is now being tested. There are certain conclusions that may, however, be drawn from our own experience with computer-aided instruction and from the reports of others.

There are some scientific disciplines in which it is relatively easy to program subject matter for presentation by the computer. Subjects involving the display of mathematical formulas, chemical reactions, graphs, and molecular models are particularly suited to this technique. It has, for instance, been used with success in the training of radar operators in simulated radar centers.[13] There are many teaching situations in which this method of presentation could provide a useful and versatile instrument of self-instruction.

The development of a computer-controlled program that requires the free use of dialogue poses a problem of a different order. In our experience, the punishing amount of programming that is required to construct and control such a dialogue may prohibit its use as a practical teaching method. This does not imply that it is impossible to create problem-solving instructional programs with dialogue, since this has been accomplished.[14, 15] But the few that are in existence operate in model situations using a limited number of programs. This means that the cost is very high and indicates that future development should be concentrated in a few centers. In this way, it may be possible to produce good programs for dissemination on national and international networks in the future.

The computer is now being utilized with success in research and teaching to: 1) do something that no other method can; 2) do something much faster; and 3) facilitate the use of present techniques.

The third of these uses is pertinent to our discussion. At present, an instructor spends many hours assembling data for his lectures, seminars, and laboratory sessions. For example, the pathologist retrieves his information from the library, the autopsy records, and the biochemistry laboratory. Rapid access to this data could prove to be a greater stimulus to education than the replacement of a lecture or tutorial by programmed instruction.

The techniques for the presentation of information that we have used in our computer-controlled program are particularly suited to the display of data on a screen in a classroom. This could provide the instructor with instant access to information when he needs it most—while the class is actually in session. In this way, the computer would be used to improve the efficiency of traditional methods of instruction and to free the instructor for the type of teaching that only he can do.

With the continuing trend of medical education towards the use of the "core curriculum" and more free time for the student, it becomes imperative to provide, in readily accessible form, self-instructional material that the student can use in his own time. The role of the computer in the development of these programs remains to be defined, but we would anticipate that it would not be insignificant.

References

1. Little, J.K. Results of use of machines for testing and for drill upon learning in educational psychology. *Reprinted in* Teaching Machines and Programmed Learning. Washington, D.C., National Education Association, 1960, Vol. 1.
2. Pressey, S.L. Development and appraisal of devices providing immediate automatic scoring of objective tests and concomitant self-instruction. *Reprinted in* Teaching Machines and Programmed Learning. Washington, D.C., National Education Association, 1960, Vol. 1.
3. Coulson, J.E., and Cogswell, J.F. The effects of individualised instruction on testing. Professional Paper SP-1829, System Development Corporation, Santa Monica, California, 1965.
4. Miller, G.E. University of Illinois, College of Medicine, Office of Research in Medical Education, Report to the Faculty, 1967.
5. Spolsky, B. Some problems of computer-based instruction. Behav. Sci., 11:487, 1966.
6. Crowder, N.A. Automatic tutoring by intrinsic programming. *Reprinted in* Teaching Machines and Programmed Learning. Washington, D.C., National Education Association, 1960, Vol. 1.
7. IBM Computer-Assisted Instruction Author and Proctor Manual, Form C24-3384-1. Endicott, N.Y., IBM, 1965.
8. Starkweather, J.A. University of California, San Francisco Medical Center, San Francisco, California. Personal communication, 1967.
9. Silvern, G.M., and Silvern, L.C. Computer-assisted instruction: Specification of attributes for CAI programs and programmers. Proc. Ass. Comp. Mach., 57-62, 1966.
10. Bowden, D.H. Computer-aided instruction in pathology. Canad. Med. Ass. J., 97: 739, 1967.
11. Skinner, B.F. Teaching and the Technology of Education. New York, Appleton-Century-Crofts, 1968.
12. Holland, J.G. Teaching machines: An application of principles from the laboratory. J. Exp. Anal. Behav., 3:275, 1960.
13. Bushnell, D.D. Applications of technology to the improvement of learning. *In* The Computer in American Education. New York, John Wiley & Sons, 1967.
14. Swets, J.A., and Feurzig, W. Computer-aided instruction. Science, 150:572, 1965.
15. Schorow, M. University of Illinois, College of Medicine. Personal communication, 1967.

General References

1. Teaching Machines and Programmed Learning, I. A Source Book, Lumsdaine, A.A., and Glaser, R., eds. Washington, D.C., National Education Association, 1960.
2. Teaching Machines and Programmed Learning, II. Data and Directions, Glaser, R., ed. Washington, D.C., National Education Association, 1965.
3. Programmed Instruction and Computer-Based Instruction, Coulson, J.E., ed. New York, John Wiley, 1962.
4. The Computer in American Education, Bushnell, D.D., and Allen, D., eds. New York, John Wiley, 1967.

PREPARATION OF ANATOMIC PATHOLOGY DATA FOR AUTOMATION†

DIANE W. CROCKER*

The use of automation continues to expand rapidly in the hospital field. A beginning is usually made in a hospital comptroller's office and then is introduced into other areas, such as the pharmacy, diet kitchen, and record room. Automation is essential in these parts of the hospital today, since it introduces greater efficiency and more rapid and accurate reporting and billing. Its cost is readily justified because computer use, in accelerating the application of automation, results in the saving of time, labor, and space. The outlook, therefore, is for *more* automation through computer usage with eventual total hospital information systems. Without discussing the merits and debits of having a medical information system represent a by-product of a comptroller's office, the consideration here will be for that part of such a system which pertains primarily to anatomic pathology.

For the present, efforts should be concentrated on anatomic pathology with the prospect of adding ultimately to a data base of anatomic pathology, information derived from clinical laboratory reports, radiology reports, and the clinical portion of the hospital record. A concentration on anatomic pathology is suggested because more time and effort are required for the development of an automated system for the collection, retrieval, and analysis of these data than for the data generated in the clinical chemistry, hematology, and other divisions of a clinical laboratory. Furthermore, there are now a number of systems being developed primarily for the recording, analysis, and transmittal of chemical and other clinical pathology data. The progress here will be of interest, since the prospect of combining one of these clinical pathology systems with one designed for anatomic pathology data will

* This study has been supported in part by the Elsie T. Friedman Fund at Harvard Medical School.

† Presented at International Academy of Pathology meeting, San Francisco, March, 1969.

be welcomed by every pathologist who directs a large and active laboratory service.

This paper is written for the pathologist who may not have ready access to a computer but who would like to organize his anatomic pathology data so that they may be ready for subsequent analysis by a computer. The file organization proposed should prove useful also to those pathologists whose volume of data may not require the use of a computer. At the same time, if a group of hospitals utilize a similar file organization, their combined experience may constitute a volume which would justify the use of a computer.

This author believes that a hospital's medical information storage and retrieval system should have its origin in, and be developed by, its laboratory service. Whether this project involves the use of the hospital comptroller's computer or a separate computer will depend upon the organization of the hospital and its laboratory service and the support available for such a system. The pathologist should be the decision-maker regarding the choice of methods for automation of his department's data. This is an important consideration if data from anatomic and clinical pathology are to form the core of an efficient reporting system and if the hospital laboratory service is to develop an intellectually useful compendium of information for analysis and for the training of residents, fellows, and students.

How can one best proceed, particularly when funds may be limited and there is no ready access to a computer? The start should be the organization of the information one wishes to study, with careful consideration given to the type of information one would like to retrieve and the various uses to which the data might be put. These are fundamental requirements of any information retrieval system. In fact, the meticulous organization of data required *before* embarking on a computerized study constitutes one of the major dividends of the overall undertaking. Having catalogued the data from surgical and autopsy pathology files and having applied a nomenclature system, one is in a position to conduct simple although useful analyses with hand or machine sorting. When poorly planned, the expression of the computer trade applies—"GI-GO," which stands for "Garbage In, Garbage Out." In this discussion of procedure and in the presentation of our approach to data collection, an effort has been made to avoid the specialized terms used in the more complex fields of automation. There is a need for bringing the computer closer to everyday life, and this can best be speeded by using the language most of us understand, namely English.

There are many ways of proceeding. The desired output and availability of funds will help make the decisions. For the pathologist who wishes to order his files for data storage and retrieval, the approach we have found eminently successful is presented.

Purpose

In anticipation of a computer facility, it is important to establish and maintain a suitable data base. This involves the organization of data collection, the accurate selection of diagnoses, and the collection and storage of these data in computer-readable form. Of course, the form in which the data are collected for retrieval and analysis will depend in part on the capacity of the computer to be used and also on the sophistication of the programming. The accuracy and completeness of the output would be dependent on the input.

One of the greatest difficulties in preparing a computer study is the requirement of establishing in advance what one wishes to determine from the data. Thus, the careful preselection of input material is necessary for a data base from which many studies can be performed. We are concerned here with the establishment of a suitable data base in pathology. The establishment of such a data base need not interfere with ongoing file maintenance; indeed, the maintenance and usability of files should be greatly enhanced by the methods described herein which are applicable to any pathology department whether or not the use of a computer is envisioned. The eventual likelihood of more time-sharing and pooled data on a central computer facility makes the availability of a computer more likely even for the smaller community hospital. Many choices between alternate ways of proceeding are available. Rather than presenting each of these, we will discuss the method which we have found works well and requires a limited expenditure of department funds. We have not yet sought grant support for this undertaking.

Coding

There are two alternate languages for data collection in pathology. Computer systems using natural language are complicated and involve sophisticated programming. We have therefore decided to use an alternate, simpler, but more restricted method which involves coding. The selection of the Systematized Nomenclature of Pathology (SNOP)[1] coding scheme was made only after detailed study of the many other available codes. The SNOP code was selected for its intentional adaptability to computer usage, its great detail, its grouping into four areas of information, and its specific relevance to pathologic terminology. Furthermore, the codes are current and reasonably well-selected, and the first volume will soon be updated. Retrieval of pathology data using this code has already been achieved at the National Institutes of Health.[2] Parenthetically, our Kodachrome Teaching Slides and Reprints are also filed according to two-digit Topographic codes of SNOP.

The SNOP code consists of four-digit coding for each of four categories. For example, "Lung, acute bronchopneumonia due to staphylococcus aureus with respiratory failure": T2800, M4101, E1601, F7109. Where no diagnosis applies in a category, those entries consist of zeros. For example, "Adrenal gland, diffuse cortical hyperplasia with Cushing syndrome" T9310, M7304, E0000, F4633. E0000 also means "etiology unknown." For simplicity, in the beginning, we have used a two-digit Topographic code, retaining space for four digits which might be used at a later date. The two digit codes include only the first two digits and represent the broader categories of anatomic locations. The coding is done externally, and, although the computer would have its dictionary for translation of code numbers, the queries would be given in code form and the output would consist of codes as well as the English equivalent.

To insure uniformity of coding, we have given this task to an experienced, full-time Coding secretary rather than leave it in the hands of multiple individuals. In the past, the code numbers had been assigned by the residents for their respective surgical and autopsy cases. There was great variation among the residents in interpretation and selection of codes used, sometimes for the same disease entity. A secretary who is well-versed in the SNOP code does all the coding. This not only insures uniformity of the coding but accuracy as well. She also keypunches, verifies, and files the cards.

Files

Presently, the main file consists of a combined Topography-Morphology file which includes the bulk of the diagnoses. In addition, there are separate color-keyed files each for Etiology, Function, and Tumors. Each file contains color-keyed cards for surgical and autopsy diagnoses. The diagnoses are filed behind index cards prepared from the SNOP code book. The basis of the main file is topographic, with morphologic diagnoses as subclassifications within each topographic category. These files are made available to the hospital staff who submit requests to the Coding secretary. She answers specific requests for a case, groups of cases, or combinations of diagnoses. If the number of cases retrieved from the file is small, then a list can be prepared from the cards. When a large number of cases is retrieved, the cards are duplicated and interpreted and the duplicate set is provided to the clinician. These cards could also be put through a Lister-Printer to obtain a listing of all the information on the cards. Once a good data base has been established, the number of requests for cases increases.

Equipment

It is useful to have the necessary peripheral equipment at hand near the files (see Table 1). However, we have made use of keypunch, interpreter, duplicator,

Table 1.   Materials and Equipment

Essential	Optional
Punch cards: less expensive if purchased in bulk, i.e. through a local computer facility or the business office.	*Verifier:* It is always best to check on the accuracy of keypunching by using a Verifier. We spot check cards rather than verifying each one.
SNOP Code Book and accompanying Visual Aid—if this is the code to be used.	
SNOP Codes on Index cards.	*Sorter:* This unit is useful for sorting large numbers of cards. The types which record the tallies per bin are most helpful.
File: We favor locked 22-drawer full-suspension files. Cards accumulate rapidly. The larger files are therefore preferable. Secretaries will find it easier to file in full-suspension drawers which do not have to be lifted out.	*Printer-Lister:* To prepare printed lists of cases.
Files containing punch cards should be in a low humidity environment preferably air-conditioned. The cards should be closely packed. If they get warped or wet, they may not pass through a duplicating machine or be usable for computer input.	*Duplicating machine:* Duplicates a deck of cards by punching holes in the proper column but does not print out the information at the top of the card.
	Interpreter: Prints at the top of the card the explanation for the punched holes.
Keypunch: Noisy. Should be in an air-conditioned room.	*Wired Board for Interpreter:* We keep a board wired to our specifications for use in the Interpreter.

and printer in various locations of the hospital, but this is time consuming. It would be preferable to have a central location, such as adjoining the record room, where all of this work could be done. The central location should be within a reasonable distance of the pathology files. Usually much of this equipment is present in the payroll office, if billing and payroll are automated. Our billing office is presently located in a separate building and the equipment is not always available when we need it. The leasing of such equipment probably could not be justified for a small scale operation within a pathology department.

Data Collection

The collection of autopsy data for keypunching has been greatly facilitated by the use of a specially devised form (Fig. 1). This form accommodates 80 numbers to correspond with the 80 columns on a punch card. Most of the entries are made by the resident who performed the necropsy. The resident lists the autopsy number, the unit or hospital number, the organs, the diagnoses, and any weights, measurements, and previous surgical numbers that are pertinent. Each diagnosis is listed in a separate space. The resident provides the Topographic (T) code numbers in columns 1 and 2 and the identification numbers in columns 21 and 22. Identification numbers 01, 02, and 03 correspond to the three major diagnoses. Some cases have only one major diagnosis, and few may have more than four. The number allowed is flexible, but in general it is held to three. These diagnoses are taken out of Topographic order, but the remainder of the diagnoses are listed in ascending Topographic order.

The Morphology (M), Etiology (E), and Function (F) codes are inserted

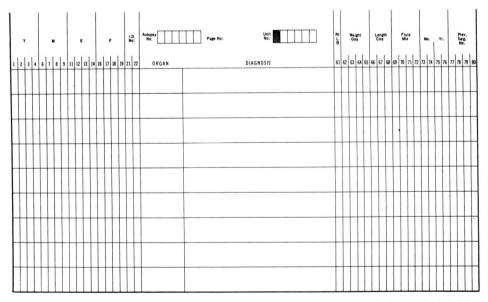

Fig. 1.   The work-sheet is filled in by the resident except for the Morphology (M), Etiology (E), and Function (F) codes which are added by the Coding secretary. This form contains 80 columns to correspond with the punch cards which are prepared from the entries on the form.

by the Coding secretary. The form, when complete, is checked by one member of the staff (the author) and subsequently is used for keypunching, each diagnosis being put on a separate punch card. This form is also used by the typist to prepare the autopsy face sheet (Fig. 2).

The information listed under Diagnostic Summary in Figure 2 represents the data transferred by the typist from the autopsy work-sheet (Fig. 1). It is not necessary to indicate which codes represent Topography, Morphology, Etiology, and Function, since the order is always the same and the clinicians and pathologists rapidly become aware of the code locations. The three major diagnoses are typed in capitals. There are 15 diagnoses in this case, but there would be 16 punched cards for diagnoses since one of the diagnoses has two different Etiology codes.

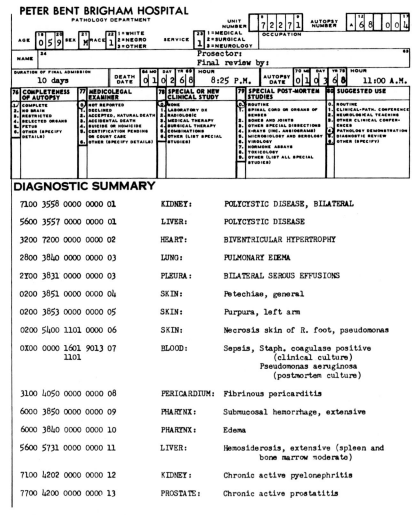

Fig. 2.   The autopsy face sheet has blocked entries for keypunching of the Master Card. The Diagnostic Summary is taken by the typist from the work-sheet (Fig. 1). The numbers to the left represent the SNOP codes. The major diagnoses are capitalized.

The upper part of this face sheet has blocked areas for data entry. The blocked areas, when keypunched, make up the Master Card of which there is one per autopsy. The information on the Master Card includes first the unit number, then the autopsy number, the patient's age and sex, his race, and the hospital service. The column numbers are listed at the top of the blocks. All blocks must be filled in. Any blocks that do not have numbers are filled in with zeros, for example autopsy number A68-4 would be listed as A68-004. If the number were entered as A68-4 with the four in the first of the three squares, that number would be interpreted as 400. There are three blocks for age so that children could be accommodated, it would thus be possible to enter the age of a child, for example, of 1.6 years. The initial M or F is used for the sex and the numbers 1, 2 and 3 for White, Negro, and Other, respectively. The Service likewise is entered numerically; 1 represents the Medical service, 2 the Surgical service, and 3 the Neurology service.

A large block of numbers is then reserved for the patient's name, the first name being typed first and then the last name. It would be possible to make use of the last 20 or more columns reserved for name for some other entry. We have not chosen to do so at the moment. The date of death and autopsy date are then keypunched in the corresponding columns. January would appear as 01, whereas October would be 10.

The specific needs of the department would determine the type of ancillary information which would be useful to have available on a Master Card. We have found that the information listed in the lower five blocks is of greatest use for our purposes. The pertinent significant information under "Completeness of Autopsy," column 76, would be circled by the resident. The number circled becomes the number to be keypunched in the corresponding column. Medical Examiner cases are likewise listed. In a hospital where many special studies are performed, both in the clinical setting and at postmortem examination, it is useful to have this type of data available for reference.

The last column lists suggested use of the case, which for our purposes consists of various teaching categories. Space is provided at the bottom of each column to add any other information of value.

A work-sheet identical to this form is useful. We had one prepared by offset printing. It has a copy of the face sheet on one side and a copy of the weight sheet on the opposite side. These are filled in by hand by the resident and transferred by the typist to the final forms. Our final face sheet has three carbons built in, as does the weight sheet (Fig. 3). This is done because copies must be sent to the patient's chart and to the physician who cared for the patient. Additional copies are sometimes needed and are obtained by adding carbons at the time of typing or by making a copy on a copying machine.

Since the number of diagnoses in our autopsies ranges from 20 to 60, with an average of 40 diagnoses per case, we run an average of 40 punch cards per case plus the Master Card. A duplicate set of each deck of autopsy cards is prepared. the duplicate deck is stored, and, when a file consisting of one year's autopsies in ascending numeric order is complete, the information on the cards is put on magnetic tape, for less bulky storage and for computer input. This updating could be done at shorter intervals. Subsequently, all the data will be transferred to a disc.

Diane W. Crocker

PETER BENT BRIGHAM HOSPITAL
PATHOLOGY DEPARTMENT

NAME   PATIENT NO. 72271   AUTOPSY NO. A68-4

WEIGHTS AND MEASUREMENTS
(NE) – NOT EXAMINED (NW) – NOT WEIGHED (A) – ABSENT

	ACTUAL WEIGHT	AVERAGE NORMAL WEIGHT
BODY WEIGHT	[19] [N W] [21 Kg] [22]	
BODY LENGTH	[N W] [24 Cm]	
STATE OF DEVELOPMENT	Normal	
STATE OF NUTRITION	Normal	
PUPILS R	_____ mm	
PUPILS L	_____ mm	
HEART	[25] [7 0 0] [27 gm]	270 – 360 gm (M) 250 – 280 gm (F)
CIRCUMFERENCE OF TRICUSPID RING	150 mm	120 – 127 mm
CIRCUMFERENCE OF PULMONIC RING	90 mm	85 – 90 mm
CIRCUMFERENCE OF MITRAL RING	100 mm	105 – 115 mm
CIRCUMFERENCE OF AORTIC RING	70 mm	77 – 80 mm
THICKNESS OF RIGHT VENTRICLE	[28] [0 • 3] [30 cm]	0.25 – 0.3 cm
THICKNESS OF LEFT VENTRICLE	[31] [2 • 0] [33 cm]	0.9 – 1.5 cm
PERICARDIAL FLUID	_____ ml	
RIGHT LUNG	[34] [0 0 0] [36 gm]	680 gm (M) 480 gm (F)
LEFT LUNG	[37] [7 5 0] [39 gm]	600 gm (M) 420 gm (F)
RIGHT PLEURAL FLUID	625 ml	
LEFT PLEURAL FLUID	475 ml	
HEIGHT OF DIAPHRAGM R	_____	
HEIGHT OF DIAPHRAGM L	_____	
PERITONEAL FLUID	0 ml	
LIVER	[40] [2 0 5 0] [43 gm]	1400 – 1900 gm (M) 1200 – 1700 gm (F)
SPLEEN	[44] [3 0 0] [46 gm]	125 – 195 gm
PANCREAS	NW gm	60 – 180 gm
RIGHT KIDNEY	[47] [3 0 0] [49 gm]	125 – 170 gm (M) 115 – 155 gm (F)
LEFT KIDNEY	[50] [4 0 0] [52 gm]	
UTERUS	_____ cm	
PROSTATE	NW gm	22 gm (M)
RIGHT TESTIS OR OVARY	NW gm	20 – 25 gm (M) 4 – 8 gm (F)
LEFT TESTIS OR OVARY	NW gm	20 – 25 gm (M) 4 – 8 gm (F)
PITUITARY	[53] [0 • 5] [55 mg]	300 – 600 mg
THYROID	[56] [0 2 0] [58 gm]	20 gm
COMBINED PARATHYROID WEIGHTS	[59] [N W] [61 mg]	35 mg
RIGHT UPPER NW RIGHT LOWER NW		
LEFT UPPER NW LEFT LOWER NW		
RIGHT ADRENAL	[62] [0 9 • 0] [65 gm]	5 – 6 gm
CORTEX	_____ cm	0.7 cm
LEFT ADRENAL	[66] [0 8 • 5] [69 gm]	5 – 6 gm
CORTEX	_____ cm	0.7 cm
THYMUS	NW gm	15 – 30 gm
PINEAL	NW mg	200 mg
BRAIN	[70] [1 6 4 0] [73 gm]	1250 – 1400 gm (M) 1200 – 1300 gm (F)

Fig. 3. Those weights and measurements appearing in blocks are punched onto a separate card. The first 18 columns correspond with the Master Card. The numbers adjacent to the blocks indicate the columns on the punch card where the information will appear. When a weight exceeds the number of blocks available, the actual weight is entered, but, for example, the keypunch operator enters 999 for numbers of 1000 or greater.

The Coding secretary keeps the files up-to-date by keypunching and filing new cases on a daily basis. In her spare time, she works back over previous years in sequential order. The older cases had previously been coded according to the Standardized Nomenclature of Disease. These are recoded in SNOP and keypunched by the Coding secretary. We now have accumulated a total of four complete years of autopsy cases with approximately 400 autopsies per year, representing a total of 1600 autopsies and 65,600 punch cards (64,000 Diagnosis Cards and 1600 Master Cards).

42   AORTA
    Extent of AS
    Degree of
      calcification
      ulceration
      elasticity
    Caliber
    Aneurysm
    Anomaly
    Thrombosis
    Dissection

45-47
    SYSTEMIC ARTERIES

45   Innominate
   Carotids

   Patency to water

46   Celiac

46   Superior mesenteric

4660   Renal
4661   R
4662   L

47   Iliacs

47   Femorals

   Other

49   SYSTEMIC VEINS

   Superior vena cava

   Inferior vena cava

   Renals

   Other

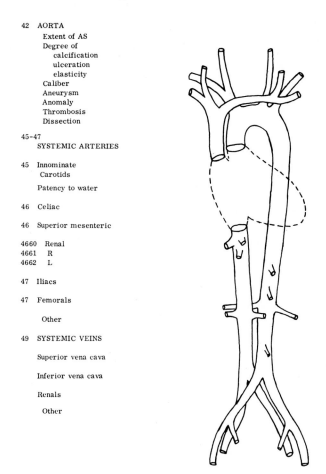

Fig. 4.   A page from the Gross Autopsy Protocol illustrates the Topographic two-digit codes beside the corresponding vessels to facilitate the resident's task of entering these numbers on the work-sheet.

All weights and measurements are entered on a form which is included in the autopsy protocol and is also used for keypunching (Fig. 3). This information, when accumulated for a sufficient number of cases, will provide a suitable data base for acquiring random curve distributions of normal as well as diseased organs. It furthermore provides ranges of measurements for various tumors, cardiac valves, and adrenal cortex. The first 18 columns of each punch card contain information identical with that in the first 18 columns of the Master Card. Unit number and Autopsy number are the two most important numbers if multiple correlations of data are to be done.

The remainder of the gross autopsy protocol is based on diagrams with space for inserting changes from the normal. A sample of one page from the protocol is shown in Figure 4. Alongside the diagrams are listed the various structures which should be commented upon. It is sufficient to list an N for normal where there are no pathologic alterations. Where there are changes, these are stated and the location drawn into the diagram. Note that numbers are present to the left of the anatomic site. These numbers represent the SNOP code which is limited in most instances to the first two digits. In certain instances, where there is particular interest in a lesion or retrieval of specific lesions, a four digit Topographic code may be required, as is shown for the renal artery. By using Topography code numbers in the gross autopsy protocol, the resident's task of inserting the Topographic code on the work sheet is thereby facilitated. Furthermore, the numbers in the protocol are organized so that they go in ascending fashion. This is a requirement for the autopsy work sheet after the first three or major diagnoses.

Because the files are used daily to retrieve cases precomputer, the cards have been color-keyed. The autopsy punch cards are white, the surgical cards are blue, and both are ordered in a similar fashion with the code numbers appearing first, then the surgical number, the Unit number, the patient's age and sex, and the diagnosis in English. The surgical pathology diagnoses are coded, keypunched, and filed on the day the case is signed out. Thus both the surgical and autopsy cases can be retrieved from the punch card file as current case material for study.

There is no reason why keypunching of diagnoses need entail an inordinate delay or jeopardize file maintenance. Whenever a tumor diagnosis is encountered, the information is duplicated onto a red card and put into the Tumor file. In this way anyone wishing to search for liposarcomas for example, rather than looking under the various sites where liposarcomas may occur, such as in soft tissue, retroperitoneum, etc., he can search the Tumor file specifically for all liposarcomas. The same applies to Etiologic diagnoses such as bacterial, viral, and mycotic infections. These are colored-keyed in purple. The Function file is maintained in much the same way with yellow cards; one could look in this file, for example, for all cases of diabetes mellitus or specific clinical syndromes such as the adrenogenital syndrome or Cushing's disease. We also maintain a separate small file for various systemic diseases which might be difficult to retrieve in a topographically oriented file. These include such diseases as polyarteritis nodosa, amyloidosis, lupus erythematosus, and Marfan's syndrome.

The above information forms the nucleus for a data base in pathology to which can be added clinical laboratory data, radiologic data, and clinical signs, symptoms, and diagnoses. There is no reason why the pathologic diagnoses should not form the basic nucleus for a hospital information retrieval system concerned with patients' records. It is certainly a good place to begin the automation of useful data when no computer is readily at hand. The preparation of such data can take considerable time and effort. If the computer is obtained before the data base has been built up, a great deal of computer time will be wasted.

Conclusions

When the organization of data collection, the accurate selection of diagnoses, and the collection and storage of much of these data in computer-readable form have been accomplished, then adequate data will be ready when a computer becomes available. The type and extent of data collection will in part depend on and be limited by the computer selected and the sophistication used in programming.

Decisions must be made wisely to protect the dollar investment as automation progresses. Since an on-line system providing almost immediate response to queries is the most useful and best for teaching purposes, we plan to install a console to the SDS 940 at the Harvard Computing Center for these purposes. This decision having been reached, we can now put all our data on SDS compatible tape and start working with a retrieval program for the SDS 940, a program which a well-automated medical center is generously giving us after having successfully tested our data. The four and a half years of autopsy diagnoses and ten years of surgical pathology diagnoses which have been coded on punch cards during the past three years should provide an adequate data base for retrieval and for training of residents in the use of automation in Anatomic Pathology.

References

1. Committee on Nomenclature and Classification of Disease. Systematized Nomenclature of Pathology, College of American Pathologists. Chicago, 1965.
2. Thomas, L.B., and Pratt, R.W. An information processing system for pathology data. *In* Pathology Annual 1966, Sommers, S.C., ed. New York, Appleton-Century-Crofts, 1966, Vol. 1, pp. 1-21.

THE INTENSIVE CARE UNIT
AND THE PATHOLOGY OF PROGRESS

G. A. FATTAL
JOHN P. WYATT*

The time has been, that when the brains were out, the man would die, and there an end. But now they rise again. . . .

MacBeth, Act III, Scene IV, line 68.

Pathology and Intensive Care

One contemporary viewpoint expressed about pathology as a discipline in the investigation of disease has been that it is bankrupt; it can offer nothing further through the autopsy room. Such a viewpoint, nihilistic at its worst and erosive at its best, clearly neglects the knowledge that the evolution of disease processes is constantly being altered by developments in medical care. It is our viewpoint that the Theatre for Information in analyzing the changing faces and masks of disease is the pathologist's atelier. This is particularly so in the consideration of the functions of a modern intensive care unit. This unit is a new center of hospital activity in which an investigative autopsy can play a most important role in the recognition, analysis, and communication of changing trends in our medical care environment.

What is an intensive care unit? It has been said that one should not speak of a ward as being allocated to intensive care unless there is continuing mortality of at least 25 percent. This trenchant comment reflects the desperate nature of the condition of the patients admitted, and, like Polyphemus, the unit exacts a daily toll. Historically, the intensive care units have developed from the head injury wards of the

* This contribution would not have been possible without the cooperation and interest of Dr. Brian Kirk, Physician-in-Charge, Intensive Care Unit (I.C.U.), Winnipeg General Hospital.

late 1930's. The significant reduction in the tragic complications of decerebrate rigidity and "lame brains"[1, 2, 3] has been a major impetus in extending the use of these specialized facilities to other conditions associated with a high incidence of grave complications.

The intensive care unit (I.C.U.) is the resuscitative care area in a hospital in which there is the maximum concentration of the most sophisticated therapeutic procedures and the minimum time for the evaluation of their effect. This unit is constantly concerned with decisions involving Homeric salvation procedures and the meticulous supervision of bioelectronic channels monitoring the critically ill. But it is not our intention to leave the impression that intensive care is a recent development. Toulouse-Lautrec has depicted a common emergency procedure of the late nineteenth century in his painting *The Tracheotomy* (Fig. 1).[4] (Unfortunately, either the title is incorrect or the physician is committing an error in anatomical judgement!)

The careful clinical study during life of deranged organs requires a matched

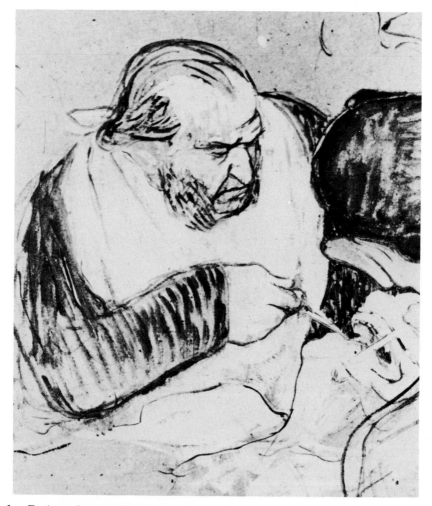

Fig. 1.   Toulouse-Lautrec: *The Tracheotomy*. (Courtesy of Sterling and Francine Clark. Institute of Art, Williamstown, Mass.)

performance from the autopsy teaching unit. The clinicians expect a comparable and ongoing analysis from the investigative autopsy unit to complement the precise physiologic studies of cardiorespiratory function, cerebral state, and hepatic and renal behavior measured during the life of the critically ill patient. Coupled with artificially supported respiration, precise electrolyte balance, and instant monitoring of vital organ systems, the rewards of the I.C.U. are now more readily perceived clinically.[5] To validate these clinical impressions, it is imperative that an investigative aura dominate the autopsy performance. To do this, a distinction should be made between the investigative autopsy and the "routine" autopsy, which contributes solely to hospital statistics.

The orientation of intensive care units varies. Where cardiologists dominate, the emphasis is on the cardiac pump; if the unit leadership is from the respiratory division, the diffusion of gases into the tissues is of paramount concern. One contribution that the pathologist can make is the prevention of polarization of therapeutic efforts into a single avenue of endeavor; he is the ballast against subdiscipline bias.

Although this essay is primarily concerned with a delineation of patterns of pathology that are characteristically related to intensive care areas, the emotional charge of therapeutic "pyrrhic victories" is not being levelled.[6] Some of the patterns of pathology are often unavoidable complications which follow Aesculapian inter-

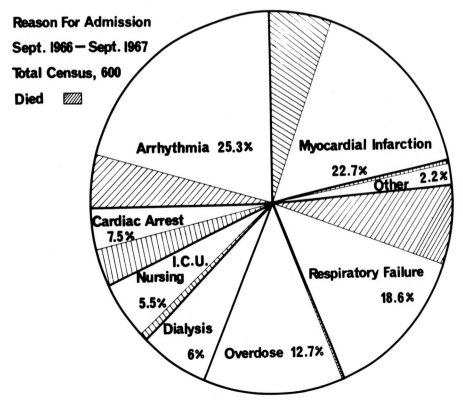

Fig. 2.   Case Distribution in the I.C.U.

ventions, obligatory in any operation concerned with intensive care. The physician may walk the I.C.U. with the "two-edged sword—Iatrogenesis" in his hand,[7] but all its ills are not necessarily of his making.

Case Distribution and a Prototype

The nature of the cases admitted to our unit reflected a broad variety of primary pathologic disorders (Fig. 2), but the admission diagnosis was of necessity a physiologic one. As a practical point, for example, preliminary information from earlier biopsy studies may restrain expensive therapeutic undertakings. One of our cases, showing diffuse radiographic infiltration of the lung fields, was unsuccessfully but intensively treated for acute respiratory failure. If the pathologic diagnosis of disseminated malignant reticulosis based on the lung biopsy performed a few days before final admission had been forwarded earlier, three days of intensive care might have been avoided.

In the two years of the I.C.U. operation (1966-1968), approximately 1,200 cases of critically ill patients have been admitted. Of these, 200 were directly from casualty. Sixty were transferred from hospital wards in their first 24 hours. An equal number were transferred from the general hospital beds as long as two weeks after their initial entry into hospital. Eight percent of the total number of patients were

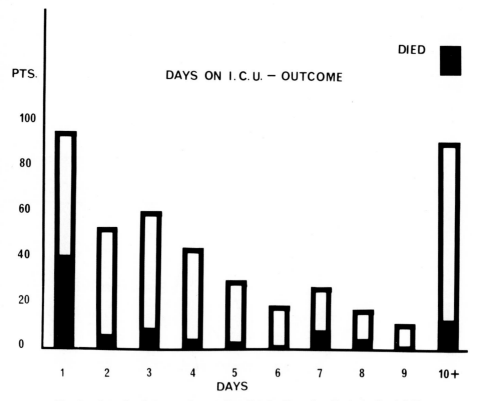

Fig. 3.   Length of stay and mortality distribution of patients in the I.C.U.

from the recovery room. The majority of patients were males, except for the third and fourth decade, where the male:female ratio was approximately one (Fig. 3).

In the year 1967, for example, 134 patients with respiratory failure were admitted; 70 percent of these were diagnosed as having acute pulmonary insufficiency uncomplicated by a previous lung disorder. In the same interval, 80 patients with myocardial infarction were seen; the three commonest physiopathologic diagnoses applied to their mode of death were shock, cardiac arrhythmia, and severe cardiac failure. One-half of the deaths in these coronary catastrophes were due to a refractory rhythm disturbance. Of the patients with myocardial infarction coming to the intensive care area, a large proportion died in the first 24 hours from irreversible cardiogenic shock (Fig. 2).

The following case represents a prototype of the patients admitted to the I.C.U. and illustrates the interwoven complexities of disease processes and therapy. The unravelling of the multiple factors involved in these case makes the unitary concept of understanding the physiopathologic derangements often difficult, always frustrating, and certainly subject to challenge.

CASE 1.   This 20-year-old, white female, a known diabetic who had been on 60 U of NPH Insulin daily, was brought to the casualty ward cyanosed and in a comatose state. A blood glucose determination of 50 mg/100 ml led to the admitting diagnosis of hypoglycemic shock. A spinal tap was done on admission without any significant findings being noted in the fluid. Support of the circulation, administration of antibiotics, correction of metabolic state, hypothermia, tracheostomy, curare relaxation, and mechanical ventilation were instituted. X-ray film of the chest showed diffuse bilateral pulmonary infiltration. Acidosis persisted and signs of renal failure were noted. From the third day on, 100 percent oxygen was used continuously. The patient was never hypercarbic. Marked bronchial breathing was heard over both lungs. The patient remained comatose and died on the fourth day. Three consecutive EEGs showed diffuse slow activity of very low amplitude. The postmortem showed multiple organ involvement, particularly cerebral, respiratory, cardiovascular, and renal.

These pathologic alterations have been seen separately or combined in many of our I.C.U. patients. This essay deals, at some length, with three of the structural changes as delineated in Case 1. They are dealt with under the following headings: respiratory, cardiovascular, and central nervous system derangements.

Respiratory Derangements

Ventilator Cuff Necrosis

The endotracheal passage of any artificial ventilatory tube almost invariably creates some degree of tracheitis,[8] with loss of epithelium and progressive degrees of metaplasia probably related to the length of time the tube is retained.[9]

The use of endotracheal intubation, particularly with cuffed tubes, has aroused clinical discussion because of its frequent association with a circumscribed, indolent form of erosion ulcer. At the level of the cuff, probably due to continuous or intermittent pressure (Figs. 4 A, B) there is an ischemic loss of mucous membrane. The cuff or the end of the plastic tracheotomy tube excoriates the trachea and produces

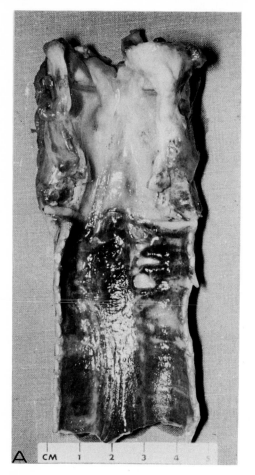
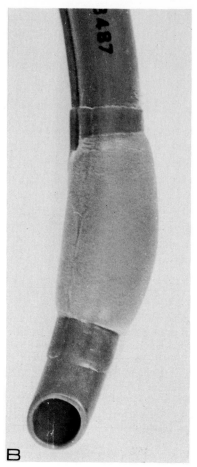

Fig. 4.   A. Trachea showing circumscribed ulceration, ecchymoses, and edema. B. Ventilator tube with pressure cuff.

a large, deep ulcer. This circumscribed lesion is often on the anterolateral surface of the trachea. The piston-like motion of the tracheotomy tube induced by IPP respirators may be an additive factor, producing shearing forces between the inflated cuff and the partially fixed trachea. The semirigidity of the tracheal cartilaginous plate obviously offers a resistance to the inflated pressure cuff. This lesion is much more frequently observed in elderly patients with circulatory difficulties. In some ways, this tracheal erosion is a symbol of unrelieved tissue compression, like buttock bed sores were for so many years.

Serious and chronic complications, such as tracheoeosophageal strictures, arising from the plastic tube have been documented in the literature.[10]

The "Respirator Lung"

Prior to a more specific discussion of the "respirator lung," comments on the deranged physiopathology and the multiple influences which can operate within a single pair of lungs are essential. Virtually 20 percent (Fig. 2) of the admission problems in the resuscitative area are of a respiratory nature. Therefore, the analysis of these lung disturbances will remain a continuing and preceptive task.

The lung, owing to its simple air-blood membrane and the relative ease of cell migration into air spaces, most effectively reflects the influence of therapeutic agents. The suppressive action of antibiotics, protracted perfusion through maintenance of cardiac action, and the countervailing effect of assisted respiration facilitating gas diffusion are influences long maintained by intensive care measures. The lung is, therefore, an excellent field to study the impress of prolonged care upon reparative responses to injury and the natural history of respiratory diseases.

The variety of pathologic problems, both of pulmonic and extrapulmonic nature, which present themselves to the unit are often well advanced down a final common pathway. The term "respiratory insufficiency," used by the I.C.U., may actually have a morphologic reflection. The concept is gaining credence that a common lung reaction may be observed in autopsy material, and yet the causative factors are widely divergent. In patients who have suffered from shock, severe trauma, sepsis, extensive burns, and prolonged extracorporeal circulation, or who have absorbed large amounts of degenerating tissue products, the lung often showed the common pathologic picture of "congestive atelectasis," capillaries packed with erythrocytes, and a heavy mononuclear and histiocytic infiltrate.

A second montage of linked factors within the lung are the often neglected physiologic considerations which are operative in the critically ill. Chronic airway obstruction, for example, is a common clinical entrance diagnosis, but its pathologic causative mechanisms may be many. A most important factor in airway obstruction is the underlying physiologic change. From the rare tracheal stricture[10] to the common bronchitis-emphysema complex, it is the "physiologic" derangements which are of importance to the gravely ill. Patients with peritonitis or upper abdominal surgery develop diaphragmatic or thoracic limitations of motion impeding ventilation. Small dosages of narcotics, curare (frequently used in the I.C.U.), and barbiturates, as well as cerebral infarction, will precipitate respiratory center depression, particularly in the patient with antecedent chronic airway obstruction. Equally profound ventilatory/perfusion ($\dot{V}/\dot{Q}$) inequalities (Fig. 5 B) may follow lung collapse or induced hyperventilation, due to the adaptive physiologic shunting which ensues. These physiopathologic deviations may gravely alter the normal cascade relationships that exist from the apex to the base of the lung.[11] Pathologists should be concerned with these $\dot{V}/\dot{Q}$ derangements rather than the putative I.Q. value of static morphology.

Disturbances in cardiac force and rhythm will seriously compromise the pulmonary circulation and produce physiologic diversions of blood and dramatic changes in the ventilation:perfusion ratio. Such physiologic alterations may precipitate hypoxia and acidosis and thus induce further compromise of the vascular bed. Significant changes in the rheologic behavior of the blood follow and lead to an abrupt increase in the blood viscosity and erythrocyte packing in the pulmonary capillaries. The "congestive atelectasis" seen at the autopsy table may be an expression of altered blood viscosity as well as cardiac perfusion.

These background comments lead us now to consider a contemporary lung derangement that plagues all intensive care units. In the last 18 months we have

G. A. Fattal and John P. Wyatt

observed 14 patients who were treated in the I.C.U. for severe respiratory difficulties and at autopsy had distinctive, noncompliant, heavy, indigo-blue lungs. We have labelled these "respirator lungs"; the I.C.U. physicians favor the term "solid lung syndrome." The principal reason for our colloquial label was that, regardless of the

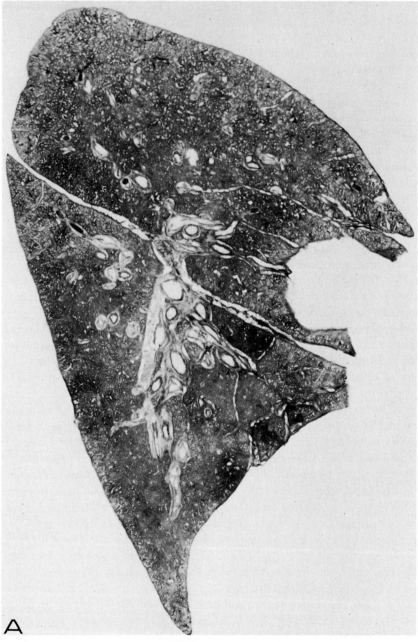

A

Fig. 5.   A. Whole lung (left) paper section. Case 1 illustrates an example of "respirator lung." The changes are homogeneously distributed throughout the lung. One-fourth actual size.

nature of the disease leading to admission, its complications, or the therapy received during the intensive care period, all of these patients had assisted ventilation for varying periods of time.

The recognition of the "solid lung syndrome" has been equally distinctive for the I.C.U. physician. The progressive solidification of the lung was clinically recorded by the progressive development of diffuse bronchial breathing, matched by generalized "frothy" radiographs. Although most of these patients survived seven to ten days, they eventually succumbed to hypoxia but the pCO_2 was consistently normal. Except for the last 24 hours, the arterial oxygen saturation had been maintained close to 100 percent, but mounting increments in the inspired alveolar oxygen levels were required. To achieve this delivery of oxygen and to overcome the in-

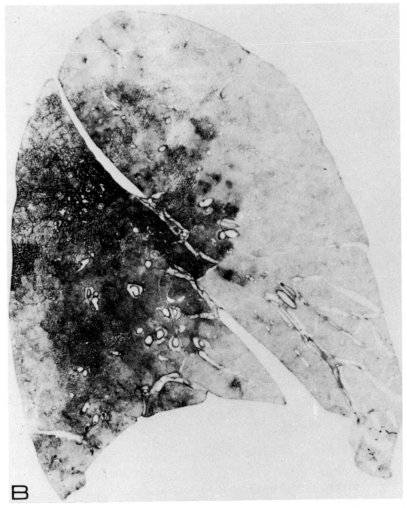

B

Fig. 5. (cont.)   B. Whole lung paper section of another "respirator lung" (left). Severe congestion and hemorrhage in posterolateral location suggest the likelihood of redistribution of pulmonary blood flow and hyperventilation in the upper and anterior parts of the lung. One-fourth actual size.

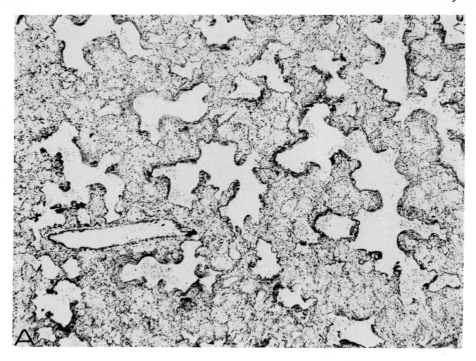

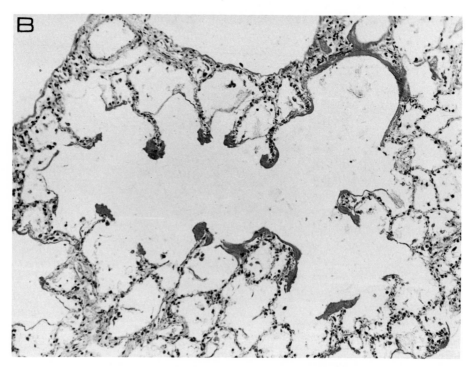

Fig. 6. Photomicrograph of "respirator lung" demonstrating the presence of hyaline membranes in terminal respiratory bronchioles. H & E. A, X25; B, X65.

creasing elasticity of the lung (noncompliance), continuing adjustments in the machine ventilatory force were needed.

Grossly, these lungs were bulky; their combined weight ranged from 1,600 to 2,200 g. The cut surfaces had a homogeneous solid appearance which was quite different from the gross impression in pneumonias and remarkably similar to the lung in hyaline membrane disease of infants (Figs. 5 A, B). Both intra-alveolar and interstitial edema was frequently observed. The most striking feature was the presence of hyaline membrane-like structures which lined the terminal respiratory bronchioles (Figs. 6 A, B), and in protracted cases there were the beginnings of organization and collagen deposition. The alveoli were, in general, fairly heavily sprinkled with macrophages (Fig. 7). Within the broadened alveolar septa, a similarly increased cell population was encountered with the occasional aggregate of polymorphonuclear leucocytes. These cells were not the major component of the infiltrate. Giemsa stains demonstrated clearly the heterogeneity of the migratory cell population (Fig. 8). The eosinophilic hyaline membrane was PAS-positive and sudanophilic. Barter, et al.[21] have emphasized the spatial relationships between these membranes and bundles of elastic fibers. Similar observations were made in our series (Fig. 6).

The location of the hyaline membranes characteristically on the elastic spurs of the air ducts infers a highly selective functional or biochemical derangement. In

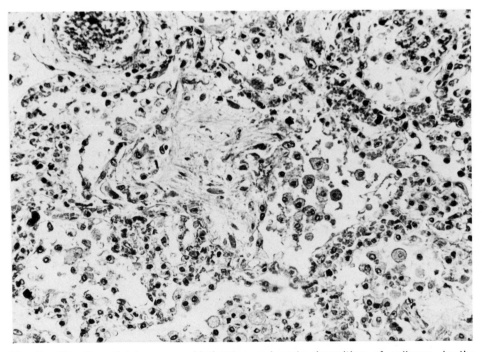

Fig. 7. Alveoli containing many histiocytes and early deposition of collagen, in the absence of significant acute inflammatory response. X160.

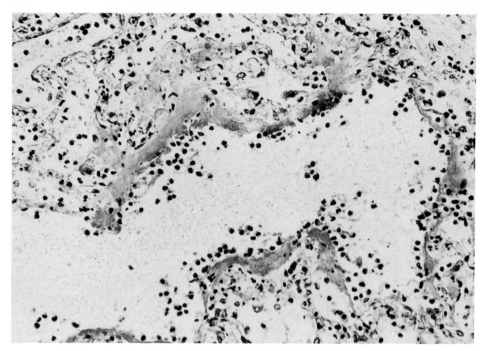

Fig. 8.   Air duct lined by hyaline membrane showing its relationship to a mixed migratory cell population. X160.

terms of clinicopathologic interpretation the concentration of the hyaline membranes at the respiratory bronchiole and air ducts probably interferes with lobular air flow. The respiratory bronchiole site and the close apposition to the lobular artery is a strategic physiologic control area, and, as in certain special pathologic conditions, derangements at this centrilobular level may influence perfusion.[19] The progressive thickening of the septa with fluid and cell infiltrates, as well as air sac filling, means impaired oxygen diffusion.

Case 1 in this essay is an example of the "respirator lung," but it also emphasizes the variety of factors (hypotension, shock, and other conditioning mechanisms) which complicate the understanding of the causation of this distinctive lung disorder.

One of the commonest therapeutic agents utilized in the intensive care ward is oxygen.[12] In 1899, Lorrain Smith[13] experimented with oxygen at several atmospheres of pressure, indicating that the lung may undergo an imperceptible transition from the physiologic to the pathologic, but this early warning was unheeded. Lung tissular effects have been searched for only since the recent therapeutic enthusiasm for hyperbaric oxygen and the appreciation of the vasospastic effects of oxygen on the developing retrolental tissues of the neonate. From the early report of capillary proliferation[14] to the more recent and widely bruited effects of oxygen upon the premature lung,[15, 16] investigative studies have now been redirected to the air-blood membranes of the adult lung and, more specifically, to the characteristic endothelial capillary damage.[17, 18, 19] Several groups of investigators[20, 21, 22] have clearly implicated high concentrations of oxygen as being the primary noxious agent producing distinctive morphologic alterations both in the newborn and the adult lung requiring oxygen assistance.

The use of oxygen, at present an irreplaceable therapeutic agent in the I.C.U., usually means that perfusional or ventilatory difficulties existed in the critically ill patient. It is our contention that to single out oxygen as the sole toxic agent responsible for new respiratory distress syndromes neglects the existence of pre-conditioning factors in the lung.

In the neonate requiring mechanically assisted ventilation, immaturity of the lung and altered vascular permeability are the two main abnormalities present which antedate the use of oxygen. Shanklin and Wolfson[15] refer to hemorrhage as being another manifestation of damaged vasculature in premature infants. The eclectic premise of Northway, et al.[16] is that the "respirator lung" in infants receiving oxygen therapy is a prolongation of the healing phase of hyaline membrane disease (respiratory distress syndrome: R.D.S.) combined with generalized oxygen toxicity.

In the adult, the conditioning factors existent in the lung before oxygen therapy are legion in number and polyvalent in character. The adult respiratory distress syndrome of Ashbaugh,[22] Barter's[21] adult cases of "oxygen poisoning" developing in the Bird respirator, and Nash's[20] large series of a similar pulmonary disability, emphasize the frequency, divergence, and overlapping nature of antecedent pathodynamic factors operating in I.C.U. patients. Direct chest trauma, hypotension, impaired cardiac function, multiple bone fractures with pulmonary fat embolism, metabolic and biochemical imbalance, uremia, hypoxia, and tracheobronchial infections are all conditioning factors[23] of major significance in the development of adult hyaline membrane disease.

The premature lung is vulnerable due to its tissue immaturity and ventilatory-perfusional difficulties induced by the pathologic alterations of R.D.S. prior to oxygen therapy. Similarly, disparate conditioning factors have an equally prominent preparative and synergistic role in the so-called "respirator lung" of the adult.

Cardiovascular Derangements

Vascular Manipulations

The introduction of various inert materials into vascular channels for a variety of diagnostic and therapeutic purposes is a well-established procedure.[24] This practice is particularly common in the intensive care unit. The desperate nature of the illness being treated usually means a large variety of intravascular manipulations.

In a large proportion of the patients, the central venous pressure (C.V.P.) is monitored through a catheter introduced into the superior vena cava usually via the basilic vein. Following catheter introduction, thrombosis in this vein is fairly common; however, extension of this thrombosing process into the great veins of the neck and superior vena cava is extremely rare. We have encountered three such cases. In all three, the catheters had been left in place for unusually long periods of time. One such example of massive intravascular thrombosis is illustrated in Figure 9.

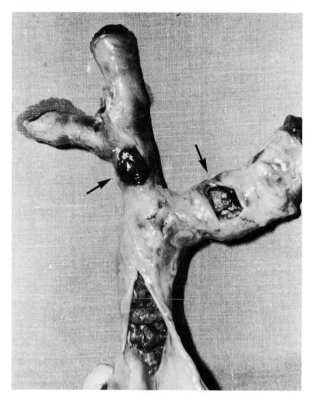

Fig. 9. Thrombosis of superior vena cava and tributaries
(arrows point to windows
made in right subclavian and
innominate veins).

CASE 2. A 31-year-old woman was admitted to the hospital for multiple and
severe injuries sustained in a car accident. The traumatic lesions were corrected surgically,
but she remained seriously ill and was transferred to the I.C.U. because of cardiorespiratory complications. A C.V.P. catheter was inserted into the left basilic vein, and
a thrombus developed. This catheter was removed and another one was introduced into
the right basilic vein. A progressive and eventually massive edema appeared in the
upper extremities, neck, and face. The prothrombin time was 16 sec (control 12 sec),
and circulating macromolecular fibrinogen breakdown products were demonstrated.

Despite heparin and antibiotic therapy, she died 10 days after admission. At autopsy
there was a massive thrombosis of the superior vena cava and its immediate tributaries
(Fig. 9). Multiple small and peripheral pulmonary thromboemboli were also found,
presumably a direct result of the thrombotic phenomenon described. The thrombi around
the catheters were bland. No inflammatory reaction was found in the vein walls. There
appeared to have been in this patient an increased propensity for intravascular clotting;
the cause of this hypercoagulability is outside the scope of this essay.

Polyvinyl tubing is the material most commonly used in the manufacture of
C.V.P. and intravenous infusional catheters. In severely ill patients who require
frequent analyses of arterial blood or the direct monitoring of arterial blood pressure, a teflon tube is introduced into a medium-sized artery. Transvenous cardiac
pacing electrodes are sheathed in silicon rubber tubing, which is alleged to be more
inert than other synthetic materials used in medicine.

Teflon tubing was associated with arterial thrombosis in only one case. Nine
patients with cardiac pacemakers came to autopsy; seven had permanent subcu-

taneous pacemakers, while in the other two the electrodes had been introduced for temporary pacing in severe acute myocardial infarction. In the seven, the pacemaker catheter was enveloped in a synovia-like sheath in the subcutaneous and deeper connective tissues of the body, and throughout its intravascular and intracardiac course it was invariably accompanied by some degree of thrombosis. The thrombotic material was the conventional layered red thrombus (Figs. 10 A, B). All seven cases of permanent pacemakers exhibited small "red sleeve thrombi" loosely investing the intracardiac portions of the catheters. The tips of four out of seven catheters were deeply embedded in the apical muscle of the right ventricle, passing obliquely through secondary trabeculae carnae and enclosed in an endothelial lined fibrous canal. The superior vena cava was extensively thrombosed and occluded in three patients with permanent pacemakers. Out of nine patients, three showed multiple small pulmonary thromboemboli. An example of massive intravascular thrombosis associated with a permanent pacemaker in a 70-year-old man with Stokes-Adams syndrome is illustrated in Figure 10A.

In spite of the possibility of triggering a thrombotic event, vascular manipulations unquestionably remain a mandatory component of the I.C.U. operation. Notwithstanding the development of more and more allegedly inert synthetic materials and the ultrarefinement of the intravascular techniques, thrombosis will remain an occasional annoyance to the I.C.U. physician.

There appears to be a great deal of individual variability in catheter-related thrombogenicity. I.C.U. physicians have noted many times that some patients develop venous thrombi almost immediately following the insertion of a polyvinyl C.V.P. catheter, while others tolerate this intravascular tubing for many days or weeks. The association of distal peripheral thrombi with intravascular catheters is common; the development of deep major vessel thromboses is uncommon. In the latter instance the centripetal spread of the thrombotic phenomenon does not appear to be directly related, either to phlebitis or embolism. This is borne out by the absence of thrombophlebitis in the juxtapositional deep veins and by freedom of the distal vein segments from propagated thrombus. This suggests that the thrombosing phenomenon is an in situ process throughout the intravenous or intracardiac course of the catheter. Further evidence for this postulate was the development of thrombi in two patients who had temporary pacing devices and were on anticoagulant therapy.

Our concern with iatrogenesis has been, up to this point, with catheter-related thromboses, but on rare occasions other vascular complications are encountered. Case 3 demonstrates a rare arterial catastrophe associated with angiography.

CASE 3.   During a parade, a 43-year-old soldier suddenly experienced dizziness and blurring of vision. Twenty-four hours later his speech became slurred and he had a questionable right-sided hemiparesis. These symptoms persisted, and unequal pupils were noted. In an effort to localize the cerebral lesion, a carotid angiography was attempted, but some difficulty was encountered and repeat punctures proved necessary. The films eventually showed some filling of the cerebral arteries. The patient suddenly became comatose, and an emergency tracheostomy was performed. After transfer to the I.C.U. the following day, another angiography was attempted. This time good filling was obtained in the external carotid system but none in the internal carotid artery. The patient remained in a deep coma and succumbed 36 hours after the second angiography.

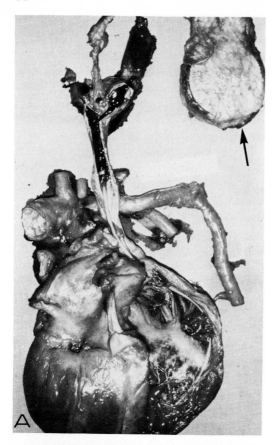

Fig. 10. A. Pacemaker (indicated by arrow) and catheter. The latter is encased in a thrombus within the superior vena cava. B. Same case. A view of the intracardiac portion of the catheter. Sleeve thrombi are clearly visible (arrow A). The tip of the catheter (arrow B) is embedded in the right ventricular myocardium and is surrounded by thin endothelialized fibrous sheath.

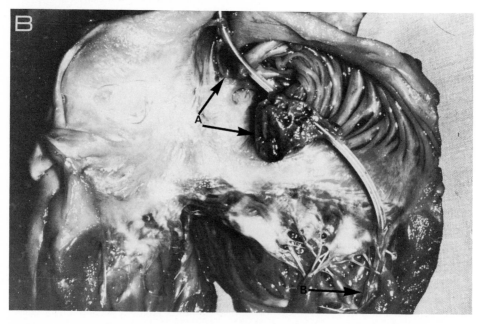

At autopsy several needle puncture marks were noted in the wall of the carotid artery at the point of bifurcation. Microscopic examination revealed an intimal tear which communicated with an intramural hematoma. The dissection of the media of the internal carotid artery had progressed upwards into the region of the carotid siphon, and the corresponding cerebral hemisphere had been recently infarcted. A postmortem radiograph of the excised arterial specimen revealed the presence of contrast medium within the intramural hematoma. The findings indicated that the initial angiographic attempt was responsible for the introduction of contrast medium in the wall of the vessel and its subsequent dissection.

Of much greater import than rare vascular catastrophies are the existence of intravascular thromboses associated with indwelling catheters, the influence of catheter materials on blood coagulability, and the clinical impact of these adventitious thrombi.

Cardiac Massage

The technique of external cardiac massage (E.C.M.) has been widely adopted as an emergency resuscitative measure. In the I.C.U. a significant proportion of cases with circulatory arrest received compressive cardiac stimulation. A smaller proportion (12 percent) received E.C.M. on the general hospital wards or the casualty department before admission to the I.C.U.

Our primary objective with those cases who had had cardiac massage was the morphologic reflections of this act as observed in tissues. The major complications (fractures of the ribs, marrow embolism, myocardial contusions, pneumothorax, pneumomediastinum, ruptures of the liver and diaphragm) are well known hazards.[25] In this essay we have confined our analysis to marrow and fat embolism.

In a retrospective review of patients who had received E.C.M., we reexamined the autopsy protocol and microscopic slides (Table 1). For contrast purposes, we

Table 1.   Incidence of Marrow Emboli in "Routine" Autopsy

	CASES
E.C.M.	24
Rib fractures	12
Emboli	1

analyzed in greater detail a prospective study group of 12 cases. The technique was as follows: multiple histologic sections with appropriate fat stains from each lobe of the lung; radiography of the excised fourth, fifth, and sixth ribs; and thick histologic sections of the latter. All of these patients had been subjected to closed-chest massage by a physician (Table 2).

Table 2.   Incidence of Marrow Emboli in a Prospective Study

	CASES
E.C.M.	12
Fracture or cartilage dislocation	3
Emboli	6

In the retrospective series of cases, a cursory examination of one histologic section from each lung, the incidence of marrow embolism was approximately 4 percent, even lower than the early survey of Baringer.[26] In the prospective group of 12 consecutive (E.C.M.) autopsies, six cases of marrow embolism were encountered, three without evidence of gross fracture. These findings are comparable to those of Yanoff.[27]

In analyzing the mechanism of closed-chest massage and the pathologic finding of pulmonary fat embolism, the fourth, fifth, and sixth grossly nonfractured ribs of each patient were examined in greater detail. Radiographic examination of the ribs was not helpful in the search for fractures in the diploe. Multiple sections of these ribs revealed trabecular fractures associated with intramedullary ecchymoses. Jagged irregular margins of these broken fragments and longitudinal splits of the trabeculae were found in situ in the areas of hemorrhage. Small fragments of recognizable bone marrow were found in blood vessels at the sites of the microtrabecular fractures. These changes were not present in a control group. Our observations suggest a cause-effect relationship between these microtrabecular fractures and pulmonary marrow and fat embolism.

The vigor of the external cardiac massage and the reestablishment of blood circulation probably are the two most important components of this "marrow pumping mechanism" (Fig. 11). Although it is apparent that a high proportion of patients undergoing closed-chest cardiac massage develop pulmonary fat and marrow embolism, the functional effects in surviving patients are difficult to appraise.

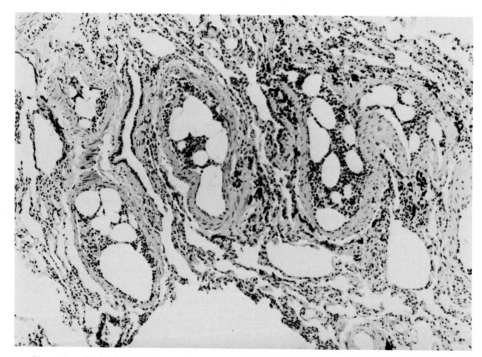

Fig. 11.   Multiple pulmonary blood vessels plugged with bone marrow emboli. X60.

Central Nervous System Derangements

One of the major system disturbances of cardinal concern to the I.C.U. physician is the functional assessment of the central nervous system in the comatose patient. Meaningful interpretations of electroencephalographic evidence of cortical function and the current inability to analyze deep ganglionic centers electronically have contributed to the physician's hesitancy in pronouncing somatic death. The final diagnosis—death—has thus become more difficult to establish, due largely to the new worship given to sophisticated instrumentation. The I.C.U. physician is still in as great a dilemma as was William Congreve, who in 1697 wrote, "Is he then dead? What dead at last, quite, quite forever dead."[28]

This fresh uncertainty in the recognition of somatic death has created a new problem for the pathologist. At autopsy certain organs show surprising degrees of advanced autolysis even though autopsy is performed soon after the final diagnosis. The pathologist's most dramatic evidence of this "premortem" autolysis is in the central nervous system—the "melted brain syndrome." Because of this observation we have introduced in the morgue the practice of infusing fixing solutions into the carotid arteries of dead I.C.U. patients. This procedure is routine if scrutiny of the hospital chart reveals extremely low amplitude in electrical activity of the brain or bursts of equipotentiality.

Twenty-four examples of EEG cases with prolonged irregular or absent electrical activity were studied. The pattern of most of these corresponded to the C and D profiles reported by Pampiglione and Harden.[29] Our current effort is directed at a search for a temporal relationship between severity of morphologic changes in the brain and the monitored parameters of patient care. In Table 3 the data from 10 randomly selected cases out of the 24 are reported. As prototypes, Case 5 and Case 8 in Table 3 are presented in greater detail.

CASE 4. (No. 5 in Table 3). A 53-year-old man was admitted unconscious from carbon monoxide poisoning. Despite hyperbaric oxygen, he remained flaccid and areflexic. Throughout the seven day period in the resuscitative area, the electrolytes and the blood urea nitrogen were always within normal range. At autopsy an unsuspected recent large myocardial infarction of the left ventricle was discovered, as well as bilateral extensive laminar necrosis of the cerebral hemispheres.

CASE 5. (No. 8 in Table 3). A 50-year-old man, a known psychotic, had been on barbiturates (long- and short-acting) and tofranil for at least three years. Two previous hospitalizations had been due to overdose of barbiturates. He was found unconscious and readmitted. Respiration was shallow and rapid (40 to 50 per min), and the patient was cyanosed (blood gas measurements showed moderate hypoxia but no hypercarbia). Assisted ventilation was started and continued until his death two weeks later. X-ray examination of the chest showed progressive infiltration of both lungs. One of the major problems in this patient was maintaining sufficient oxygen tension. Neither carbon dioxide retention nor abnormalities in electrolyte balance were recorded throughout his course. Temperature remained high (102 to 105° F), and the patient gradually deteriorated and died in shock.

At autopsy, apart from the extensive cortical liquefaction of the brain, both lungs were extremely heavy, noncompliant, and solid. There was a generalized stuffing

Table 3. Correlative Study Between C.N.S. Lesions and Electroencephalogram: March 1967-1968

		CLINICAL DATA				LESIONS*			
No.	Diagnosis	Age	Days In I.C.U.	E.E.G.	Cerebral Cortex	Globus Pallidus	Hippocampus	Cerebellar Cortex
1	Diabetic, delayed death from hanging	58	6	0/2 days	Focal laminar	–	+	0
2	Multiple bone and visceral injuries	32	3	0/1 day	0	0	++	0
3	Congestive heart failure	62	6	0/4 days	+	+	+	0
4	Myocardial infarction	70	10	0/4 days	+	++	+	0
5	CO poisoning; Myocardial infarction	53,	5	Arythmic, irregular for 4 days; 0 for 1 day	Generalized multilaminar ++++	++	++	+++
6	Nicotine sulphate poisoning	19	4	0/1 day	++	++	+	++
7	Gouty nephritis, congestive failure	68	4	0/2 days	+	0	+	+
8	Barbiturate overdose and coma; 2 episodes 3 days apart	50	7	0/4 days	++	+	+	+
9	Diabetic; hypoglycemic shock	20	4	Low amplitude 2 days; 0/1 day	+++	0	++	++
10	Chronic bronchitis-emphysema with hypoxia; renal failure	57	10	0/3 days	+	+	++	+

* 0 represents lack of phasic activity or absence of morphologic lesion.

of the air sacs with hyaline membranes interwoven with fibroblasts, histiocytes, and collagenous matrix. This lung alteration, already discussed in an earlier section, clearly contributed to generalized cellular hypoxia, with extremely vulnerable tissues (brain) showing greater degrees of structural damage.

An extensive and severe postmortem dissolution of the brain, particularly the cerebral cortex, is not infrequent in individuals who have been deeply unconscious for a week or more (Figs. 12 A, B). The persistence of cardiac action would suggest that stimuli to the sinoatrial conducting bundle continue to arise from the deep ganglionic brain centres which are spared ischemic and autolytic changes for a

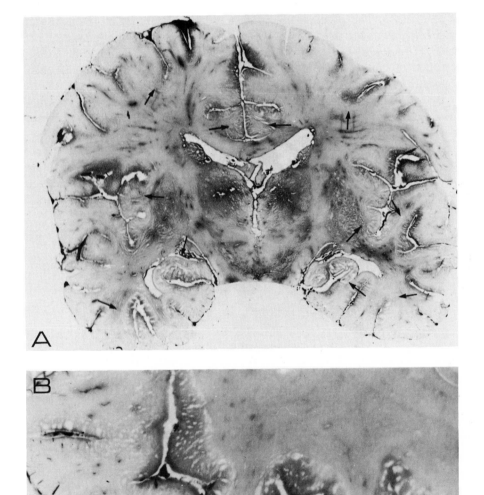

Fig. 12.   A. Whole brain paper section, 300 μ in thickness, demonstrates patchy laminar necrosis of cortex and patchy tinctorial irregularities of white matter. One-half actual size. B. Same section as shown in A. X 3.

greater period of time. These brains, particularly their cortices, often have a "tooth-paste" appearance, and give off a rather distinctive odor, probably related to anaerobic tissue breakdown. The greater the degree of breakdown of cerebral lipo-proteins (Fig. 13), the less successful the fixation with formalin.

Edema and liquefactive necrosis of the brain may be quite pronounced, al-though the interval of time between the clinician's decision to withdraw all forms of mechanical assistance and the performance of the autopsy may only have been one or two hours. The greatest concentration of dissolution is usually cortical, with punctate mottling at the base of the convolutions the most prominent feature. With progression of the liquefactive necrosis, the extent of laminar necrosis is more notice-able (Fig. 12B). The selective erasure of the middle neuronal strata in the sesqui-laminated cortex is observed in the hypoxic as well as hypoglycemic brain. Extreme degrees of pericellular edema and perivascular dissolution without the histologic companion of granulocytic infiltration are morphologic hallmarks of this form of brain death.

Budd,[30] as early as 1852, indicated that organ changes appear to become aggravated after death. Loss of cytoplasmic structure and nuclear karyorrhexis are now well recognized as tissue effects often associated with postmortem change.

The degree of dissolution in I.C.U. cases suggests that there has been a pre-mortem liberation of lysosomal enzymes which brings about colliquation while the pumping action of the heart is still effective. Investigations into autolysis have indi-cated that factors other than the release of hydrolytic enzymes influence cell dis-

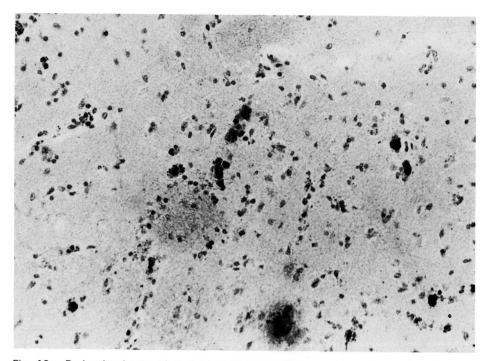

Fig. 13.   Brain showing multiple lipid droplets, mostly perivascular in location, free and intracellular. Oil red O. X160.

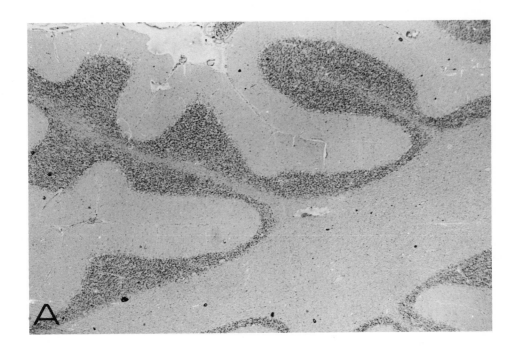

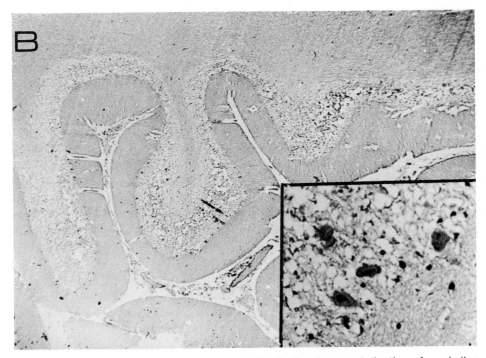

Fig. 14. A. Normal cerebellar folia. H & E. X10. B. Massive conglutination of cerebellar folia. H & E. X10. Inset demonstrates neuronal degeneration. X125.

solution. For example, the dependence of autolysis on oxygen tension is well recognized.

In the patient on IPP and without activity in the electroencephalogram for several days, a consideration of the factors concerned in brain necrobiosis, although speculative, is of current interest. Since subnormal oxygen tensions would be present in the hypoxic brain fields, carbon dioxide, due to its rapid diffusability, might not influence the acidity of the tissues which favors autolysis. The total effect may be a form of controlled autolysis. Diffusion of oxygen and amino acids would be impaired in the hypoxic fields. The integrative action of these factors would further control autolysis by inhibiting the production of —SH groups. Inhibition of —SH groups favors the liberation of the intracellular proteolytic enzymes and accordingly enhances tissue liquefaction.[31]

Selective vulnerability of cell fields to disintegration is a distinguishing feature of tissue hypoxia. Older theories contended that this tissue susceptibility to hypoxic injury was related to the distance of the circulatory pathway, or certain cell fields with specialized intracellular metabolic cycles were more readily influenced by lack of oxygen. In rare events, the substrates of the cell involved in oxygen usage might be lacking (oxyachrestic hypoxia). A recent postulate[32] is that the neurones of the cortex, due to their large surface area (cell + axon + dendrites) are readily susceptible to minor degrees of hypoxia. This built-in susceptibility would foster, after the cell membrane has been injured, an early liberation of proteases and cathepsins, thus advancing tissue necrosis. The cerebellum seems to be peculiarly prone to conglutinative changes probably due to altered metabolism induced either by ischemia or electrolyte derangements (Figs. 14 A, B).[33, 34]

Experimental work on the blood flow to a rabbit brain has revealed that certain areas remain ischemic, even after restoration of circulation. In as short a period as five minutes obstruction, no reflow develops in these areas. A spastic narrowing of the vascular lumen, not microcirculatory thrombosis, appears to be the pathogenetic mechanism. The prompt development of glial swelling, a central nervous injury of polyvalent etiology, may impinge upon capillaries and produce the irreversible phenomenon of no reflow.[35, 36] Failure of electrolyte transfer and accumulation of extravascular water increase blood viscosity and compound the microcirculatory cerebral problem.

Certain of our cases had greater destruction of the central nervous system than others. A comatose state, provoked by selective hypnotics or cellular poisons such as nicotine, seems to be associated with a limited neuronal damage. Case 5, a combination of cardiac failure (circulatory hypoxia) and carboxyhemoglobin poisoning (anemic hypoxia), showed the greatest degree of cerebral damage (Figs. 12 A, B). An interesting feature of this case was that the EEGs, although arythmic and irregular, always revealed some evidence of electrical activity. This case illustrates the synergistic action of two forms of hypoxia. To some extent, this is an anatomic recapitulation of earlier experimental studies by Scholz and Schmidt.[35]

Selective vulnerability of brain matter was not clearly demonstrated in our 10 cases (Table 3). This morphologic disparity may well represent a blurring of the traditional patterns of hypoxia—the result of sustained care.

Summary

In dealing with problems arising from the I.C.U., the hospital pathologist quickly becomes aware that there is no retreat into the sanctuary of factual morphology. He cannot ignore the pathobiologic derangements which developed during the period of sustained life. The morphologic alterations observed by the pathologist in the morgue are the culmination of complex, interwoven but often disparate, functional, biochemical, and physical phenomena. The nature of these changes is further compounded by the multiple, active, and continuous lines of medication, along with other iatrogenic efforts by the I.C.U. staff.

To decipher the maze of available information and constantly to devise ways and means of increasing the interpretative values of pathology at the autopsy table are the tasks of the hospital pathologist. "The alveoli are filled with granulocytes." Is this enough evidence to state that pneumonia was the cause of death if the patient was afebrile, receiving appropriate antibiotics, on a balanced fluid intake, with normal blood gases and satisfactory cardiac action? Are other pathways of death being overlooked?

The pathologist must ask fundamental questions about the mechanisms of death, time of visceral and somatic death, criteria for viability of tissues, and other changing parameters of life and death. As the intensive care unit is an ever changing one, the hermeneutics of morphology must be reflective of that change.

Due to the glamorous nature of intensive care units, numerous efforts to compare mortality rates, salvable ratios, and resuscitative procedures have produced a deluge of reports.[37, 38, 39] Beginning with the admission policy of the unit to the codification of pathology findings on the fatal cases, there is a clear need for the establishment of common methods of reporting. Both from the clinical and morphologic viewpoints, conscientious quantitation of the disease process, the procedures, and the pathology should be the dominant theme of the hospital record.

To those of us convinced of the necessity of a new educational approach to the postmortem examination, it is apparent that the traditional routine autopsy is all but inadequate for the purpose at hand. To achieve this aim, we suggest a prospective collaboration between the I.C.U. physician and the autopsy teaching unit staff on a few fatal cases selected each week. In the intensive care unit clinical and morphologic translations can be analyzed to provide an understanding not only of the progress of disease but also the diseases of progress.

References

1. MacIver, I.N., Lassman, L.P., Thompson, C.W., and McLeod, I. Decerebrate rigidity reduced from 80 percent to 40 percent. Lancet, 2:544, 1958.
2. Editorial. Severe head injuries. Lancet, 1:514, 1968.
3. Lewin, W. Mortality of head injuries fall from 9 percent to 3.5 percent over eight years. Proc. Roy. Soc. Med., 60:1208, 1967.
4. Henri de Toulouse-Lautrec: The Tracheotomy. (Courtesy of Sterling and Francine Clark, Institute of Art, Williamstown, Mass.)
5. Lown, B., Fabhro, A.M., Hood, W.B., and Thorn, G.W. Coronary care unit: New perspective and directions. J.A.M.A., 199:188, 1967.

6. London, P.S. Survival after head injury: A pyrrhic victory producing lame brains. Ann. Roy. Coll. Surg. Eng., 41:460, 1967.

7. Hildreth, E.A. The significance of iatrogenesis. J.A.M.A., 193:386, 1965.

8. Yarington, C.T., and Frazer, J.P. Complications of tracheotomy. Arch. Surg., 91:652, 1965.

9. Friedberg, S.A., Griffith, T.E., and Hass, G.M. Histologic changes in the trachea following tracheostomy. Ann. Otol., 74:785, 1965.

10. Gibson, P. Aetiology and repair of tracheal stenosis following tracheostomy and intermittent positive pressure respiration. Thorax, 22:1, 1967.

11. West, J.B., Glazies, J.B., Hughes, J.M.B., and Maloney, J.E. Recent work on the distribution of pulmonary blood flow and topographical differences in alveolar size. *In* Form and Function in the Human Lung. London, E. & S. Livingston, 1968, Sec. 3, pp. 111-124.

12. Schiff, M.M., and Massaro, D. Effect of O_2 administration by a Ventura apparatus on arterial blood gas values in patients with respiratory failure. New Eng. J. Med., 277:950, 1967.

13. J. Lorrain Smith. The pathological effects due to increase of oxygen tension in the air breathed. J. Physiol., 24:19, 1899.

14. Pratt, P.C. The reaction of the human lung to enriched oxygen atmosphere. Ann. N.Y. Acad. Sci., 121:809, 1965.

15. Shanklin, D.R., and Wolfson, S.L. Therapeutics O_2 as a possible cause of pulmonary hemorrhage in premature infants. New Eng. J. Med., 277:883, 1967.

16. Northway, W.H., Jr., Rosahn, R.C., and Porter, D.Y. Pulmonary disease following respirator therapy of hyaline-membrane disease: Bronchopulmonary dysplasia, New Eng. J. Med., 276:357, 1967.

17. Kistler, G.S., Caldwell, P.R.B., and Weibel, E.R. Development of fine structural damage to alveolar and capillary lining cells in oxygen-poisoned rat lungs. J. Cell Biol., 32:605, 1967.

18. Buckingham, S., and Sommers, S.C. Pulmonary hyaline membranes. Amer. J. Dis. Child., 99:216, 1960.

19. Bowden, D.H., Wyatt, J.P., and Adamson, I.Y.R. The reaction of the lung cells to a high concentration of oxygen. Arch. Path., 86:671, 1968.

20. Nash, G., Blennerhassett, J.B., and Pontoppidan, H. Pulmonary lesions with oxygen therapy and artificial ventilation. New Eng. J. Med., 276:368, 1967.

21. Barter, R.A., Finlay-Jones, L.R., and Walters, M.N.I. Pulmonary hyaline membrane: Sites of formation in adult lung after assisted respiration and inhalation of oxygen. J. Path. Bact., 95:481, 1968.

22. Ashbaugh, D.G., Bigelow, D.B., Petty, T.L., and Levine, B.E. Acute respiratory distress in adults. Lancet, 2:319, 1967.

23. Clowes, G.H.A., Zuschneid, W., Turner, M., Blackburn, G., Rubin, J., Toala, P., and Green, G. The pathogenesis of pneumonitis associated with severe infections in other parts of the body. Ann. Surg., 167:630, 1968.

24. Comparative Study on Cardiac Catheterization. Braunwald, E., and Swan, H.J.C., eds. Circulation, Vol. 37, Suppl. 3, 1968.

25. Saphir, R. External cardiac massage. Medicine (Balt.), 47:73, 1968.

26. Baringer, J.R., Salsman, E.W., Jones, W.A., and Friedlich, A.L. External cardiac massage. New Eng. J. Med., 265:62, 1961.

27. Yanoff, M. Incidence of bone marrow embolism due to closed chest cardiac massage. New Eng. J. Med., 269:837, 1963.

28. William Congreve. The Mourning Bride. 1697.

29. Pampiglione, G., and Harden, A. Resuscitation after cardiocirculatory arrest. Lancet, 1:1261, 1968.

30. Budd, G. Diseases of the Liver, 2nd ed. Philadelphia and London, J. Churchill, 1852.

31. Bradley, H.C. Autolysis and atrophy. Physiol. Rev., 18:173, 1938.

32. Dixon, K.C. Cerebral vulnerability to ischemia: An hypothesis. Lancet, 2:289, 1967.
33. Olsen, S. Acute selective necrosis of the granular layer of the cerebellar cortex. J. Neuropath. Exp. Neurol., 18:609, 1959.
34. Ikuta, F., Hirano, A., and Zimmerman, H.M. An experimental study of postmortem alterations in the granular layer of the cerebellar cortex. J. Neuropath. Exp. Neurol., 22:581, 1963.
35. Scholz, W., and Schmidt, H. Durchblutungsstorungen bei Hypoxamie (Asphyxia). Arch. Psychiat. Nervenkr., 189:231, 1952.
36. Chiang, J., Kowada, M., Ames, A., Wright, R.L., and Majno, G. Cerebral ischemia: III. Vascular changes. Amer. J. Path., 52:455, 1968.
37. Lawrie, D.M., Greenwood, T.W., Goddard, M., Harvey, A.C., Donald, K.W., Julian, D.G., and Oliver, M.F. A coronary-care unit in the routine management of acute myocardial infarction. Lancet, 2:109, 1967.
38. Yu, P.N., Imboden, C.A., Fox, S.M., and Killip, T. Coronary care unit: I. A specialized intensive care unit for acute myocardial infarction. Mod. Conc. Cardiovasc. Dis., 34:23, 1965.
39. Partridge, J.F., and Gedees, J.S. A mobile intensive-care unit in the management of myocardial infarction. Lancet, 2:271, 1967.

NORMAL VALUES IN PATHOLOGY

ROLAND E. BERRY

Normal values in clinical pathology have posed a difficult problem ever since laboratory tests were used in clinical medicine. Most clinical laboratories formerly accepted the normal limits established by the people who developed and published the various tests. During the period when our instruments were not very precise, this acceptance was not too serious. As our instruments improved, however, it became increasingly evident that the range of normal values is dependent on many things, including the instruments used and the methodology of the test itself. It also became evident, particularly in chemistry, that the range of normal values differs in different population groups.

Many people began to wonder whether it was entirely valid to establish a range of normal values on a group of medical students and assume that this range of values could be used on the medical wards to evaluate patients such as elderly females or infants. The dictum that each laboratory should establish its own range of normal values for each test became more widely accepted during the past decade. The mechanism for doing this, however, remained as confused as before. How does the laboratory in a 150-bed hospital in a community of 20,000 population establish a range of normal values for blood glucose? How many "normal" people should such a laboratory use to determine the range of normal values? Even if a valid number of individuals were available for each of the many clinical tests, and if the laboratory were capable of doing this much additional work, there were no well-defined rules for handling the data from these individuals to arrive at a range of normal values. Finally, how would such a laboratory know that the individuals were "normal" with respect to any specific laboratory test?

In a brief paper read before the Clinical Chemistry Council session at the meeting of the American Society of Clinical Pathologists in 1962, R. G. Hoffmann out-

lined a statistical method which he subsequently published and which provided the
first sound approach to the problem of normal values in the individual laboratory.[1]
In 1964, our laboratory reported initial studies with this method.[2] We have subsequently applied the method successfully to a wide variety of tests in the clinical
laboratory and to various weights and measurements in autopsy pathology.

Clinical Chemistry

To illustrate the mechanism of Hoffmann's method, we can use recent data from
the St. Francis Hospital at Escanaba, Michigan for the serum sodium determination.
Between December 29, 1966, and April 19, 1967, at the request of physicians this
laboratory did 187 sodium determinations on various hospitalized patients. The reported values on these 187 tests ranged from 106 mEq/l to 160 mEq/l. Table 1
gives the distribution of the values. In this table, a reported value of 119 mEq/l is
entered in the 120 group, and a value of 121 is entered in the 122 group. The second column gives the number of patients for each group of reported values. The
third is the percentage of patients in each group, and the last column is the cumulative percentage of patients with increasing levels of sodium. Thus 5.9 percent of the
187 determinations had a serum sodium of 120 mEq/l or less, and 90.3 percent of
the results were 140 mEq/l or less.

How the reported values are grouped depends in part on the expected range of
normal values. In the case of the glucose determination with a normal range of 70
to 100 mg/100 ml, grouping in 5 mg steps (e.g., 60, 65, 70) is adequate. For

Table 1. Serum Sodium Determination

MEQ/LITER	NUMBER OF PATIENTS	PERCENT	CUMULATIVE PERCENT
Less than 116	5	2.7	2.7
116	3	1.6	4.3
118	1	0.5	4.8
120	2	1.1	5.9
122	1	0.5	6.4
124	5	2.7	9.1
126	6	3.2	12.3
128	12	6.4	18.7
130	17	9.1	27.8
132	17	9.1	36.9
134	32	17.1	54.0
136	29	15.5	69.5
138	27	14.4	83.9
140	12	6.4	90.3
142	3	1.6	91.9
144	2	1.1	93.0
146	6	3.2	96.2
148	3	1.6	97.8
150	0	0	97.8
Over 150	4	2.0	99.8
Total	187	99.8	

potassium, on the other hand, where the range of normal values is approximately 4.0 to 5.0 mEq/l, grouping by 0.2 mEq has proven satisfactory. Whether the values need to be grouped at all depends largely on the calibration curve. With the glucose determination in our laboratory, a 1 percent T change on the calibration curve is read as a change of 3 mg/100 ml in concentration. Ungrouped tabulation of the reported results in this case would not give a satisfactory curve when the cumulative percentages are subsequently plotted on probability graph paper. The necessity of grouping, therefore, depends on the sensitivity of the final measurement. We will see the effect of this again in the measurement of heart valves at autopsy (see p. 80).

In Figure 1, the cumulative percentages from Table 1 are plotted on the proba-

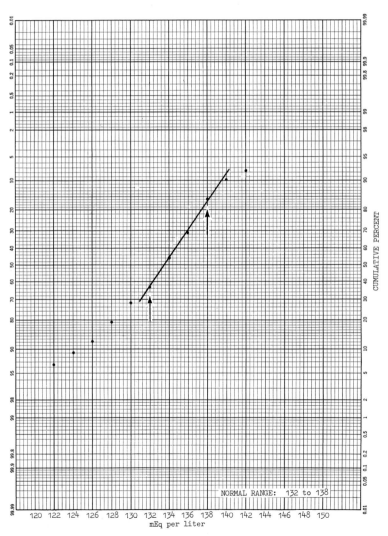

Fig. 1.   Serum sodium determination: 187 consecutive patient values taken from December 29, 1966 to April 19, 1967; St. Francis Hospital, Escabana, Michigan. Graph paper is Keuffel & Esser Co., probability type, X90 divisions, number 46 8003.

bility (vertical) scale of probability graph paper against the group value on the linear (horizontal) scale. The curve obtained by so plotting the cumulative percentages has a straight-line segment from 132 mEq/l to 140 mEq/l. This means that between these two extremes, the patient values have a random distribution. If we assume that normal values have a random distribution in a given normal population, then these values are at least part of the range of normal values. In his original paper, Hoffmann was concerned with establishing the range of normal values for the general population on the basis of 200 to 300 individual values. To do this, the straight-line segment of Figure 1 must be projected downward to the 5 percent level on the probability scale and upward to the 95 percent level, giving a range of normal values for sodium of 126 to 142 mEq/l (Fig. 1). In the biologic sense, this is statistically correct. In medicine, however, we are concerned primarily with determining whether the results of a laboratory test indicate possible derangement of the physiologic function that the test is intended to evaluate.

A serum sodium, for example, of 142 mEq/l may be normal in a given patient, but, since 90 percent of the values obtained in this series of 187 consecutive determinations on patients were 140 mEq/l or less, one should consider 142 mEq/l abnormal until proven otherwise. In the same manner, since 65 to 70 percent of the sodium values were 132 mEq/l or more, values below 130 mEq/l should be considered abnormal until proven otherwise, even though in a small percentage of individuals values lower than this may indeed be normal.

Following the above reasoning, our laboratory considers only the straight-line segment of the probability curve as the range of normal values and refers to it as the *clinical* range of normal values. For sodium, then, we use 130 to 140 mEq/l as our stated range of *clinically* normal values. We prepare probability curves on every 200 to 400 consecutive reported values for all chemistry determinations whenever a sufficient number of values have been accumulated. We therefore have a number of probability curves for many of the more common chemical determinations. Table 2

Table 2.   Representative Ranges of Normal Values at St. Francis Hospital

DATE	NUMBER OF PATIENTS	CALCULATED RANGE	DATE	NUMBER OF PATIENTS	CALCULATED RANGE
Fasting Glucose			SGOT		
7/27/66	532	75-105	4/28/65	191	8-12
12/15/66	607	80-105	3/10/66	376	10-18
4/19/67	371	85-100	7/27/66	232	10-18
			4/20/67	355	12-18
Urea Nitrogen			Sodium		
3/10/66	235	10-18	11/11/65	206	134-138
7/27/66	270	10-14	6/15/66	332	134-138
10/25/66	228	12-24	12/28/66	258	134-142
4/19/67	356	12-20	4/19/67	187	132-140
Postprandial Glucose			CO_2 Content		
7/27/66	324	100-140	3/10/66	199	16-32
7/21/67	421	105-140	4/19/67	215	20-30

gives some of the ranges which have been calculated at St. Francis Hospital in recent years.

On July 27, 1966, we had accumulated 532 consecutive glucose determinations on patients and calculated a range of 75-105 mg/100 ml. Between July 27 and December 15, 1966, we accumulated another 607 determinations with a calculated range (as described above) of 80 to 105 mg/100 ml. There is obviously a slight shift in normal limits by the modified Hoffmann method. This may, in part, be due to shifts in technique. With our frozen serum pool program, we are continuously striving for better reproducibility, and we change our technique of performing the test if our reproducibility appears to be getting less than we feel is adequate, i.e., one standard deviation of 4 to 5 mg/100 ml.

The ranges of normal values for CO_2 content (Table 2) are an excellent example of the effect of quality control measures on the range of normal values, as well as on reproducibility. Prior to March, 1966, it was evident that the CO_2 content determination was not as good as it should have been, and much effort was spent in improving our techniques for all of the electrolyte determinations, including the CO_2 content. As of March 10, 1966, it was obvious that we were getting too many low values, and we recognized that a range of normal values of 16 to 32 mM/l was probably due in part to faulty techniques. Our performance between March 10, 1966, and April 19, 1967, was perceptibly better, and the range of normal values calculated from consecutive patient values was clearly more reasonable during this period.

From Table 2, it is relatively easy to provide the clinician with practical limits for normal values based on data that are readily available from the daily log book of patient values. While there are slight shifts in these limits, the calculated ranges for any specific determination are remarkably close, considering the wide range of values obtained from a patient population in which wide deviations from the normal are found.

For the less frequently performed chemistry procedures such as serum bilirubin, calcium, and amylase, Hoffmann's method also can be used, but the period of time necessary to accumulate sufficient numbers of consecutive patient values is considerably longer. At St. Francis Hospital, the clinical chemistry results were not recorded in a daily log book prior to January 1, 1965. Tabulating the consecutive patient values for calcium from that date to May 19, 1967 yielded 159 values. During this period, the calcium procedure had not been significantly changed, so the range of normal values could be calculated by the Hoffmann method and gave a range of 3.8 to 5.0 mEq/l (7.6 to 10.0 mg/100 ml). In the case of the amylase determination, we still do not have enough values from consecutive patients to calculate a normal range.

In introducing a new test for routine use in diagnosis and therapy, we first of all standardize the procedure using our frozen serum pools. Once this is done, we do the test on a series of random serum samples from the daily patient serums until we have accumulated sufficient values over a period of time to draw a probability curve (usually 150 or more) and derive the range of normal values from the curve. At this point, we can provide the clinicians with a range of normal values applicable to our laboratory. We can also provide them with a reproducibility in terms of standard deviation at the time we begin to do the test on patients at the physician's request. In general, it is our policy to subject every new test to this procedure prior to doing the test for clinical information.

At the time we obtained our instruments for blood pH, we spent several weeks working part time with the technique itself. Having familiarized ourselves with the operation of the instruments, we performed 4 to 8 pH determinations a day on random patient bloods until we had accumulated 86 pH readings on miscellaneous patients on whom various tests (other than pH or electrolytes) were ordered. Table 3 gives the distribution of pH values on these 86 patients, and Figure 2 gives the probability curve for the data in Table 3.

Table 3.   Distribution of pH Values in Random Patient Bloods

pH	NUMBER OF PATIENTS	PERCENT	CUMULATIVE PERCENT
7.30	0	—	—
7.32	2	2.3	2.3
7.34	1	1.1	3.4
7.36	7	8.1	11.5
7.38	23	26.8	38.3
7.40	13	15.3	53.6
7.42	18	21.0	74.6
7.44	13	15.3	89.9
7.46	5	5.8	95.7
7.48	3	3.5	99.2
7.50	0	—	99.2
7.52	0	—	99.2
7.54	1	1.1	100.3
	86	100.3	

Since the series is small, the segment between pH 7.38 and 7.46 is not perfectly straight, but it is clear that this is the portion that approaches a straight line. It is also clear that this normal range coincides very closely with the range of 7.35 to 7.45, which is generally accepted as the range of normal values. Our probability curve could not, in this case, give a normal range of 7.35 to 7.45 because our grouping at 0.02 intervals does not allow us to recognize the point for pH 7.35 or pH 7.45. With these facts in mind, we have used the blood pH for diagnostic and therapeutic purposes with a stated range of normal values of 7.35 to 7.45. To date, we have accumulated only 51 values on patients on whom the pH has been requested, but we feel fairly confident that after 100 or 200 consecutive patient values, the calculated range of normal values will not be very far from this range.

Other Clinical Laboratory Tests

After working with the Hoffmann method in clinical chemistry, we began to try the method in other areas of the laboratory where the final reports were numerical values. The most obvious place to begin was with the hemoglobin determination in hematology. The range of normal values calculated on various dates from the consecutive patient data prior to that date are given in Table 4 for hemoglobin,

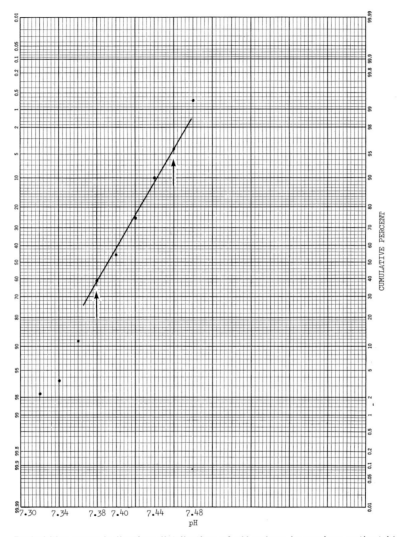

Fig. 2.   Probability curve indicating distribution of pH values in random patient bloods.

hematocrit, and the mean corpuscular hemoglobin concentration (derived from simultaneous hemoglobin and hematocrit determinations). Establishing the range of normal values for hemoglobin was somewhat difficult when the values were grouped at 0.2 g intervals, and, as seen in Table 4, the range of values showed some shift-

Table 4.   Calculated Ranges of Normal Values in Hematology

DATE	NUMBER OF PATIENTS	RANGE	DATE	NUMBER OF PATIENTS	RANGE	DATE	NUMBER OF PATIENTS	RANGE
	Hemoglobin			*Hematocrit*			*M.C.H.C.*	
11/30/64	512	11.8-14.4	7/31/64	444	35-41	8/ 3/66	200	32-35
8/15/66	200	12.2-15.0	9/30/64	395	33-40	2/13/67	213	32-35
8/26/66	200	12.6-15.2	11/ 1/64	458	32-43	3/27/67	211	32-35
2/13/67	224	11.6-14.8	8/15/66	200	37-44			

ing. It was hoped that the hematocrit, being less subject to technical error, would prove to be more stable, but it showed some degree of variation also. Only when the hemoglobin and hematocrit were correlated in the mean corpuscular hemoglobin concentration (M.C.H.C.) did we obtain easily read probability curves with stable ranges of normal values. Since the M.C.H.C. is stable, we are inclined to attribute the difficulties with the hemoglobin and hematocrit curves to biologic, rather than technical, factors. If technical errors occurred in the hemoglobin and hematocrit determinations, one would have expected some shifting of the M.C.H.C., unless the errors occurred in the same direction in each of the determinations the majority of the time. This problem probably deserves more study.

While we have not done so, there is no reason to suppose that ranges of normal values could not be done for such things as urine specific gravity or number of cells per cubic millimeter in spinal fluid. It would be of interest to see what range of normal values one would obtain for urine specific gravity done by the hydrometer as compared with urine specific gravity done by the refractometer. The two methods almost certainly would not yield the same range of normal values, since the potential technical errors with the hydrometer are considerably greater than with the refractometer.

Organ Weights and Measurements

In anatomic pathology, the weighing of organs is a well-established part of the autopsy procedure. It is rare, however, that the scales used for weighing organs are checked to assure that they are equally sensitive in all portions of the graduated scale over an extended period of time. All degrees of care (or carelessness) are seen in removing excess tissue before weighing is done. Various scales are graduated differently, and consequently, the weight is read with different degrees of precision.

Table 5.   Distribution of Spleen Weights

WEIGHT IN GRAMS	NUMBER OF SPLEENS	PERCENT	CUMULATIVE PERCENT
Less than 50	2	0.9	0.9
50	6	2.8	3.7
75	17	7.9	11.6
100	39	18.0	29.6
125	22	10.2	39.8
150	28	13.0	52.8
175	26	12.0	64.8
200	15	7.0	71.8
225	10	4.6	76.4
250	15	7.0	83.4
275	3	1.4	84.8
300	8	3.7	88.5
325	5	2.3	90.8
350	6	2.8	93.6
375	0	0.0	93.6
400	3	1.4	95.0
Over 400	11	5.1	100.1
Total	216	100.1	

Clearly these problems make weighing of an organ quite comparable, though less complex, to doing a blood glucose determination. Establishing ranges of normal values for organ weights can, therefore, be done by the Hoffmann method.

Between October, 1961, and April, 1964, at the Veterans Administration Hospital at Iron Mountain, Michigan, 216 spleens were weighed at consecutive autopsies. In Table 5, the weights of these 216 spleens are tabulated. Since the autopsy room scale was graduated at 25-gram intervals, the recorded weights are multiples of 25, with no attempt to estimate weights between successive graduations. If the scale indicator fell between two graduations, the weight was recorded as that of the next highest graduation. In Table 5, the recorded weights are tabulated directly from the report without grouping.

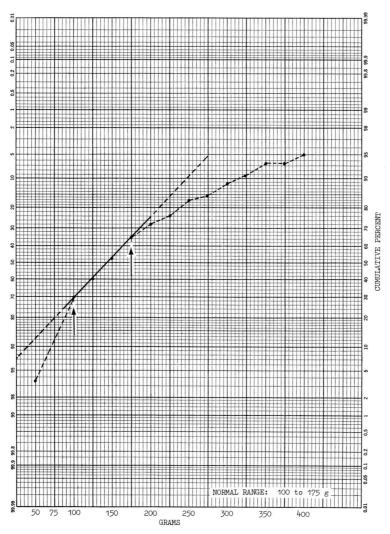

Fig. 3.   Probability curve for spleen weights: 216 consecutive autopsies taken from October 21, 1961 to April 28, 1964; Veterans Administration Hospital, Iron Mountain, Michigan.

In Figure 3, the cumulative percentages are plotted on probability graph paper in the same manner as described earlier. The straight-line segment of the curve is 100 to 175 g. It is of interest that the upper limit of normal in *Gray's Anatomy*[3] is 170 g based on quite different criteria, since the Hoffmann method was not available at the time *Gray's Anatomy* was published.

In working with Hoffmann's method, the results are not always as clearly evident as in the case of the spleen weights. This is presumably due to the fact that the mixed population of consecutive patient values contains homogenous groups, other than the "normals," in which the values have a random distribution. Such a circumstance is seen with the 218 heart weights taken in the same consecutive autopsies from which the spleen weights were taken. Table 6 and Figure 4 were derived in the same manner as described for the spleen.

Table 6. Distribution of Heart Weights

WEIGHT IN GRAMS	NUMBER OF HEARTS	PERCENT	CUMULATIVE PERCENT
175	2	0.9	0.9
200	2	0.9	1.8
225	4	1.8	3.6
250	14	6.4	10.0
275	12	5.5	15.5
300	20	9.2	24.7
325	15	6.9	31.6
350	11	5.1	36.7
375	15	6.9	43.6
400	22	10.1	53.7
425	8	3.7	57.4
450	11	5.1	62.5
475	15	6.9	69.4
500	15	6.9	76.3
525	7	3.2	79.5
550	4	1.8	81.3
575	8	3.7	85.0
600	4	1.8	86.8
625	4	1.8	88.6
650	4	1.8	90.4
675	4	1.8	92.2
700	3	1.4	93.6
Over 700	14	6.4	100.0
Total	218	100.0	

The probability curve for the heart weights shows two straight-line segments (300 to 400 g and 425 to 525 g). Thus, there are apparently two groups of patients in this series that show a random distribution of heart weights in two distinctly different ranges. This curve does not give us the range of normal values unequivocally as in the case of the spleens (see above). Without consideration of other factors than the curve alone, the range of normal values may be taken as 300 to 400 g, 425 to 525 g, or 300 to 525 g. The curve does not help us decide which should be taken as the range of normal values, other than indicating that 55 percent of the weights are 400 g or less. In this particular case, one is inclined to take 300

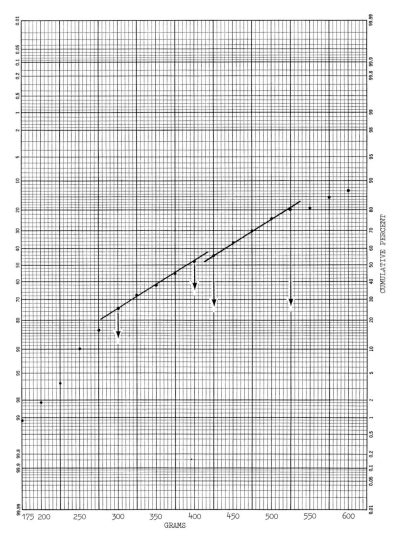

Fig. 4.   Probability curve for heart weights: 218 consecutive autopsies taken from October 21, 1961 to April 28, 1964; Veterans Administration Hospital, Iron Mountain, Michigan.

to 400 g as the range of normal values, since this range includes the 50 percent cumulative level. Since *Gray's Anatomy* gives 280 to 340 g as the range of normal male hearts, our calculated range would at least appear reasonable.

If, for the moment, we accept 300 to 400 grams as our range of normal heart weights, we are then required to offer some explanation for the second group in which the heart weights have a random distribution between 425 and 525 grams. The patients in this series were all males, largely past the age of 50 years, and many had signs of cardiac failure of various degrees from chronic passive congestion of the lungs to pulmonary edema. It is entirely conceivable that the heart weights of 425 to 525 g represent the range of "normal" values for males with moderate cardiac failure. To prove this, one would need to do probability curves using only the consecutive heart weights from autopsies showing ancillary findings of cardiac failure with and without hypertension. If, in so doing, the random distribution between 300 to 400 g disappeared (or accounted for much less than fifty percent of the series) and the random distribution between 425 to 525 g shifted to include the 50 percent level, then we would have statistical support for the cardiac failure hypothesis in explaining this second group of random values of heart weights.

Some of the interesting information that can be obtained from these probability curves is demonstrated by the weights of the kidneys obtained at autopsy in the Veterans Administration series. There were 428 kidneys from 214 consecutive autopsies in which each kidney was present and was weighed separately after removal of the perinephric tissues. The distribution of weights is given in Table 7, together with the data necessary for the probability curve. The probability curve is shown in Figure 5.

Table 7. Distribution of Kidney Weights

WEIGHT IN GRAMS	NUMBER OF KIDNEYS	PERCENT	CUMULATIVE PERCENT
Less than 50	3	0.7	0.7
50	3	0.7	1.4
75	15	3.5	4.9
100	54	12.5	17.4
125	73	17.0	34.4
150	86	20.0	54.4
175	83	19.3	73.7
200	54	12.5	86.2
225	21	4.9	91.1
250	21	4.9	96.0
275	5	1.2	97.2
300	6	1.4	98.6
Over 300	4	0.9	99.5
Total	428	99.5	

As in the case of the spleen, the range of normal values is readily identified as being 100 to 200 g (as compared with 125 to 170 g in *Gray's Anatomy*). If separate probability curves are drawn for the 214 left kidneys and the 214 right kidneys, the range of normal values for the left kidney is 75 to 175 g, while that for the right kidney is 100 to 200 g. This suggests the possibility that the right kidney tends to be somewhat heavier than the left kidney. Whether this is indeed true in the general population requires further study of other patient groups, including both males and females as well as patients of younger age groups than those used for the present series. If there is a difference in the normal weight of the two kidneys, then the practice of weighing the two kidneys together and reporting a combined weight may not be entirely valid.

In Figure 6, the probability curve for 71 kidneys from 36 consecutive autopsies at St. Francis Hospital, Escanaba, Michigan (August, 1966, to May, 1967) is shown. Clearly the range of normal values is 125 to 225 g as compared with 100 to 200 g for the Veterans Administration series. There are several possible interpretations of

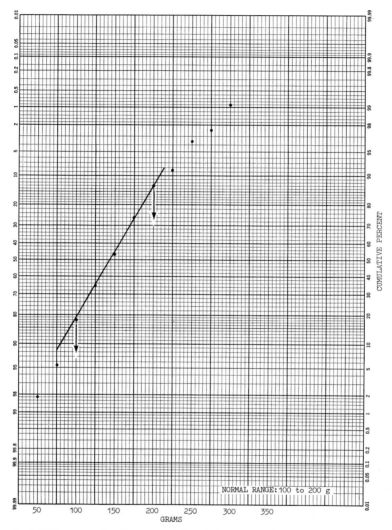

Fig. 5.   Probability curve for kidney weights: 215 consecutive autopsies taken from October 21, 1961 to April 28, 1964; Veterans Administration Hospital, Iron Mountain, Michigan.

these two results. First of all, the St. Francis Hospital series is small. One must be careful not to draw conclusions too readily from the Hoffmann method when the series is less than 150 to 200 individual readings. Another possibility is that the mechanical characteristics of the two autopsy scales were sufficiently different to account for the shift. Finally, there may indeed be biologic differences in the two groups, such that the kidneys of the St. Francis Hospital group were generally heavier.

Turning our attention to measurements in autopsy material, the use of Hoffmann's technique is equally applicable. Among the routine measurements made in our laboratory is the thickness of the adrenal cortex in the final microscopic sections

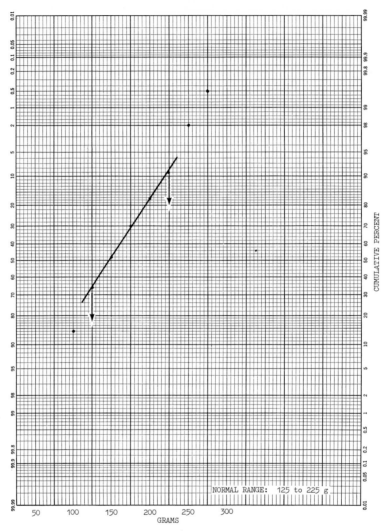

Fig. 6. Probability curve for kidney weights: 71 kidneys from 36 consecutive autopsies taken from August, 1966 to May, 1967; St. Francis Hospital, Escabana, Michigan.

as described by Parker and Sommers.[4] This measurement is done in our laboratory with a glass slide marked with a 2.0 mm line graduated at 0.1 mm and 0.01 mm intervals. This slide is superimposed on the adrenal section, and the measurement of the cortex read through the scanning (3.5x) objective to the nearest 0.1 mm. Figure 7 gives the probability curve for 134 adrenals from consecutive autopsies at the Veterans Administration Hospital and Figure 8 gives the similar curve from 112 adrenals from consecutive autopsies at St. Francis Hospital. In both series, the range of normal values for practical purposes can be taken as 1.0 to 2.0 mm, although there is some suggestion that the adrenals from the Veterans Administration Hospital tended to have a slightly thicker cortex than those from the mixed male and

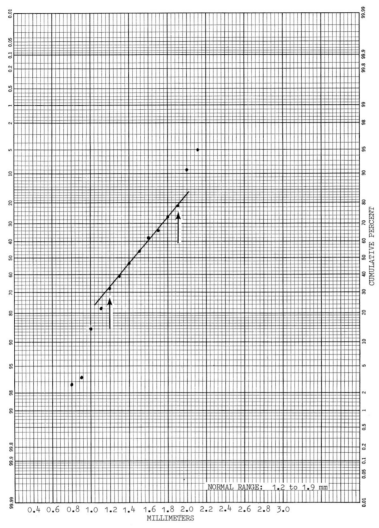

Fig. 7. Thickness of adrenal cortex measured on prepared slide: 134 consecutive autopsy measurements (all male) taken from January 30, 1962 to August 1, 1964; Veterans Administration Hospital, Iron Mountain, Michigan.

female population at the nongovernment hospital. In both series, the upper limit of normal coincides with that established by other criteria by Parker and Sommers[4] in 1956. With a larger series of cases, the St. Francis Hospital data could be divided into consecutive male and consecutive female cases to determine whether the range of normal values in these two groups were different and whether the range of normal values in the male coincides with that at the Veterans Administration Hospital.

Another measurement done routinely at our autopsies is the circumference of each of the four heart valves at the time the cardiac chambers are laid open at the autopsy table. The measurements are recorded to the nearest 0.1 cm. If the circum-

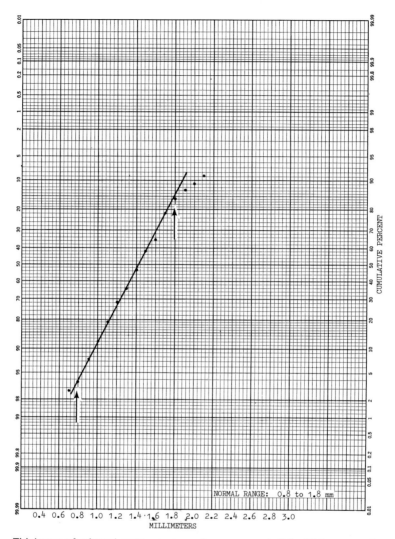

Fig. 8. Thickness of adrenal cortex measured on prepared slide: 112 consecutive autopsy measurements (male and female) taken from August 25, 1964 to August 1, 1967; St. Francis Hospital, Escabana, Michigan.

ferences are tabulated by 0.1 cm intervals, the resulting probability curve has no meaning because no clearly defined straight-line segment can be discerned. If, however, the circumferences are tabulated by 0.5 cm intervals, a meaningful curve is obtained, as seen for the tricuspid valve in 194 consecutive autopsies at the Veterans Administration Hospital (Fig. 9). In grouping the measurements into 0.5 cm intervals, a measurement of 13.4 cm would be placed in the 13.5 cm group, and a measurement of 13.6 cm would be placed in the 14.0 cm group.

The range of normal values thus obtained is 11.0 to 13.0 cm for the tricuspid valve. Figure 9 is also of some interest in relation to Figure 4. In the discussion of

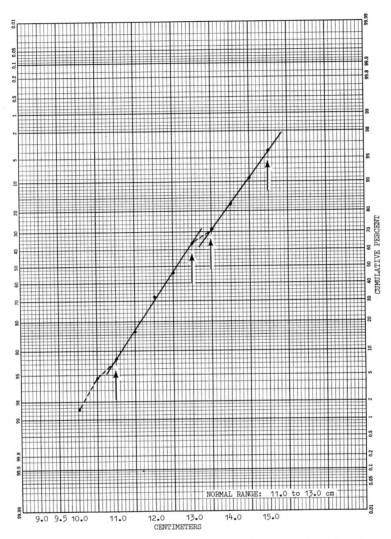

Fig. 9. Tricuspid valve circumference: 194 consecutive autopsies taken from October, 1961 to April, 1964; Veterans Administration Hospital, Iron Mountain, Michigan.

the probability curve for heart weights at the Veterans Administration Hospital, it was noted that cardiac failure may account for the random distribution of weights between 425 and 525 grams. Twenty percent of the heart weights were in that group. In Figure 9, it can be seen that 25 percent of the 194 tricuspid valves were dilated if 11.0 to 13.0 cm is taken as the range of normal values. The next step, if one were to further investigate whether this relationship was significant, would be to take all of the hearts with weights between 425 and 525 g and prepare a probability curve of their tricuspid valve measurements, do the same with the hearts of 300 to 400 g weight, and compare the two curves. Unfortunately, neither the series at the Veterans Administration nor at the St. Francis Hospital is as yet sufficiently large to give subgroups that can be considered meaningful.

From the data here presented, it is clear that the statistical method which Hoffmann presented for the clinical laboratory has application in the pathologic anatomy laboratory. The results of this type of analysis are reasonable in the light of our general experience in pathologic anatomy. The method can be used as an experimental tool by calculating ranges of "normal" values for measurements in specifically selected populations, e.g., valve circumference in male hearts weighing over 500 g.

In both the clinical laboratory and the anatomic pathology laboratory, we have been impressed by the potential information that this statistical technique seems capable of providing. Since it utilizes consecutive patient data, the accumulation of sufficient data is no problem in the average laboratory, even if one subdivides the patient data into specific groups for comparison. Furthermore, since the method is based on numerical values, adaptation of the method to computer analysis should be possible in order to examine large volumes of consecutive patient data with numerous group selections over various intervals of time.

References

1. Hoffman, R.G. Statistics in the practice of medicine. J.A.M.A., 185:864, 1963.
2. Sparapani, H., and Berry, R.E. The range of normal values in the quality control of clinical chemistry. Amer. J. Clin. Path., 42:134, 1964.
3. Gray, H. Anatomy of the Human Body, 24th ed. Philadelphia, Lea & Febiger, 1942.
4. Parker, T.G., and Sommers, S.C. Adrenal cortical hyperplasia accompanying cancer. Arch. Surg., 72:495, 1956.

REPAIR BY REGENERATION

EDWIN R. FISHER*

Repair by regeneration is a biologic phenomenon experienced in varying degree by all members of the phylogenetic series. It signifies the replacement or restoration of lost parts, including cells, by structurally, and often functionally, similar units. Although it is customary to connect the process of repair with antecedent injury, regeneration may also ensue in its apparent absence. Thus Lüscher (1955) designated regeneration as accidental when it represents the consequence of injury, and physiologic when overt evidence of the latter is lacking.

Physiologic regeneration encompasses the familiar phenomenon of cellular replacement encountered in growth and ageing. This form of regeneration increases and assumes greater significance with differentiation in the phylogenetic scale, being greatest in mammals (Masshoff, 1955). It is similarly axiomatic that the ability of tissues to exhibit such physiologic regeneration is inversely proportional to their degree of differentiation.

Some confusion exists concerning the applicability and analogy between the terms "compensatory hypertrophy" and "regeneration." Cameron (1952) considers the healing of a traumatized part as regeneration and that following extensive destruction as compensatory hypertrophy, whereas increased function per se represents adaptive hypertrophy. Linzbach (1955) recognized *"strukturelle"* and *"funktionale" Anpassung*. He suggested that the tissue first increases its performance to meet demands, resorting only to structural activity when performance fails in this regard. Yet, in the strict sense, hypertrophy refers to increase in unit size and hyperplasia in unit number. It must be considered, however, that, even in instances of hypertrophy, there may be hyperplasia of subcellular units accommodating in-

* This study was supported in part by USPHS Grant C-5195.

creased functional demands. The validity of this possibility awaits further investigations of the subcellular nature of hypertrophy. Despite the potential significance of this broader application of a definition or understanding of regeneration, it is customary to relate this phenomenon to those responses characterized by an increase in unit number rather than size.

Regenerative Capacity of Cells and Kinetics

The variation in physiologic regeneration has prompted several classifications of adult mammalian cells, utilizing their mitotic ability as an index for this capacity (Bizzozero, 1894; Cowdry, 1942; Masshoff, 1955). Generally, three major categories of cells may be appreciated on this basis. In some, such as neurons and cardiac and smooth muscle, cell division is rare or nonexistent. Those of solid viscera or organs, including liver, kidney, as well as connective tissue in general, exhibit a low mitotic index, perhaps no greater than that necessary to account for normal increases in body weight. Such cells, however, do exhibit the capacity for more accelerated renewal following partial removal. Lastly, there are those tissues and cells with evidence of continuous regeneration. In this group are hemopoietic tissues, epidermis, intestine, and gonads.

The application of such techniques as labelling with tritiated thymidine and mitotic arrest by colchicine has provided accurate estimates of the renewal velocity of various cell populations. Edwards and Klein (1961) extensively studied the relative renewal rates of 34 different types of cells in normal adult mouse with tritiated thymidine. They concluded that rigid categorization of cell types according to mitotic index is unwarranted, since all cells, save neurons and cardiac muscle, exhibit DNA synthesis at a fairly steady state above that required for normal growth.

Bertalanffy (1964), who has concisely presented the technical details of the tritiated thymidine and colchicine techniques, as well as their comparative merits, has tabulated the turnover times of cell populations of a variety of species. He has also indicated the four principal phases of cell renewal through which cells pass in this process. The M, or mitotic, phase in most tissues lasts between 40 to 70 minutes. This is followed by a more variable period of differentiation and metabolic activity, or postmitotic gap, designated as G_1. Cells of nonproliferating populations are considered as being persistently in this phase. Renewing cells pass invariably into the S phase, or period of DNA synthesis, which appears fairly constant in mammalian cell populations, lasting 6 to 8 hours. A second gap, or G_2 stage, lasting from less than 1 to 4 hours, intervenes between the completion of DNA synthesis and the onset of mitosis. In renewing cell populations, some cells, as well as their daughters, pass continuously through all phases of this cycle. Others, however, differentiate at G_1, assume their specific function, and eventually are lost, only to be subsequently replaced by the mitotic division of cells comprising the generative fraction of the cell population. Modifications of cell renewal kinetics as observed under normal conditions are also profoundly influenced in pathologic situations. Unlike physiologic regeneration, accidental regeneration decreases in the course of phylogenesis. The phenomenon of limb regeneration in lower forms, attendant with its complexities of spatial organization and patterns, is legend. Recently it has been comprehensively reviewed by DeHaan and Ebert (1964).

General Biochemical Features

Generally, many of the biochemical features of regeneration are comparable, regardless of tissue involved. Needham (1960) categorized the events into two phases. An R, or regressive, phase following the initial trauma, which is understandably accompanied by proteolysis, increases in sulfhydryl groups and lactic acid and notably decreases in RNA concentration. The P phase of progressive growth and differentiation is characterized by marked synthetic activity with its accompanying increase in RNA and DNA concentrations and reversal to preexisting pH.

Theories of Regenerative Stimulus

There has been perhaps no greater subject of extensive biologic investigation as well as controversy than that concerned with establishing the pathogenetic mechanisms of regeneration. Weiss (1939, 1952, 1955) has considered two tissue-specific antagonists to influence tissue growth: *template,* an intracellular, nondiffusible growth-stimulating factor, and an inhibitor designated as *antitemplate,* which is diffusible. Tissue destruction is visualized as resulting in a decrease in the latter, providing for unopposed growth activity mediated by template.

Teir (1951) invoked the concept that a variety of organ-specific wound hormones are available for liberation from tissues which exert a stimulating effect on homologous tissue, but that these are subordinated to the secretions of the endocrine system. Abercrombie (1957) suggested the occurrence of both local and systemic hormones which might influence growth.

These concepts are at least in large measure based upon previous demonstrations, albeit in many instances subject to criticism, of humoral factors purportedly released following cell damage. Evidence relating to such factors has been presented in the plant kingdom as long ago as 1910 by Boysen-Jensen and later by English, et al. (1939). Carrel (1924) considered such a mechanism operative in animal tissues. In 1943, Davidson designated such humoral factors as hormones. Teir (1951) considered that such hormones were not only organ-specific, but that specific inhibitors were also operative simultaneously. Examples of tissue-specific growth-promoting hormones have been purportedly demonstrated for liver, orbital gland (Teir, 1951), skin (Nettleship, 1943), and thymus (Roberts and White, 1949).

Glinos (1956) considered an inhibitory factor to reside in the albumin fraction of plasma with decreased concentrations occurring during hepatic regeneration. Growth promoters lacking organ specificity have also been claimed (Paschkis, 1958). Yet, Washburn (1960) asserted that no chemical substance compatible with that of a hormone was identifiable in healing wounds. In many instances, identification of growth-promoting hormones has not been verified by other investigators, and, consequently, they have not been unequivocally accepted.

Linzbach (1955) has stated that regeneration in paired organs is the result of increased functional requirements or is a form of structural adaptation. Bollman and Mann (1935) demonstrated regeneration of the kidney resulting from accumulation of nitrogenous waste products in the blood. However, again absolute support relating regeneration to functional demand is lacking. Halsted (1909) provided the axiomatic concept that regeneration in an endocrine organ is dependent upon a deficiency of physiologic need for its secretions.

Endocrine regeneration appears more clearly related to hypophyseal control, and the action of pituitary tropic hormones in this regard has been the subject of much investigation. The role of the pituitary in other instances of regeneration is less well established. There is accumulating evidence that erythropoiesis may, at least in part, be regulated by the anterior pituitary as well as by the kidney (Jacobs, 1958).

Adrenalectomy of the rat (Teir and Carpén, 1959) has been noted to stimulate mitoses in the skin and forestomach, and cortisone administration has the converse effect on mitotic activity (Needham, 1960), suggesting a possible adrenal role in mitotic activity. However, this view is not substantiated by subsequent findings of Räsänen and Teir (1961), who observed ACTH to stimulate mitosis in several rat tissues of intact but not adrenalectomized members.

Another hypothesis concerning regeneration, unrelated to a humoral factor, has been more recently proposed by Büchner (1961) and also related to carcinogenesis by Oehlert (1961, 1963). It suggests that there is a regulatory mechanism between cytoplasmic and nuclear structures. Cytoplasmic differentiation, particularly of endoplasmic reticulum, represents a brake on DNA synthesis. Damage or destruction of the cytoplasm, such as following administration of diethylnitrosamine or when subject to an increased metabolic load during hepatic regeneration, leads to loss of this braking system with augmented DNA synthesis, polyploidy, and cell division. This concept pertinently indicates the similarities and possible analogies and interrelationships among regeneration, hyperplasia, and neoplasia.

This article shall deal principally with the regenerative phenomena encountered under accidental or pathologic situations in organs and tissues which normally exhibit limited cellular renewal. Indeed, repair following injury in such tissues is in large part by regeneration.

Hepatic Regeneration

Much information has accumulated concerning hepatic regeneration. Most attention has been directed toward the phenomena resulting from surgical removal of variable amounts of the liver. Comprehensive reviews dealing with many of the parameters involved following partial hepatectomy are available (Fishback, 1929; Bollman and Mann, 1936; Mann, 1944; Wilson, 1951; Mann and Mann, 1953; Davidson, 1957; Harkness, 1957; Abercrombie, 1957; Paschkis, 1958; Glinos, 1958a; Brauer, 1958; Weinbren, 1959; Doljanski, 1960; Novikoff and Essner, 1960; Leevy, 1960; Bollman, 1961; Bucher, 1963). Fewer studies have been made concerning the regenerative process following hepatic insult not attended by overt loss of hepatic mass. Cameron (1936) considered regeneration to occur 36 to 72 hours following necrosis induced by moderate amounts of carbon tetrachloride, with complete restoration evident at 120 hours. DNA synthesis and increased mitoses indicative of regeneration are evident in parenchymal as well as ductal cells two days following ligation of the bile duct (MacDonald and Pechet, 1961). A similar situation is noted in hepatic cells in rats subjected to choline deficiency (MacDonald, et al., 1960).

Most investigations of regeneration have been performed utilizing young adult rats following removal of the median and left lateral lobes of liver, according to the technique and procedure described by Higgins and Anderson in 1931. The findings which follow refer to observations made under such circumstances.

Morphologic Changes

LIGHT MICROSCOPY.   During the initial 8 hours following partial hepatectomy, there is a dispersion of cytoplasmic basophilia within hepatic cell cytoplasm, particularly in the periphery of hepatic lobules (Glinos, 1958b) which may be appreciated by light microscopy. Intracytoplasmic droplets also occur during this early period (Aterman, 1961). Glycogen depletion and lipid accumulation are also encountered at this time. An increase in size of hepatic cells, nuclei, and nucleoli is noted between 12 and 24 hours following partial hepatectomy. Mitoses appear at 24 hours. Their number increases rapidly to about 28 hours, followed by a rapid decline and subsequently more gradual decrease during the next several days (Brues and Marble, 1937; Harkness, 1957). The number of binucleate cells also falls rapidly following cell division. Hepatic cells may appear histologically normal as early as three to four days following partial hepatectomy, although restoration of hepatic mass is not complete until 10 to 15 days. Harkness (1957) has indicated that the number of hepatic nuclei are never restored to normal, although estimates of nuclear DNA are within normal range, indicating increase in polyploidy. Sinusoidal and ductular cells also participate in the regenerative process, although their growth activity apparently lags behind that noted in the parenchymal cells (Grisham, 1960). Connective tissue is restored at even slower rates, and collagen content remains low even after six weeks.

ELECTRON MICROSCOPY.   Relatively few electron microscopic studies of hepatic regeneration have been performed. The apparent dispersion of basophilia and cytoplasmic vacuolation observed by light microscopy clearly appear related to dilation of granular endoplasmic reticulum, as well as apparent relocation of granules from the endoplasmic membranes to the cytoplasm (Fig. 1) (Davis, 1962; Fisher and Fisher, 1963). It has been suggested by Porter (1954) and Scott, et al. (1962) that free ribosomes are concerned with protein synthesis for intracellular processes, whereas those associated with membranes are related to the protein synthesis necessary for secretion. Although Davis (1962), as well as Bernhard and Rouiller (1956), indicated early loss of endoplasmic reticulum with subsequent repletion at approximately 16 hours, Fisher and Fisher (1963) were less certain about the validity of such quantitation of these structures. The latter authors also concluded that the disposition of the granular endoplasmic reticulum during early phases of regeneration was, in large part, dependent upon the glycogen content of hepatic

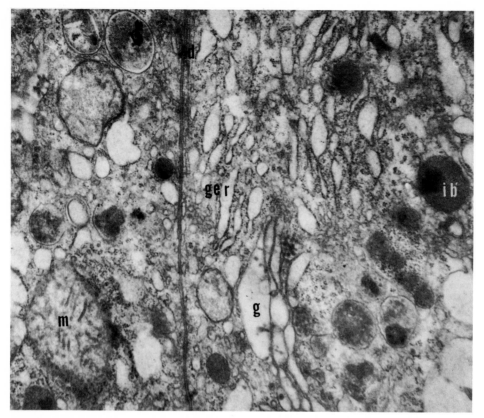

Fig. 1.   Areas from two adjacent hepatic cells 6 hours following partial hepatectomy. Cell membranes are distinct, containing occasional desmosomes (d). Granular endoplasmic reticulum (ger) is dilated. Golgi apparatus (g) containing dense bodies also appears distended. Mitochondria (m) are swollen. Many inclusion bodies (ib) are noted in the glycogen-free cytoplasm. X 18,500. (From Fisher, E. R., and Fisher, B. *Lab. Invest.*, 12:929, 1963.)

cells. It was poorly oriented during the phase of glycogen depletion encountered in the immediate post hepatectomy period. Smooth profiles of endoplasmic reticulum also appeared quantitatively related to the amount of intracytoplasmic glycogen being most abundant prior to reaccumulation of glycogen within hepatic cells (Fig. 2).

Cytoplasmic inclusions, most often comprised of solitary limiting membranes and a variable matrix corresponding to microbodies, multivesicular bodies, and cytosomes, are increased during the first 18 hours following partial hepatectomy. The lysosomal nature of many of these structures is confirmed by their acid phosphatase content (Essner and Novikoff, 1961), and their increase is coincident with an increase in lysosomal enzymes demonstrated biochemically in vitro during regeneration (Adams, 1963). Generally, no abnormality in Golgi structures is appreciated during the regenerative process, except for lacunar dilation during its early phase (6 hours). Qualitative changes in mitochondria are lacking, except for

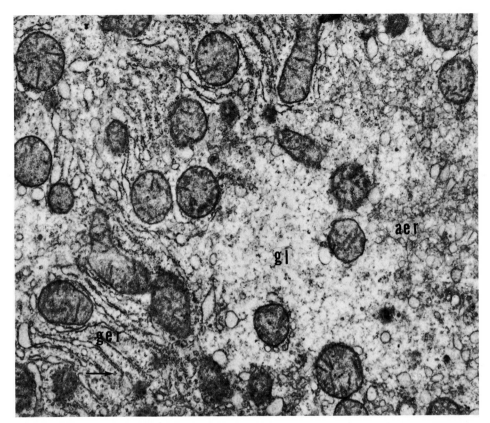

Fig. 2.   Portion of hepatic cell 24 hours after partial hepatectomy. Granular endoplasmic reticulum (ger) appears less dilated than at earlier intervals. Many smooth profiles of endo-plasmic reticulum (aer) are observed in a well-glycogenated focus (gl). Some polyribosome rosettes are noted (arrow). X 13,760. (From Fisher, E.R., and Fisher, B. *Lab. Invest.*, 12:929, 1963.)

some swelling of these organelles during the first 6 hours. At 72 hours following partial hepatectomy, hepatic cells appear ultrastructurally normal (Fig. 3). Similar ultrastructural changes have been noted following partial hepatectomy in rats sub-jected to prior portacaval shunt (Fisher and Fisher, 1963). Cytoplasmic changes in sinusoidal or ductal cells comparable to those noted in parenchymal cells have not been observed. It appears significant that the cytoplasmic changes noted fol-lowing partial hepatectomy were also encountered in pair-fed sham controls (Fig. 4) (Fisher and Fisher, 1963). These changes have been recounted in other in-stances of hepatocellular damage induced by a variety of modalities (Bassi, et al., 1960), minimizing the specificity of the changes cited to the posthepatectomy regen-erative process per se.

Biochemical Changes

A rise in glutamic and aspartic acids as well as lysine has been observed within 6 hours after partial hepatectomy, with their subsequent decrease at 20 to 30 hours.

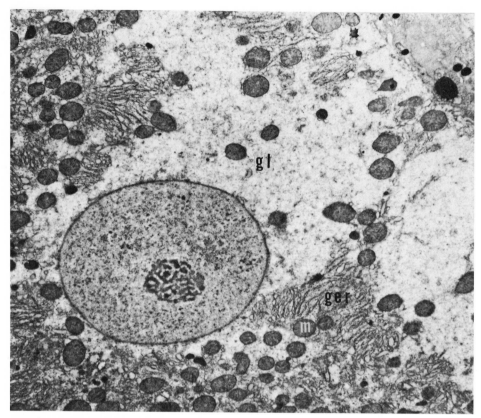

Fig. 3.   Normal-appearing hepatic cell 72 hours following partial hepatectomy. Abundant glycogen (gl) is evident, and compressed granular endoplasmic reticulum (ger) is arranged in parallel arrays in proximity to mitochondria (m). X 5,100. (From Fisher, E. R., and Fisher, B. *Lab. Invest.,* 12:929, 1963.)

Other amino acids appear increased at this time (Christensen, et al., 1948). Incorporation of amino acids into protein has been considered to be most pronounced by the third day (Harkness, 1957). It is of interest that the increase in amino acid incorporation into protein occurs without a parallel increase in aerobic formation of high energy phosphates (Clerici, et al., 1960). Increased sulfhydryl levels have been observed at the time of the mitotic burst in the regenerating liver (Smith, 1962).

Extensive variations in parenchymal cell enzymic patterns accompany the regenerative process. ATPase activity has been noted to be decreased in microsomal fractions of liver coincident with rapid growth (Morgan and Leon, 1963). Histochemical studies have disclosed a prompt decrease in succinic dehydrogenase, which recovers to normal by 96 hours. On the other hand, alkaline phosphatase is increased up to 48 hours and then reverts to normal (Bartok, et al., 1962). Alterations in lysosomal enzymes have been previously cited. A net increase in RNA is seen by 24 hours, with original amounts being restored by two to five days (Nygaard and Rusch, 1955).

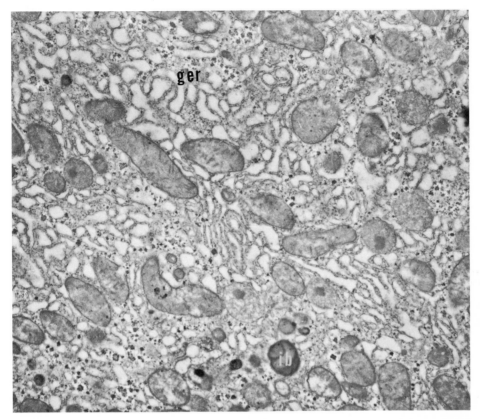

Fig. 4.   Portion of hepatic cell from sham-operated control, pair-fed for 24 hours to rat subjected to partial hepatectomy. Food intake was approximately one-half normal. Dilation of granular endoplasmic reticulum (ger) is apparent. A few rare aggregates of glycogen are noted, appearing black in this preparation. Inclusion bodies (ib) are also evident. X 12,900. (From Fisher, E. R., and Fisher, B. *Lab. Invest.*, 12:929, 1963.)

Factors Influencing Hepatic Regeneration

A number of anatomical, hormonal, pharmacologic, and environmental factors appear to influence the regenerative process. Recognition of many of these factors appears mandatory when comparing results from one laboratory with another. Apparently, they represent a source of differences noted in the literature. Differences encountered in various species have been attributed to anatomical variations of their respective livers (Brauer, 1963). The strain of rat also appears to influence many of the parameters of regeneration (Harkness, 1952). Although the liver of the mouse, another species widely utilized for such studies, duplicates the findings in the rat, the process appears somewhat delayed (Wilson, et al., 1953). Restoration of liver is more rapid in young adult rats than in older members, a situation also noted in mice (Bucher and Glinos, 1950).

Although some endocrines appear to modify the response to partial hepatectomy, Harkness (1957) has indicated that none appears critical. Weinbren (1959) has further indicated that many of the studies relating an endocrine influence to regeneration have been inadequately controlled, since changes following endocrine manipulation may also occur in a normal liver. Further, a small hepatic fragment as following hepatectomy may respond more profoundly to such influence, since the normal fragment, with its attendant normal functional capacity, is in large measure capable of inactivating many endocrine-derived substances.

Regeneration of the liver in the rat appears unaffected by hypophysectomy (Harkness, 1957; Weinbren, 1959); but in the dog it appears inhibited (Astarabadi, et al., 1953). Although liver mass is restored following cortisone administration, this appears to be the result of fatty change and increased glycogen deposition induced by this agent. RNA synthesis does not appear affected by cortisone, but DNA synthesis and mitotic activity are (Roberts, et al., 1952). Effects of thyroidal influences have been conflicting, although Nazario and Cohen (1961) recently found that thyroidectomy impairs regeneration in rat liver and that this inhibition is overcome by the administration of thyroxine. Splenectomy has been noted to accelerate the regeneration of liver mass, but the precise mechanism concerned is uncertain (Perez-Tamayo and Romero, 1958). No gonadal influence on hepatic regeneration has been observed (Bucher, 1963).

The quantity of tissue removed by partial hepatectomy may alter the rate of restoration. Generally, the less removed, the slower the response (Pack and Islami, 1956; Glinos, 1958a). MacDonald, et al. (1962) concluded from their studies that at least 9.4 to 12.3 percent or more of liver had to be removed to initiate the regenerative process. Bucher and Swaffield (1964) observed that DNA labelling in 1- to 15-month-old rats increases logarithmically in proportion to the amount of liver excised. The percentage increments were the same for all quantities, except if the liver loss exceeded a certain amount, which differed with age, when higher levels of DNA synthesis occurred. Ingle and Baker (1957) noted that multiple monthly partial hepatectomies over a 1-year period did not interfere with the regenerative capacity of the liver. Similarly, the induction of cirrhosis does not interfere with the regenerative capacity. Indeed, Rabinovici and Wiener (1961) noted that restoration occurs more rapidly in rats exhibiting the most severe cirrhotic changes.

Interference with DNA synthesis and mitosis by the administration of irradiation (Holmes and Mee, 1955; Albert and Bucher, 1960) or such drugs as fluorouracil (Paschkis, et al., 1959) inhibits the regenerative capacity.

Environmental factors, such as crowding of the animals subjected to partial hepatectomy, appear to retard regeneration. Interference with the diurnal cycle by altered schedules of illumination and darkness may also affect this process (Bucher, 1963). Generally, dietary factors appear to play little role in the regenerative process.

Nature of the Regenerative Stimulus

Considerable interest and investigation have been directed to the identification of the regenerative stimulus in the liver following partial hepatectomy. There is little evidence to support earlier considerations that this phenomenon resulted from an overloading of the excretory function of the remaining segments of liver following partial hepatectomy. Similarly, the primacy of portal blood flow as proposed by Bollman and Mann (1936), Mann (1944), and Child, et al. (1953) has been contradicted by the considerations offered by Weinbren (1955), Harkness (1957), and Brauer (1963). Indeed, unaltered regeneration follows partial hepatectomy in rats with portacaval shunts (Weinbren, 1955; Fisher, et al., 1962). Also, increasing hepatic blood flow by arterialization of the liver does not result in greater regenerative growth (Fisher, et al., 1954).

Most attention has been directed toward the identification of a humoral-stimulating substance or an inhibiting factor which is depressed, destroyed, or overbalanced by the former. Since 1954, when Friedrich-Freksa and Zaki reported that injection of serum from hepatectomized rats into normal animals resulted in increased mitoses in the livers of the latter, there have been numerous attempts to confirm and elaborate on this observation. Much of the results have been conflicting. Hughes (1960) could confirm these findings only after utilizing large amounts of posthepatectomy serum, whereas Glinos (1958a) was unsuccessful. Zimmerman and Cellozzi (1960) noted that injection of plasma from partially hepatectomized donors stimulated mitoses in livers of normal members, but they subsequently found that it was the heparin utilized in the collection of the blood which was essential in producing this effect (Zimmerman and Cellozzi, 1961). Further, recognition that injections of plasma from normal donors may have a similar mitogenic effect (Glinos, 1958a; Fisher, et al., 1963) invalidates many previous studies in which such control injections were not utilized.

A divergence of findings likewise exists concerning the effect of post-hepatectomy serum or plasma on the regenerative process in partially hepatectomized recipients. Although Stitch and Florian (1958) found that normal serum inhibits mitoses in such animals and post-hepatectomy serum augments this phenomenon, Glinos (1958b), Bucher, et al. (1961), and Fisher, et al. (1963) could not confirm these observations. Utilizing parabiotic members to demonstrate humoral factors in regeneration, Christensen and Jacobsen (1949) noted more mitoses in the liver of the untouched parabiont when the contralateral member was subjected to partial hepatectomy than were observed in unoperated single rats. This finding was confirmed by Wenneker and Sussman (1951) and Bucher, et al. (1961). The latter authors also noted greater mitotic activity in parabiotic triplets in which two members were subjected to hepatectomy. However, Islami, et al. (1959) and Rogers, et al. (1961) failed to confirm these findings and indicated the necessity for utilizing sham-operated parabiotics as controls. A similar view was presented by Fisher, et al. (1963).

It would appear that the major difficulties in identifying a humoral factor or factors concerned with the regenerative process revolve about the lack of standardized procedures from one laboratory to another, particularly in the selection of suitable controls. Reliance on mitotic activity as a parameter of regeneration appears inconvenient because of the wide range of variations encountered. The results thus far fail to provide unequivocal evidence for the existence of a stimulating or inhibiting factor.

Another experimental model has recently been described to evaluate controlling factors of hepatic regeneration. Utilizing functionally active, heterotopic, partial hepatic autografts without portal blood supply, Leong, et al. (1964) noted that, following partial hepatectomy, DNA synthesis and mitosis in such grafts were virtually identical to those occurring in the residual livers of the same animals. Moolten and Bucher (1967) have recently observed increased incorporation of C^{14} thymidine into hepatic DNA of normal partners joined by cross-circulation technique to members with partial hepatectomy. These authors have suggested that the humoral mechanism responds almost instantaneously to changes in liver mass and that the agent may be metabolized so rapidly that only prolonged and continuous exposure would demonstrate it. Indeed, synthetic changes were noted when cross-circulation was maintained for 19 hours. Exposure for 7 hours or less was ineffective.

Renal Regeneration

Most studies of renal regeneration have dealt with the compensatory increase in renal mass in the remaining kidney following unilateral nephrectomy. This phenomenon has been commonly referred to as compensatory hypertrophy, yet it is also characterized by increase in cell number as well as size, *vide infra,* therefore warranting its inclusion in a discussion of regeneration.

Macromicroscopic Changes

The weight of the remaining kidney following unilateral nephrectomy has been noted to increase about 30 percent within three days following unilateral nephrectomy. Mitotic activity is less dramatic, increasing about 10 percent within this period (Williams, 1962). Fajers (1957) has observed the mean volume of renal tubular nuclei to increase 24 to 48 hours after operation, and Sulkin (1949) considered the onset of mitosis to occur at 48 hours, with peak activity between 72 and 240 hours. Polyploid cells are notably more frequent in the regenerating than in the normal kidney. The major portion of regeneration occurs within tubular portions of the nephron (Bollman and Mann, 1935). It has been estimated, however, that glomeruli exhibit a 20 to 30 percent increase in diameter, although new glomeruli are not encountered (Lubarsch, 1925).

Biochemical Changes

Estimates of RNA:DNA ratios parallel the findings noted above. Mandel, et al. (1950a, 1950b) observed increase in RNA up to 30 days, whereas increments of DNA content were much less and occurred more slowly. Normal ratios of RNA: DNA were reestablished two months following regeneration induced by unilateral nephrectomy.

Endocrine and Other Effects

Renal regeneration following unilateral nephrectomy appears unaffected by thyroidectomy (Zeckwer, 1945), adrenalectomy (Latorre, 1959), or castration

(MacKay, 1940). Results concerning the effect of hypophysectomy in this regard are divergent (Astarabadi and Essex, 1953; Colonge, 1944; Fontaine and Veil, 1947; Winternitz and Waters, 1940). However, it would appear that with the utilization of proper controls, taking into account the loss of renal mass and impairment in DNA synthesis normally encountered following hypophysectomy, renal regenerative phenomena in the hypophysectomized animal might be more clearly visualized (Fontaine, 1948).

Regeneration has been noted to be enhanced in unilaterally nephrectomized dogs subjected to ureteroduodenostomy of the remaining member (Bollman and Mann, 1935). MacKay, et al. (1932) concluded from the results of their studies that regeneration is decreased with advancing age. On the other hand, high protein diet augments the phenomenon in the unilaterally nephrectomized rat (MacKay, et al., 1938). Yet, other functional demands as induced by pronounced salt overloading fail to influence the sequence of events noted (Allen and Mann, 1935).

Mechanisms of Renal Regeneration

FUNCTIONAL DEMAND. Investigations concerning the possible mechanisms involved in renal regeneration following unilateral nephrectomy have, in large part, conceptually paralleled those advanced for hepatic regeneration. Similarly, the results are conflicting, leading to the conclusion that no unequivocal information has been provided in elucidating the morphogenesis and other pathogenetic mechanisms involved. Braun-Mendenez (1952) has critically reviewed the evidence relating the initiation of regeneration to an increased functional load placed upon the remaining kidney, but he could find no compelling evidence to support such a view. Similarly, reduction in renal excretory function appears unlikely as an initiating factor. The results of unilateral ureteroperitoneostomy performed on one kidney instead of unilateral nephrectomy tend to militate against this view, since such a procedure purported to decrease renal excretory function is not attended by regeneration in the contralateral, intact member (Goss and Rankin, 1960; Simpson, 1961). It does appear significant in this regard, however, that ureteroperitoneostomy provokes peritonitis, decreased food and water intake, and inanition. Royce (1963) has recently demonstrated that these factors inhibit regeneration following unilateral nephrectomy. It would therefore appear that further exploitation of the possibility of impaired excretory function as an inciting factor in renal regeneration is necessary before this possibility can be eliminated from consideration.

EFFECT OF TISSUE HOMOGENATES. The inhibition of renal regeneration, induced by the administration of crude preparations of renin (Schaffenburg, et al., 1954), has provoked the consideration of a possible renal endocrine influence on this phenomenon. It would appear significant, however, to verify this finding with more refined samples of this pressor agent as well as to control more completely the effect of administration of this agent on fluid balance before considering that reduction in endocrine activity of the kidney may represent a provocative factor in renal regeneration. Further, it appears that the administration of homogenates of kidney, including preparations subjected to boiling, which should destroy renal renin content, similarly inhibit the regenerative process (Goss, 1963).

Goss (1963) has recently reviewed the findings observed following the administration not only of kidney but also other tissue homogenates on renal regeneration, and he has reported his own findings in this regard utilizing homogenates of fresh, cooked, or frozen kidneys. These and other tissue homogenates inhibited renal mitoses approximately 50 percent in unilaterally nephrectomized rats. He has concluded that the existence of growth-regulating agents related to organ mass per se and distinct from functional or other demands is problematic.

ROLE OF HUMORAL FACTOR.   Relatively little information is available concerning the possibility that renal regeneration may be induced by the elaboration of a humoral or other renotropic factor. Sacerdotti (1896) observed no enlargement of the surviving kidney of fasted unilaterally nephrectomized rats. However, injections of blood from animals in which both kidneys were removed resulted in renal enlargement in normal rats. Ogawa and Nowinski (1958) observed that serum obtained from rats 48 hours after unilateral nephrectomy increased the mitotic activity of kidney cells in tissue culture. However, Williams (1962), administering plasma both subcutaneously and intraperitoneally, could not discern any growth-promoting activity in vivo. Indeed, such injections, as well as administration of kidney macerates, resulted in inhibition of regeneration. He attributed this inhibitory effect to the depression of food intake, which also adversely affects renal regeneration, and he concluded that there was no support for the view relating renal regeneration to organ-specific factors.

Regeneration of Urinary Bladder

It has been recognized for many years that the urinary bladder exhibits the capacity to "regenerate." However, as indicated by Johnson, et al. (1962) in their excellent historical review of this subject, investigation and clinical application of this phenomenon have been infrequent. Schiller (1923) and Kretchmer and Barber (1928) observed "regenerated" bladder following subtotal resection of this structure in rabbits as comprised histologically of the usual three layers, except that it was thinner and the submucosa more vascular. The proportion of connective tissue to muscle was greater than normal.

One of the most extensive studies of vesicle "regeneration" was that performed in dogs by Bohne, et al. (1955). These investigators utilized an acrylic mold with ureteral and urethral catheters which were placed in the bladder fossa following cystectomy. This mold was subsequently removed 5 to 10 weeks later. Biopsy at 3 to 5 weeks disclosed a dense covering of the mold comprised of granulation tissue and inflammatory cells. At 6 to 10 weeks a lining of transitional epithelium was noted. This was subtended at 14 to 16 weeks by a zone of granulation tissue, a layer of fibroblasts, fibroblasts and smooth muscle cells, and, lastly, adipose tissue. Function was satisfactory in some of these dogs.

Since smooth muscle is considered to exhibit a limited capacity for regeneration, its development in the regenerated bladder is of interest. Baker, et al. (1958) believed the smooth muscle to be derived from immature mesenchymal elements rather than representing an extension from the urethra or ureters. A similar conclusion was reached by Johnson, et al. (1962) from their studies. It is also apparent

Pancreatic Regeneration

One of the earliest allusions to the regenerative capacity of the pancreas was by Kyrle (1908) who observed duct proliferation and mitoses in acinar cells in the pancreatic remnant following partial pancreatectomy. Parker (1919) was also impressed with the relatively frequent mitoses of acinar cells in foci of necrosis of glands from humans with infectious disease. A similar experience was encountered in animals exposed to chloroform or arsenic. Most of the recent investigations of the regenerative ability of the pancreas have dealt with its restitution following the administration of ethionine, an analogue of methionine (Fitzgerald and Alvizouri, 1952; Kinney, et al., 1955; Popper, et al., 1952; Wachstein and Meisel, 1953).

Morphologic and Microradioautographic Findings

Most acinar epithelium of the rat is destroyed after 10 days of administration of this agent. Islet tissue and ductal epithelium appear relatively unaffected. During this degenerative phase, labelling of nuclei with tritiated thymidine is markedly depressed or absent as compared to the normal, untreated animal (Fitzgerald, 1963). During the first several days following cessation of ethionine treatment, cells are encountered among the degenerating acinar forms which exhibit intense basal basophilia. Although the precise identification of this cell is uncertain, ultrastructural study (Herman and Fitzgerald, 1962) suggests that it represents a progenitor for regenerated acinar epithelium, and, further, that it is an acinar cell which has survived the lethal effect of ethionine. Ultrastructurally, such cells show, in addition to cytoplasmic changes characteristic of ethionine damage, small zymogen granules, a fine granularity of the nuclear matrix, decreased Golgi substance, and conspicuous whorls of rough endoplasmic reticulum (Fig. 7). The latter correspond to the basophilia observed by light microscopy. Since nuclear labelling is not increased at this time, these changes are considered to indicate that cellular protein synthesis precedes that of DNA in this situation (Fitzgerald, 1960). At eight days following cessation of ethionine treatment, the whorled endoplasmic reticulum is replaced by a normal-appearing organelle. Nucleoli and Golgi structures are enlarged, and zymogen granules are more abundant. Increased labelling of nuclei with tritiated thymidine may also be noted at this time, followed by evident mitotic activity and subsequent restitution of cell structure to normal by 18 days (Fitzgerald, 1960). Although the ultrastructural study signifies the acinar cell as the regenerating cellular constituent in this instance, it is also considered likely that small pancreatic ductules contribute to the renewed cellular population (Fitzgerald, 1960; Herman and Fitzgerald, 1962).

That the regenerative process encountered in the pancreas may not be stereotypic is quite evident from the results of Fitzgerald (1963), following ligation of the inferior splenic artery or duct to the splenic segment of the rat pancreas. Unlike the situation encountered with ethionine, degenerating acinar elements, characterized by loss of basal basophilia, presence of cytoplasmic vacuolization, and often a

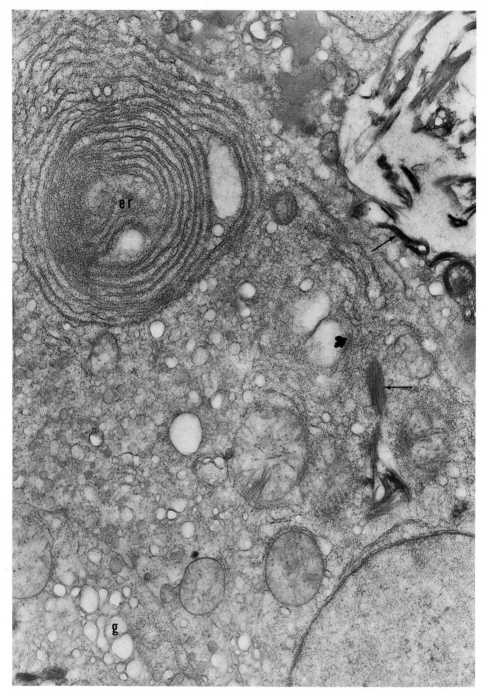

Fig. 7.   Acinar pancreatic cell of ethionine-treated rat at 12 days. Prominent whorls of regenerating granular endoplasmic reticulum are evident at upper left (er). Areas of degeneration are also noted (arrows). Many cytoplasmic vacuoles and vesicles are conspicuous as is the Golgi zone (g). X 19,000. (From Herman, L., and Fitzgerald, P. J. *J. Cell Biol.*, 12:297, 1962.)

decrease in nuclear staining, are accompanied by increased labelling of nuclei with tritiated thymidine. This information strongly indicates an asynchrony between nuclear and cytoplasmic activities and suggests the need for caution in estimating degenerative cellular change without perhaps resorting to techniques for evaluation of nuclear activity.

Salivary Gland Regeneration

Early studies concerning regeneration in salivary glands largely dealt with the effects of trauma on individual glands (Fuckel, 1896; Carraro, 1909). Although the resultant changes were largely banal scar tissue, some restoration of acinar elements purportedly from ductular elements was contended. Bizzozero (1903) observed mitotic activity in the submaxillary gland of the rabbit four days following excision of the contralateral member. Such activity reached its maximum by six days, quickly diminished, and was unaccompanied by weight gain of the organ. A similar situation was observed in the parotid gland of this species. Lacassagne and Caussé (1941) noted that denervation of one submaxillary gland resulted in its atrophy and was accompanied by increased mitotic activity in the contralateral member. Degeneration of the outer orbital gland of the rat has also been observed to produce a similar effect in the uninvolved member (Teir, 1951).

More recently, Alho (1964) has published the results of a very comprehensive and well-controlled study of the regenerative capacity of the submaxillary gland of rat and mouse following extirpation of its contralateral member. By three days mitotic activity was augmented in the acinar cells of the rat and less constantly in those of the mouse. However, gain in weight of the gland was noted in only one of several experiments in both the mouse and rat. No increase in volume of tubular and acinar elements was observed, and nucleic acids were not increased over that encountered in controls. The increased mitoses without constant increase in organ weight suggested to Alho (1964) that, for the most part, the submaxillary gland cells were simply exhibiting an increased turnover rate analogous to that experienced in physiologic regeneration. However, he considered those occasional instances in which weight gain was encountered to indicate true or compensatory regeneration. The possibility was suggested that certain external or internal factors may have been responsible for the varied responses. Since mitotic activity was also observed in the parotid gland following extirpation of one submaxillary gland, there was a possibility that the changes observed in the remaining submaxillary gland might be the result of a nonspecific organ humoral factor. Lastly, Alho found no correlation between the mitotic activity and function.

Thyroidal Regeneration

The regenerative capacity of the thyroid gland has been recognized since Halsted's classical experiments of this phenomenon following partial ablation of the dog thyroid in 1896. All species exhibit this reaction to partial removal or destruction (Marine and Lenhart, 1911). The degree of regeneration, however, appears related to the amount of gland removed or destroyed. Loeb (1919) found it necessary to remove at least one and one-half lobes of guinea pig thyroid to evoke such a response. Seasonal changes (Loeb, 1926) and changes in body weight (Loeb, 1929) similarly appear to affect this process at least in the guinea pig. Marine and Lenhart (1911) were impressed with the histologic as well as physiologic similarities between regenerating thyroid and spontaneous hyperplasias encountered within the gland. They related the degree of regeneration following ablation largely to the physiologic requirements of the animal.

One of the most complete histologic descriptions of regenerating thyroid tissue was that of Gray (1929). He noted the presence of small, basophilic epithelial cell clusters at the site of excision of the gland several days after operation. He also encountered small acini with relatively little colloid, which he interpreted as resulting from the reunion of epithelium from acinar remnants and the darkly staining epithelial clusters. Budding of such acini was noted and followed by hypertrophy, as well as some hyperplasia of the epithelial components. Mitoses were frequently observed in such acini at five to nine days following resection, and the acinar elements appeared normal by 10 to 12 days. Pituitary and thyroid extracts inhibited the process, whereas administration of KI generally did not influence the regenerative capacity of the gland (Gray, 1929; Loeb, 1926, 1929).

Gonadal Regeneration

Surprisingly, there is little information concerning the regenerative capacity of the reproductive organs. Addis and Lew (1940) noted that removal of one-half of ovarian or testicular mass in the rat resulted in growth of these tissues with a rate independent of the growth rate of these organs at the time of removal. Growth was rapid at first and then decelerated, ending at 40 days following partial ablation. In neither instance was complete restoration of mass noted. Prostatic tissue, seminal vesicles, and the uterine horns failed to exhibit any appreciable growth following partial excision.

Carmichael and Marshall (1908) considered the degree of ovarian hypertrophy in the rabbit to be dependent upon the amount of ovarian tissue removed. Hatai (1913) considered the compensatory enlargement of the remaining ovary of the rat following hemispaying to be twice that of the normal. Arai (1920) noted that enlargement of the remaining ovary following unilateral oophorectomy in the rat appeared three to five weeks following operation. If performed before puberty, the surviving ovary was 40 percent heavier than the normal at this time. Hemispaying of adult rats resulted in 100 percent increase in ovarian weight. He considered the increase in weight to be the result of a greater abundance of well-developed normal as well as degenerate follicles. Changes in ovarian stroma did not appear significant.

Lung Regeneration

It has long been recognized that removal of portions of lung is followed by enlargement of the remaining segments. It is, however, uncertain whether this represents an increase in the number of lobules (respiratory units) or increase in size.

Cohn (1939) observed that removal of two-thirds of the lung tissue of adult rats resulted in growth of remaining lung, which stopped once a normal intrapleural pressure was reached. He considered this growth response due to the mechanical stimuli involved, but he did not emphasize whether such change represented hypertrophy or true regeneration. Montgomery (1943) noted new bronchial buds and alveoli in areas of scar following wounding of the lung, but he considered dilation rather than hyperplasia to occur in adult lung, a view also expressed by Longacre and Johansmann (1940).

Endothelial Regeneration

It is commonly held that vascular endothelium regenerates. This represents an important assumption in the concept (Duguid, 1946; Crawford, 1956) of the evolution of the atheromatous plaque. There is, however, some divergence of opinion concerning the source of the regenerative elements, as well as the degree and rapidity of this phenomenon. Much of this, however, as emphasized by Cotton, et al. (1961), may represent species difference. The experiments of Poole, et al. (1958, 1959) indicate this to be a relatively slow process in the rabbit, but a fairly rapid one in the dog. Although such regeneration may completely bridge an existing defect, some abnormalities of endothelial cells, consisting principally of multinucleated forms, may appear. Gottlob and Zinner (1962) related this in large part to the type of trauma damaging the endothelial surface. "Hard" injury, as following the release of a constricting suture, resulted in a relatively normal endothelial surface. Injury following compression was accompanied by excessive evidences of regeneration characterized by "endothelial polyps" and multinucleated forms.

It is also generally agreed that the regenerating endothelium arises in the host's tissues (Fisher and Fisher, 1956; Florey, et al., 1961; Meijne, 1959). Indeed, mitotic activity may be quite prominent at the edge of denuded endothelial areas (Cotton, et al., 1961). However, two observations of endothelial regeneration occurring over vascular homografts and prostheses prompted Stump, et al. (1962) to propose another source for such cells. These investigators were impressed with the rapidity by which long segments of aortic prostheses were re-endothelialized, as well as by the presence of regeneration in such structures often appearing as isolated islands away from the host's aorta. This suggested to them the possibility that such endothelium might also arise from the granulation tissue infiltrating the prosthesis along its course, as well as from the cellular elements of the circulating blood.

In support of this latter view, they performed the ingenious experiment of suspending dacron hubs in the lumen of a prosthesis which was placed in the abdominal aorta of young pigs. The hub was endothelialized in a similar fashion to the main prosthesis, but the supporting struts of polyethylene sutures used to hold the hub in place were not (Stump, et al., 1963). O'Neal, et al. (1964) examined such structures by a variety of histologic techniques and by electron microscopy; they observed ultrastructurally normal-appearing endothelium, subtended by collagenous fibers, fibroblasts, and smooth muscle cells (Fig. 8). Although identification of the circulating cells providing this quite unconventional, yet provocative, form of differentiation is not made, these findings clearly indicate an ancillary and perhaps most

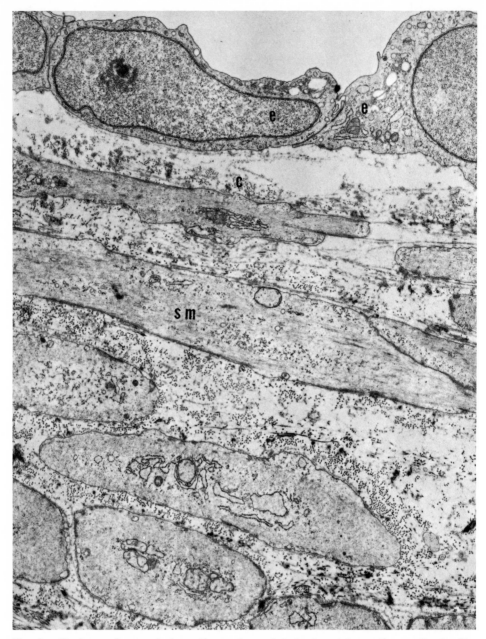

Fig. 8. Electron micrograph from the surface of hub placed in aortic prosthesis. The endothelial cells (e) have overlapping cell processes at their junctions. Collagen (c) is present beneath endothelium and between elongated cells resembling smooth muscle cells (sm). X 10,100. (From O'Neal, et al. *Exp. Molec. Path.*, 3:430, 1964.)

significant mechanism participating in the process of endothelial regeneration. They also provide information which may be highly significant in considerations of the varied capacities for differentiation exhibited by some cells.

Skeletal Muscle Regeneration

Although early observers failed to ascribe a regenerative capacity to skeletal muscle, it is now generally accepted that such a phenomenon does ensue following a variety of traumas, including separation of fibers following transection (Godman, 1958; Field, 1960; Adams, et al., 1962). The success of regeneration and establishment of continuity is dependent upon the distance of separation of muscle fibers and the preservation of the sarcolemmal sheaths which constitute a framework for the components of regenerating muscle (Adams, et al., 1962).

Morphologic Changes

LIGHT MICROSCOPY. The light microscopic features of the events of regeneration of skeletal muscle have been recounted in detail by a number of investigators (Waldeyer, 1865; Volkmann, 1893; Forbus, 1926; Millar, 1934; Nageotte, 1937; Clark, 1946; Godman, 1957; Lash, et al., 1957; Field, 1960; Adams, et al., 1962). Following simple transection, the wound is occupied by a coagulum consisting of cellular elements of the blood, as well as fibroblasts and macrophages. Degenerative changes characterized by loss of myofibrils and infiltration of such altered sarcoplasm by neutrophils and macrophages dominate the initial two days following injury. Surviving sarcolemmal nuclei in this area, as well as remote from it, become swollen and rounded, with prominent and often multiple nucleoli. Short rows of such nuclear forms appear at the site of injury within the next several days. Sarcoplasm in such cells assumes a prominent basophilia. Also noted at this time are isolated, large, basophilic cells resembling macrophages. Although mitotic figures are noted near the zone of injury in mononuclear cells, none are conspicuous in the sarcolemmal tube or in normal-appearing muscle.

By eight days the sarcolemmal tubes are occupied by abundant, granular cytoplasm and rows of prominent nuclei. Nuclear accumulation in such foci is quite rapid. Lash, et al. (1957) estimate a two-fold increase in such structures from the fifth to eighth day of regeneration. Longitudinal orientation of fibrillar material within the granular cytoplasm may be noted as early as five to eight days and cross striations at a somewhat later period. Myofibril formation first becomes evident in a subsarcolemmal position. As the buds of sarcoplasm and their nuclei from each end of the damaged fiber meet, more myofibrils become evident so that by 21 days these structures, including cross striations, are prominent. This process continues until approximately one month after transection, at which time the area of injury appears normal. The only evidence of preexisting damage is the occasional tandem arrangement of muscle nuclei, distortion, and minimal fibrosis.

It is of interest that diseased muscle, as in muscular dystrophy, in humans as well as the experimental animal, exhibits comparable features of regeneration following injury (Walton and Adams, 1956; Keeler and Young, 1962; Walker, 1962; Walker and Drager, 1962). Indeed, regeneration is considered to occur spontaneously in uninjured dystrophic muscle (Walker, 1962). Although the earlier literature refers to mitotic division of damaged skeletal muscle fibers in the regenerative process (Waldeyer, 1865; Volkmann, 1893; Forbus, 1926), it has been suggested more recently that such activity is the result of amitotic proliferation (Millar, 1934; Clark, 1946; Godman, 1957). As a result of cytophotometric analyses of Feulgen stained sections, Lash, et al. (1957) considered mitotic division to occur only in mononuclear cells in the wound coagulum, but not in the regenerating muscle per se. However, Zhinkin and Andreeva (1963) considered DNA synthesis, as estimated by the administration of tritiated thymidine as an indicator, to proceed in embryonic as well as regenerating muscle in the same manner as in other tissues where cell reproduction by mitosis occurs.

Much of the difficulty in convincingly establishing the cellular kinetics involved in regenerating muscle has apparently been the result of the inadequacy of light microscopy in resolving the true identity of those cells observed in mitosis. This shortcoming has also been reflected in the lack of unanimity expressed concerning the nature of the regenerative process. Thus, many have advocated that skeletal muscle regenerates as a result of budding of the viable fibers. This phenomenon has been referred to as "budding regeneration." Others (Volkmann, 1893; Speidel, 1938; Adams, et al., 1962) consider the possibility that new muscle cells arise from isolated or singular cellular elements which are believed to represent myoblasts, although their absolute identification by light microscopy has been uncertain. Regeneration by myoblastic proliferation has been designated as discontinuous in contrast to the continuous or budding form.

ELECTRON MICROSCOPY. Albrook (1962) and Price, et al. (1964) have described their electron microscopic observations of regenerating skeletal muscle. The more recent findings clearly establish the identity of isolated myoblastic cells in the cellular population of regenerating skeletal muscle. Since there has been little doubt concerning the occurrence of the continuous form of regeneration, it would appear that both processes may be involved. These investigators noted that initially following the injury, many large macrophages could be identified. These cells frequently had pseudopodal cytoplasmic extensions which could be observed engulfing debris and subsequently forming phagosomes. Their cytoplasm also contained microbodies, lipid, and myelin figures. Such macrophages could be distinguished ultrastructurally from another cell type which clearly appeared to represent the myoblasts, since myofibrillar development could be followed in their cytoplasm during the course of the regenerative process. These cells lacked a basement membrane and, although granular endoplasmic reticulum was poorly developed compared to fibroblasts, free RNA was evident (Fig. 9).

In some areas fine filaments, precursors of the myofilaments, were found in association with the free RNA. In addition, these cells were characterized by small mitochondria, which were more uniform than noted in normal adult muscle cells, and by prominent Golgi structures. Binucleate and multinucleate forms were apparent, and, although no mitotic figures were noted, evidence for amitotic division was also lacking. The fine filaments noted to be associated with free cytoplasmic RNA became progressively more longitudinally oriented within the cell. Subsequently noted were other thicker aggregates of filaments that had a diameter comparable to the thick myosin filaments of the A band (Fig. 10). These two types of filaments aligned themselves so that later the thicker ones represented A bands and

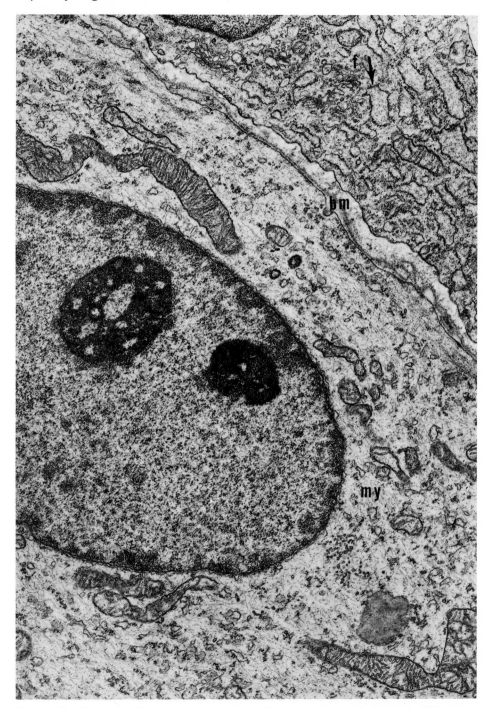

Fig. 9.   Portion of myoblast (my) from regenerating skeletal muscle located within sarco-lemmal tube adjacent to sarcolemmal basement membrane (bm). Portion of fibroblast is located in upper right corner (f). Cytoplasm of the myoblast contains fine filaments and RNA particles. X 27,400. (From Price, H. M., et al. *Lab. Invest.*, 13:1279, 1964.)

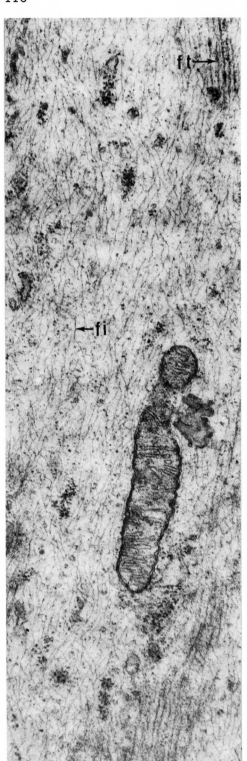

Fig. 10. Portion of myoblast from regenerating skeletal muscle containing longitudinally oriented fine filaments (fi) as well as thicker filaments (ft) in upper and lower positions. Relatively few polyribosomes are present. X 35,000. (From Price, H. M., et al. *Lab. Invest.*, 13:1279, 1964.)

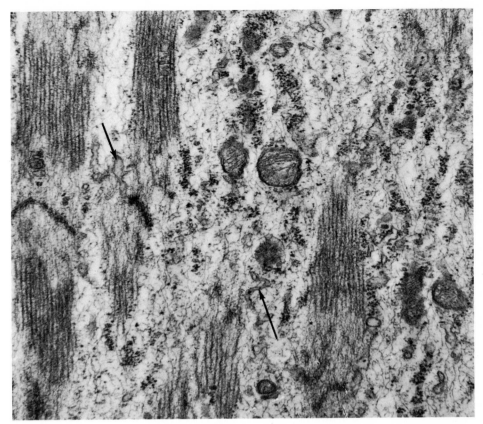

Fig. 11.   Early sarcomere formation within a differentiating skeletal muscle cell. Sarco-
plasmic reticulum (arrows) and myofibril formation appear as a random process. Fine filaments are seen between the forming myofibrils. X 33,600. (From Price, H. M., et al. *Lab.
Invest.*, 13:1279, 1964).

the thinner ones I bands. Early Z bands also appeared within such cells, and invaginations of peripheral plasma membranes gave rise to cisternae resembling sarco-
plasmic reticulum (Fig. 11). When the myoblast became mature it was encom-
passed by two basement membranes—one from the sarcolemmal tube and the other
apparently from intercellular connective tissue fibers. The results of this study provide evidence establishing the identity of the myoblast as an isolated or singular
cellular element participating in regeneration of skeletal muscle.

Origin of Myoblasts

The origin of the myoblasts has recently been explored by microradioauto-
graphic techniques. Walker (1953) injected tritiated thymidine into dystrophic mice
following skeletal muscle damage. The muscle was again traumatized, and the nuclei
of the newly formed fibers also contained the label, indicating that the myoblastic
elements arise from injured muscle fibers. To exclude their derivation from connective tissue elements, he injured the overlying connective tissue in mice treated with

the label and then injured the muscle; he found no evidence of tritium in the baso-philic myotubes of the regenerating muscle. He has thus concluded that the myo-blasts are derived from within the damaged muscle fibers by a mechanism of de-differentiation and subsequent re-differentiation.

Significant information is lacking concerning the nature of the stimulus respon-sible for the regenerative response in skeletal muscle. Similarly, the mechanism whereby the regenerating fiber is capable of reorienting its filaments into function-ally contractile units is unknown.

Nerve Regeneration

It has long been recognized that neurons lack regenerative capacity. Yet, it is also widely appreciated that following transection or such trauma as crush to periph-eral nerves, anatomical as well as functional restitution frequently occurs. The suc-cess of such an event is in large part dependent upon the viability of neuronal cells, extent of injury, and, in the case of transection, degree of separation of the fibers (Hicks and Warren, 1950; Barton, 1962). The importance of neuronal survival and axon-neuron interrelations has been vividly demonstrated by the cinemato-graphic studies of tissue cultures of sensory cells of the inner ear of the mouse and chick by Shambaugh and Orr (1963). Nutrient flow is clearly retrograde from axon to neuron as well as in the reverse direction. Thus, when the axon is severed, the former course is prevented, resulting in cell death unless a new axonal segment appears. Addition of nutrient in the form of calf serum was capable of prolonging cell life despite loss of axonal substance.

Since neurons fail to proliferate, one might justifiably question that the axonal growth observed in the proximal stump following injury represents a bona fide example of regeneration. Nevertheless, certain structural elements, notably Schwann cells, which are of unquestionable importance in the process, do exhibit proliferative activity. Further, common application of the term "regeneration" to this process would make any discussion of this field perhaps incomplete without its inclusion.

Morphologic Changes

LIGHT MICROSCOPY.   Since Waller's (1850) classic description of the events subsequent to excision of a portion of peripheral nerve, much investigation has been directed to the degenerative phenomena occurring in the distal segment of such nerves. Indeed, Wallerian degeneration has been the subject of much physiologic, morphologic, biochemical (briefly reviewed by Fisher and Turano, 1963), and, more recently, ultrastructural study (Vial, 1958; Terry, et al., 1959; Glimstedt and Wohlfart, 1960; Barton, 1962; Fisher and Turano, 1963).

Less attention, aside from histologic examination by light microscopy (Biel-schowsky, 1909; Ramón y Cajal, 1928; Nageotte, 1932; Hicks and Warren, 1950; Geren, 1954), has been directed to the events within the proximal stump. The events appear comparable in both sensory and motor nerves (Weiss, 1948). It is well recognized that, after a brief latent period, bands of Schwann cells with abun-dant cytoplasm extend from the proximal stump. Mitoses have been observed in such cells (Abercrombie, 1946; Greenfield, et al., 1960), but are relatively infrequent. Strands of axonal material may also be appreciated coursing among the proliferated Schwann cells. Histiocytic elements may contaminate the picture, but these appear essential for the removal of debris. Fibroblastic infiltration of the area also occurs and, if excessive, may interfere with subsequent development of continuity. Also, the degree of injury, whether associated with a wide hiatus, as in excision of portions of nerve, or simple crushing, profoundly influences the degree of restoration of continuity, although the regenerative process in the proximal stump appears generally comparable in both situations. By approximately three to five weeks, restitution under those conditions propitious for such an event may be appreciated.

ELECTRON MICROSCOPY.   Prior to the use of electron microscopy, the mechanism of myelinization of peripheral nerves was poorly understood, since light microscopy failed to provide sufficient resolution to assess this important aspect of nerve regeneration accurately. However, ultrastructural studies of Terry, et al. (1959) and Barton (1962) of regenerating nerve, as well as the classic studies on the embryogenesis of myelinated nerve by Geren (1954), have clarified this problem. The ultrastructural observations, which confirm previous conceptions of regeneration derived from light microscopy, signify that the myelinization of regenerated sciatic nerve of mice following transection recapitulated the process of myelinization noted in embryogenesis by Green (1954).

By 21 days following transection, invaginations of the Schwann cell cytoplasm by the naked axon can be appreciated. The plasma membranes at the site of entry are approximated, and this space, which becomes elongated, is designated as the mesaxon (Fig. 12). The latter wraps around the axon in a spiral fashion and becomes identifiable as myelin. The defect at the site of entry in the Schwann cell becomes covered by an external basement membrane acquired from the extracellular tissue. At the time of myelinization, continuity and relatively normal-appearing nerve with its outer coat of perineurim and internal endoneural fibers are evident.

Regeneration in Central Nervous System

Although there is no regeneration of central nervous system pathways in mammals, proximal stumps of the severed axons do exhibit a limited incomplete ability in this regard. After initial attempts to repair the defect, degeneration of axonal sprouts ensues (Bielschowsky, 1909; Ramón y Cajal, 1928). Lampert and Cressman (1964) have used electron microscopy to reexamine the events following the transection of the dorsal ascending tracts in the thoracic spinal cord of adult rats. They noted that terminal and preterminal axoplasmic enlargements of the proximal axoplasmic stump occur within one week. These sprouts are much richer in mitochondria, endoplasmic reticulum, and electron-dense granules than normal axons. These buds also become invested in Schwann cells and undergo myelinization. However, their growth becomes blocked by the development of glial scar tissue, which is also believed to be derived from Schwann cells, and by one month they exhibit vacuolar degeneration of their substance and subsequent phagocytosis. Lampert and Cressman suggest that the diversion of the regenerating axons from synaptic junctions may be responsible for the degeneration encountered.

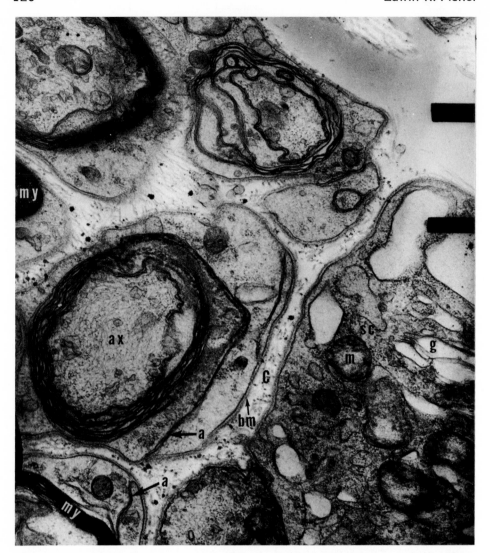

Fig. 12.   Area from proximal line of transection of sciatic nerve of rat at 21 days. Variable degrees of myelinization of axons (ax) are evident. Axolemma (a) clearly arise from the cytoplasmic membrane of Schwann cells. These latter are bounded by a somewhat amorphous basement membrane (bm). Looping of the axolemma about the axon is more evident in those fibers which appear more poorly myelinated or undergoing early myelinization as compared to those with more fully developed sheaths (my). Intercellular collagen (C) and portion of cytoplasm of Schwann cell (sc) with mitochondria (m) and prominent Golgi structure (g) are also present. X 25,000.

Splenic Regeneration

Following removal of the spleen in the dog as well as in man, hypertrophy of accessory splenic tissue is not uncommon. This phenomenon, however, does not represent an example of true regeneration. Investigations of the regenerative capacity of the spleen have been sparse. MacKay and Polland (1931) found enlargement of

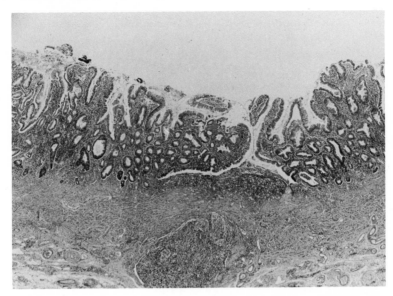

Fig. 10.   Formation of ulcer by undermining in ulcerative colitis. H&E. X60.

matically excludes that diagnosis and in conjunction with the thickened bowel wall
is highly suggestive of Crohn's disease (Fig. 14). The classical cobblestone pattern
of the mucosa is due to transverse ulcers between the rugae in addition to longitudinal ulceration, but if there is much muscular spasm the appearance may be more
polypoid than cobblestone (Fig. 15).

In the majority of cases, the pathologist has little difficulty in arriving at the
correct diagnosis. The presence of tuberculoid granulomas is usually considered
to be diagnostic. They are found in all coats of the bowel wall but are most frequently present in the submucosa (Table 1).[24] They may also be found in regional
lymph nodes and in anal skin tags (Fig. 16).

Table 1.   Crohn's Colitis: Granulomas*

	NUMBER	PERCENTAGE
Resected specimens	30	100
Mucosa	3	10
Submucosa	15	50
Muscle	10	33
Subserosa	9	30
Anal	6	20
Lymph nodes	6	20
Total	23	77

* From McGovern, V.J., and Goulston, S.J.M. *Gut,* 9:164, 1968.

In approximately 25 percent of cases, however, granulomas are either absent or
so scarce that they are not found in ordinary routine sections. In such cases, one
must rely on other criteria for diagnosis. The most helpful diagnostic features are
the characteristic lymphoid aggregates, the fibrosis, and the mode of ulcer formation.

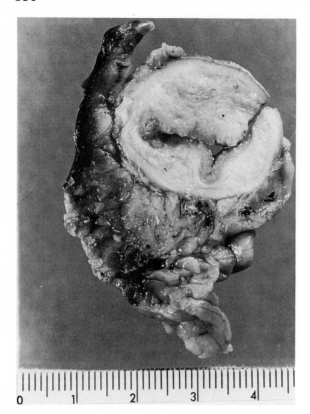

Fig. 11. "Stricture" of colon in chronic ulcerative colitis.

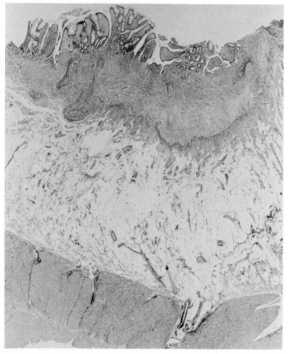

Fig. 12. Microscopic appearances of the stricture in Figure 11. The mucosa is irregular; the muscularis mucosae is greatly hypertrophied with delineation of the two layers; the submucosa is composed of adipose tissue and the muscle coat is hypertrophied. H&E. X8.

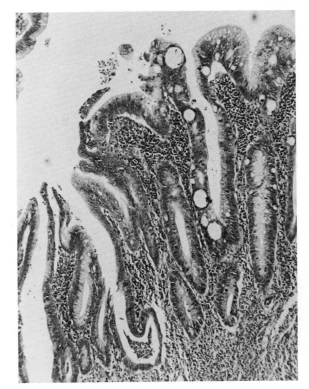

Fig. 13. Precarcinomatous focus in a patient with chronic ulcerative colitis who had an established carcinoma in the cecum and another in the transverse colon. There is epithelial atypia, and mitoses are present high in the crypts instead of being confined to the basal regions. H&E. X75.

LYMPHOID AGGREGATES. Lymphoid tissue is normally present in the bowel wall and usually consists of follicular aggregates with or without germinal centres. They may be confined to the lamina propria or they may be partly in the submucosa. In any chronic inflammatory condition, lymphoid tissue in the vicinity of the muscularis mucosae may be increased in quantity and exhibit prominent germinal centres, but in Crohn's disease the typical lymphoid aggregates are situated in the deeper portions of the submucosa and do not have germinal centres (Fig. 17). Lymphoid aggregates in Crohn's disease may be found in all layers of the bowel wall, but they are found most consistently in the submucosa (Table 2).

Table 2. Crohn's Colitis: Lymphoid Aggregates*

	NUMBER	PERCENTAGE
Resected specimens	30	100
Submucosa	30	100
Muscle	19	63
Subserosa	24	80

* From McGovern, V.J., and Goulston, S.J.M. *Gut,* 9:164, 1968.

FIBROSIS. Fibrosis is invariably present in the submucosa of affected segments but may also be found in the other coats (Fig. 17, Table 3). It does not have the dense cicatricial quality found in benign strictures of ischemic origin, but it can be fairly firm and in the resected specimen is often visible to the naked eye. Fibrotic strictures

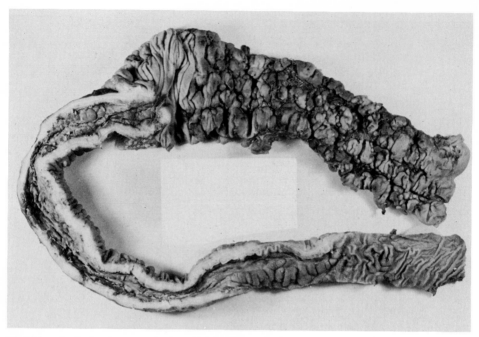

Fig. 14.   Crohn's disease of the terminal ileum and of the ascending colon. The cecum appears to be unaffected. Between the ulcers, the colonic mucosa appears normal.

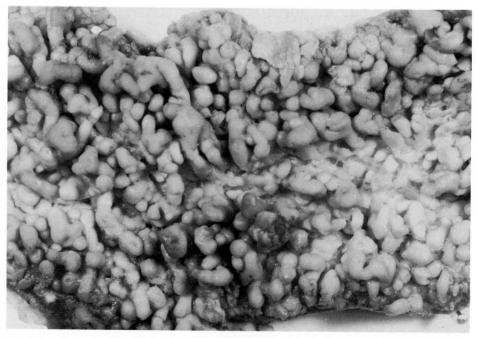

Fig. 15.   Long standing Crohn's disease of the entire colon. The polypoid mucosa simulates ulcerative colitis.

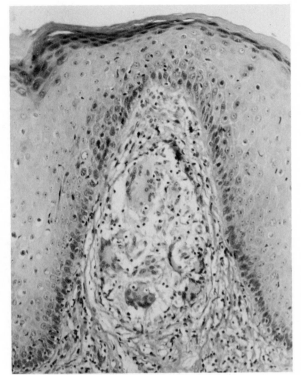

Fig. 16. Anal granuloma from the patient whose colon is illustrated in Figure 15. H&E. X150.

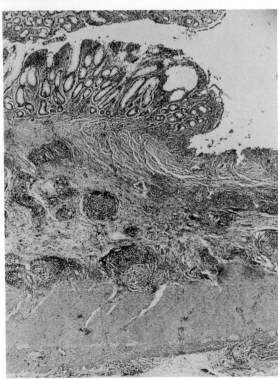

Fig. 17. Whole thickness of bowel wall in Crohn's disease showing the margin of an ulcer, fibrosis of the submucosa, and lymphoid aggregates. There are tuberculoid granulomas just above the muscle coat. H&E. X22.

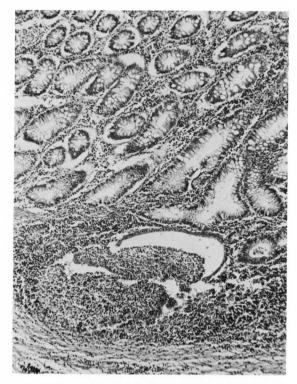

Fig. 18. Destruction of the base of a crypt with the formation of an abscess. The overlying crypt epithelium appears normal. H&E. X60.

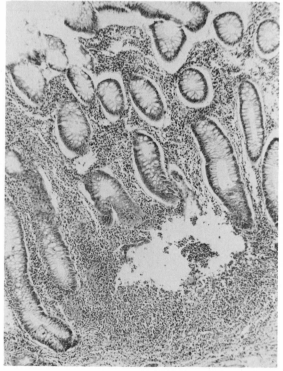

Fig. 19. Destruction of the bases of crypts with abscess formation. A granulomatous reaction is developing in the deeper portion. H&E. X60.

Table 3.   Crohn's Colitis: Fibrosis*

	NUMBER	PERCENTAGE
Resected specimens	30	100
Submucosa	30	100
Muscle	18	60
Subserosa	13	43

* From McGovern, V.J., and Goulston, S.J.M. *Gut,* 9:164, 1968.

of the colon occasionally complicate pulmonary tuberculosis. These two conditions can be differentiated from Crohn's disease because they lack the characteristic lymphoid aggregations and the typical patterns of ulcer formation.

ULCER FORMATION.   Aggregates of lymphocytes are present in the bases of ulcers in the earliest stages of formation. Whereas degeneration of crypt epithelium starts at any level in ulcerative colitis, it always starts in the basal cells of the crypts in Crohn's disease and never in the absence of lymphocytic aggregates (Fig. 18). Lymphocytes, however, are sometimes replaced by a granulomatous reaction in the base of an ulcer (Fig. 19). Neutrophils and other leucocytes accumulate around the affected crypt cells, often in the form of a "crypt abscess," while the more superficial portions of these tubules are unaffected. When a complete crypt is involved, however, an oblique cut may show only a superficial crypt abscess. The mucosal epithelium surrounding an ulcer may be quite normal in contrast to what is found in ulcerative colitis.

Once the process of cell degeneration starts, ulcers form in the same way as in ulcerative colitis, by undermining or by loss of tubules from the lamina propria. Another kind of ulceration takes the form of clefts, which extend into the submucosa in an oblique undermining fashion or penetrate directly through the bowel wall in the form of fistulas (Fig. 20). In very acute lesions, the affected portion of mucosa may be replaced by a mass of fissured leucocytic exudate from which fistulous abscesses track through the bowel wall.

When healing occurs, mucosa may grow down a fistulous track into the submucosa and produce the appearance which has been described as "colitis cystica profunda."[9]

DIAGNOSIS.   The diagnosis of Crohn's disease of the colon is readily made when the characteristic macroscopic appearances are accompanied by the presence of tuberculoid granulomas. When granulomas are absent, one can still make the diagnosis on the presence of submucosal fibrosis with lymphoid aggregates and normal mucosal epithelium in the unulcerated areas. The main diagnostic features are presented in Table 4. Irregularity of the mucosal pattern, which results from healing

Table 4.   Crohn's Colitis: Diagnosis*

	PERCENTAGE
Submucosal lymphoid aggregates	100
Submucosal fibrosis	100
Granulomas	76
Fissured ulcers	59

* From McGovern, V.J., and Goulston, S.J.M. *Gut,* 9:164, 1968.

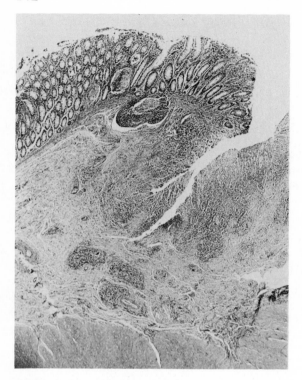

Fig. 20. Splitlike fissure extending into the submucosa.
Typical fibrosis and lymphoid
aggregates are present in the
submucosa. H&E. X17.

of an ulcer in which there had been disruption or destruction of the muscularis mucosae, may suggest the diagnosis of ulcerative colitis, but the normality of the epithelial cells is an important distinguishing feature.

Cleftlike ulcers extending obliquely into the submucosa are highly suggestive of Crohn's disease when they are present, but the most characteristic features of ulcer formation are the collections of lymphocytes in the deepest part of the lamina propria with subsequent degeneration of the basal cells of the overlying crypts.

Rectal biopsy is regarded by Lockhart-Mummery and Morson[21] as a valuable aid to diagnosis, and in 16 of the 19 cases in which rectal biopsy was performed, tuberculoid granulomas were found. These authors emphasize that care must be exercised in selecting the site for the biopsy. Mindful of the fact that Crohn's disease is patchy and that normal bowel is present between the affected areas, Lockhart-Mummery and Morson recommend that the edge of an ulcer is a suitable site for biopsy provided that a good deal of submucosal tissue be obtained.

Anal lesions are common in Crohn's disease, and a high percentage of these have tuberculoid granulomas.[21] Furthermore, granulomas in anal lesions such as fistulas, fissures, and tags have been found to antecede the clinical and radiologic manifestations of Crohn's disease in some cases.[13]

Ischemic Enterocolitis

Ischemic enterocolitis is the name given to a disorder which has been variously described in the past as hemorrhagic enterocolitis,[42] uremic enterocolitis,[16] acute postoperative enterocolitis,[31] and even staphylococcal enterocolitis. It is now known to be a specific entity caused by transient ischemia of the alimentary tract, which is insufficient to cause full-thickness infarction of the bowel.[23] There is an acute form which affects the whole or only a portion of the intestinal tract, and a chronic form which affects only a segment of the gut, usually in the region of the splenic flexure and upper part of the descending colon.

PRECIPITATING FACTORS. The chief precipitating factors in the causation of ischemic enterocolitis are: hypotension; splanchnic vasoconstriction; mesenteric vascular occlusion; and cardiac and aortic surgical operations.

Hypotension is a component of the shock syndrome and is encountered in a large variety of disorders both medical and surgical, the commonest being myocardial infarction. Septicemia, acute hemorrhagic pancreatitis, acute hemorrhage, and syncope are other fairly common conditions which precipitate ischemic enterocolitis through hypotension.

Splanchnic vasoconstriction occurs when there is a fall in the effective circulating blood volume, as in congestive cardiac failure. Digitalis also causes splanchnic vasoconstriction,[10] and this probably accounts for the occasional case of ischemic enterocolitis in patients under treatment for congestive cardiac failure. Other agents causing splanchnic vasoconstriction are catecholamines and gram-negative bacterial endotoxins.[41] The splanchnic blood flow is also reduced by halothane and cyclopropane anesthesia,[6] and while this is not of clinical importance in most subjects, it is possibly significant in patients who have sustained blood loss or who are hypotensive.

Mesenteric vascular occlusion occurs in a variety of ways. The commonest is atheromatous occlusion of the mesenteric vessels at their origin. Embolus is the next most frequent cause of occlusion, and thrombosis leading to ischemic enterocolitis has occasionally been observed in patients with polyarteritis nodosa and with aortic arteritis (Takayasu's disease). Ischemic enterocolitis is also seen in dissecting aneurysm and atheromatous aneurysm of the abdominal aorta.

During *cardiac operations or operations involving the aorta,* the blood supply to the gut is often temporarily suspended or reduced in volume. At autopsy, these patients frequently exhibit ischemic enterocolitis and other visceral manifestations of the shock syndrome.

Most cases fit into the categories just mentioned, but there is a small group in which there is no clear-cut history or objective evidence of a precipitating cause. Sometimes the precipitating cause is revealed at a later date by the discovery of unsuspected cardiovascular disease. A case of this type was that of a 46-year-old psychiatric patient with ischemic colitis who was eventually found to be subject to attacks of atrial fibrillation accompanied by severe hypotension. There are others, however, in which the precipitating cause remains a mystery.

PREDISPOSING FACTORS. The majority of patients who become severely hypotensive or who suffer from congestive cardiac failure do not develop ischemic disease of the intestinal tract. Conditions which predispose to ischemic enterocolitis are: atheromatous disease of the mesenteric arteries; respiratory insufficiency; anemia; and inadequate mesenteric arterial anastomoses.

In the presence of one of these factors, the gut may have insufficient reserves to withstand any further reduction of blood supply by an episode of hypotension, arteriolar vasoconstriction, or sudden vascular occlusion. Ischemic enterocolitis or even infarction of the gut may ensue.

An important predisposing factor in the development of ischemic enterocolitis is the relatively poor vascular anastomosis in some persons, in the vicinity of the splenic flexure and descending colon (Fig. 21). This area is supplied by an accessory from the middle colic branch of the superior mesenteric artery anastomosing with the left colic branch of the inferior mesenteric artery. Whereas the rest of the alimentary tract has a continuous system of vascular arcades, this is not always the case in this region which is thereby rendered particularly vulnerable to any reduction in blood supply or in oxygen tension. Reiner[35] showed that the mesenteric system can be readily filled through the superior mesenteric artery but less easily through the inferior mesenteric. Occlusion of the superior mesenteric artery is thus likely to have more far-reaching and serious consequences than occlusion of the inferior mesenteric, but, in either case, the portion of the gut most likely to be affected is the splenic flexure and the upper part of the descending colon.

In a few cases hypotension alone, without any discoverable predisposing cause, has been responsible for fatal ischemic enterocolitis.[23]

PRIMARY DISEASE. Ischemic enterocolitis complicates a variety of disorders but the most common are those of the cardiovascular system, particularly myocardial

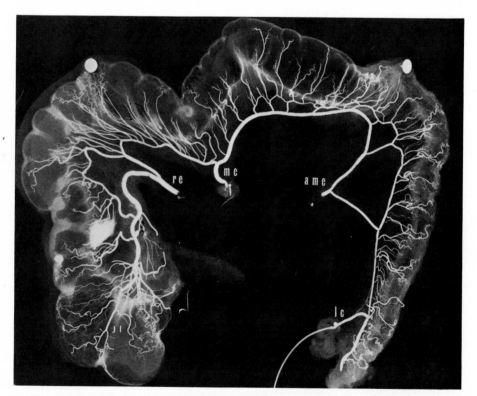

Fig. 21.   X-ray of injected autopsy specimen of large bowel showing the anastomotic pattern. The descending colon is supplied by an accessory branch (amc) of the middle colic artery (mc) which anastomoses with the left colic (lc) artery.

infarction and congestive cardiac failure. These patients often have atheromatous narrowing of the mouths of their mesenteric vessels and are thereby predisposed to development of ischemic enterocolitis by the shocked state in myocardial infarction, or by splanchnic vasoconstriction in congestive cardiac failure.

Because of its association with degenerative cardiovascular disease, ischemic enterocolitis is most frequently seen in older persons. Nevertheless, it can occur at any age, even infancy. We have seen it in a New Guinea child whose bowel was predisposed by healing polyarteritis. The precipitating factor in this case was not determined.

Other primary disorders commonly associated with ischemic enterocolitis have been rheumatoid disease and pulmonary emphysema.

PATHOLOGY.   The affected portion of gut in acute ischemic enterocolitis is intensely congested, frequently hemorrhagic, with free blood in the lumen. The serosa may be congested and discolored, but often it appears quite normal. Ulcers are very irregularly distributed and may encircle the lumen, or in the colon they may have a longitudinal orientation overlying the *taeniae coli* (Fig. 22). Perforation of ulcers is more common in the small intestine than in the large.

Microscopically, hemorrhages are found in the mucosa and, in severe cases, in the submucosa also. Fibrin thrombi in mucosal capillaries are characteristic of

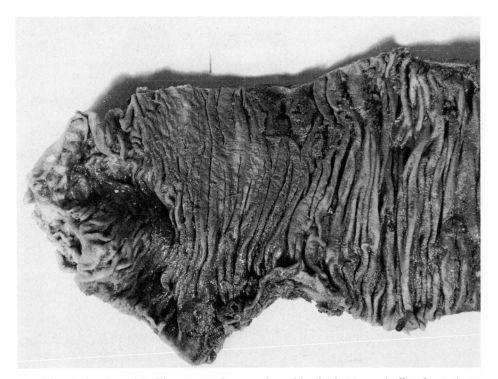

Fig. 22.   Ischemic colitis. The mucosa is necrotic and beginning to peel off to form ulcers. The patient was a 79-year-old female who had involvement of the terminal ileum, ascending colon, and part of the transverse colon ascribed to kinking of the ileo-colic artery by adhesions.

ischemic enterocolitis; in severe cases, they extend into the submucosal venules and veins. Sometimes there is actual necrosis of venules even when they do not contain thrombi. Apart from capillaries, the vessels affected are always veins and venules, never arteries or arterioles (Figs. 23, 24). The mucosa rapidly becomes necrotic

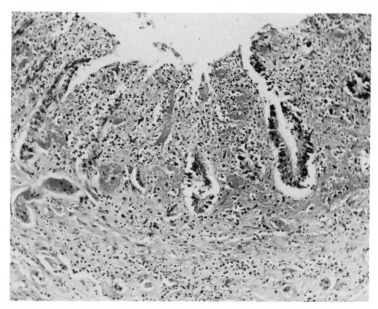

Fig. 23.   Ischemic colitis resulting from hypotension due to fatal hemorrhagic pancreatitis. There are fibrin thrombi in the mucosa which also shows inflammation and early mucosal necrosis. Hemorrhage was minimal. H&E. X150.

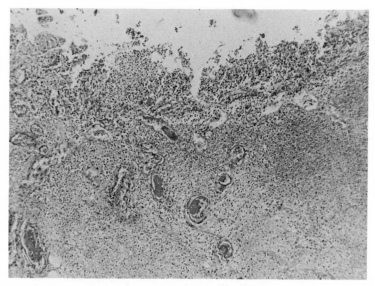

Fig. 24.   Ulcer with necrotic surface. There is hemorrhage and inflammation in the sub-mucosa. Fibrin thrombi are present in the remnants of the mucosa and in the submucosal venules. The patient had severe hypotension from myocardial infarction which occurred four days before death. H&E. X60.

and after three or four days undergoes dissolution, leaving an ulcer. Healing may be rapid if the disorder is of mild degree, but perforation may occur. When the ulceration extends through the muscularis mucosae, healing is by cicatrizing granulation tissue, and at this stage one may refer to the disorder as chronic.

Acute ischemic enterocolitis due to hypotension or splanchnic vasoconstriction usually complicates some disorder that is already likely to be fatal. Consequently, it tends to be diagnosed more frequently at autopsy than in the living patient. Should the patient survive, healing of deep ulcerations can lead to benign strictures simulating neoplastic disease when confined to single short segments.

When a vessel is occluded, there may be temporary ischemia pending the development of anastomotic compensation. In the large bowel, the segment of bowel affected is usually where the anastomoses are least effective, in particular the splenic flexure and descending colon. If infarction does not occur, a localized area of ischemic enteritis or colitis results, which may then progress to cicatricial stenosis (Figs. 25, 26, 27).

Ischemic colitis may be said to be chronic when ulcers persist beyond six weeks from the onset of the condition. By that time, if the lesion is severe enough to be causing symptoms, there should be cicatricial narrowing of the affected portion of colon (Fig. 28). The luminal surface is covered with a fibrinous exudate, and fibrous thickening of the wall can be seen with the naked eye.

Microscopically, the fibrosis is more dense than that seen in any other disease of the colon. It may be confined to the submucosa, but in some cases it will be found replacing the muscle coat. At an earlier stage, one may find organizing thrombi within veins and venules of the submucosa, but by the time stenosis of the gut has occurred, one has to rely on the criterion of Marston, et al.,[26] namely the presence of hemosiderin-containing phagocytes in the submucosa, for confirmation of diagnosis.

DIFFERENTIAL DIAGNOSIS. Sigmoidoscopic biopsy can be most helpful in distinguishing between acute ischemic colitis and acute ulcerative colitis. Ulcerative colitis almost invariably involves the rectosigmoid region, and it would be very unusual for a normal biopsy in the acute disease. Ischemic colitis sometimes affects the sigmoid colon, and the presence of hemorrhage in the lamina propria or even fibrin thrombi may then be found.

Chronic ischemic colitis is an obstructive lesion and is therefore most likely to be confused clinically with carcinoma or Crohn's disease. It is usually beyond the range of the sigmoidoscope, and the diagnosis can only be made with certainty after the specimen has been removed. The absence of granulomas and lymphoid accumulations and the presence of dense cicatrization and hemosiderin-containing phagocytes in the submucosa indicate that the stenosing lesion is of ischemic origin. The possibility of ischemic stricture of the colon should already have been suspected because of the site of the lesion and perhaps the history.

Pseudomembranous Colitis

Pseudomembranous colitis is a pathologic entity of uncertain etiology, characterized by sudden onset of profound shock due to severe watery diarrhea.

The bowel is usually dilated and has lost its normal mucosal pattern. Yellow

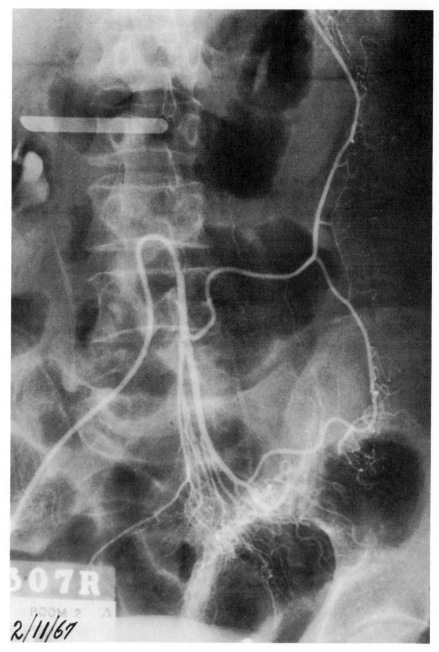

Fig. 25.   Angiogram of 67-year-old woman who was awakened by severe abdominal pain accompanied by distension and passage of blood per rectum. A catheter is in the inferior mesenteric artery. Filling of the hemorrhoidal vessels is good, but there is defective filling in the distribution of the left colic artery.

or greenish bile-stained plaques a few millimeters in diameter may be sparsely scattered over the mucosa of a small segment of the large bowel, or there may be numerous plaques involving the entire large bowel and sometimes a portion of the

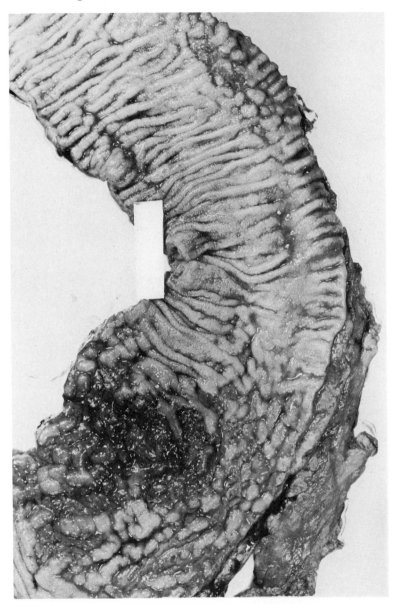

Fig. 26.   Three weeks after onset of symptoms, the patient whose angiogram is repro-
duced in Figure 25 had a left hemicolectomy. There are linear ulcers in the upper part of
the descending colon and a large irregular ulcerated area in the lower part.

small bowel. The appearance in the more florid cases has been likened to the
cracked moss-covered bark of a tree (Fig. 29). The consistency of the plaques
varies from gelatinous and semitranslucent to opaque and firm, according to the
relative proportions of mucus and fibrin in their composition. The ileum may be
involved to a certain extent, but the disease affects the colon much more frequently.
The serosa usually appears normal.

   Microscopically, there is a characteristic appearance. The earliest lesion con-

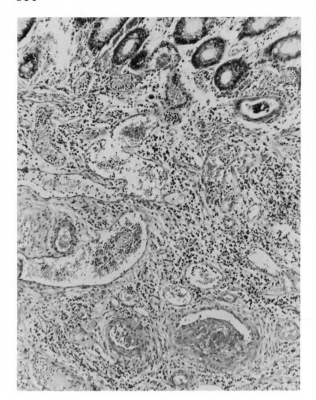

Fig. 27. The ischemic nature of the ulcers in the colon illustrated in Figure 26 is confirmed by the presence of organizing venular thrombi in the submucosa. H&E. X75.

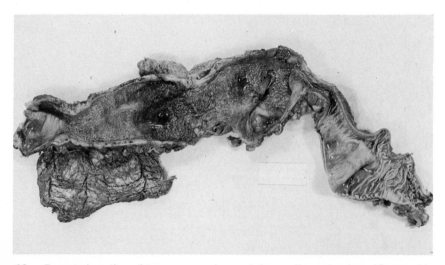

Fig. 28.   Resected portion of transverse colon and descending colon in a 46-year-old male showing stenosis, which is particularly marked in the descending colon. The colon was resected 12 weeks after the sudden onset of diarrhea. Histologically this specimen showed dense cicatrization with hemosiderin-containing phagocytes in the granulation tissue. The patient died from a cardiomyopathy of unknown cause, and an elongated thrombus attached at one end to the arch of the aorta was found at autopsy. The ischemia of the colon was presumably due to embolus.

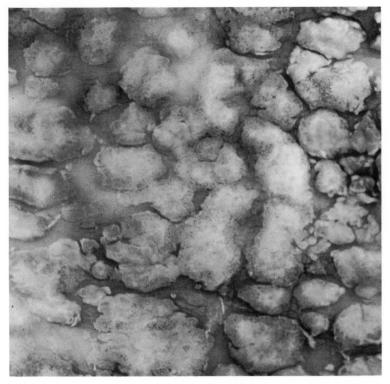

Fig. 29. Portion of the colon showing the typical plaques of pseudomembranous colitis. X 2.5.

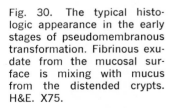

Fig. 30. The typical histo-logic appearance in the early stages of pseudomembranous transformation. Fibrinous exu-date from the mucosal sur-face is mixing with mucus from the distended crypts. H&E. X75.

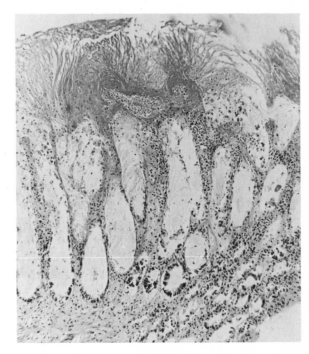

sists of foci of fibrinoid necrosis of the mucosal surface, while the subjacent crypt epithelium produces excessive amounts of mucus. Fibrin erupts from the surface and mixes with the mucus to form a jelly-like mucofibrinous exudate which fuses with the necrotic surface of the mucosa (Fig. 30). Between the plaques of pseudo-membranous transformation, the mucosa is quite normal.

There is marked edema of the submucosa, but cellular infiltration is absent. Polymorphonuclear leucocytes in moderate numbers may be found in the surface exudate only.

In the early stages the exudate can be scraped off the bowel surface with a knife, but later it is firmly incorporated into the mucosa and cannot be easily removed. Eventually, if the patient survives long enough, the affected mucosa is discarded, and ulcers may result if the whole thickness of mucosa has become necrotic.

ETIOLOGY. Pseudomembranous enterocolitis occurs most commonly in association with obstructive lesions of the colon, but it is also found in cardiorenal conditions in which it may be precipitated by uremia, cardiac failure, or pneumonia. Of 94 patients who developed the condition postoperatively, 41 were being treated for carcinoma of the colon (Pettet, et al.[32]); of 14 patients in whom the condition was not preceded by surgical operation, 5 had colonic obstruction due to carcinoma of the colon, and cardiac disease was the next most common accompanying disorder (Kleckner, et al.[19]); 5 of the 14 patients described by Goulston and McGovern[12] had colonic obstruction, while cardiac and renal disease were the commonest disorders in the remainder.

Foci of pseudomembranous change too small to cause clinical manifestations are common in obstructive conditions and have been observed by the writer even on the surface of an adenomatous polyp of the colon.

The cause of pseudomembranous colitis is obscure. Possible causes suggested by previous authors have been antibiotic therapy,[34] surgical operations,[32] staphylococcal enterotoxin,[1, 39, 40] and ischemia.[14, 25] None of these factors can be a sole cause, since the disorder occurred prior to the antibiotic era[32] and occurs in patients who have never undergone a surgical operation.[2, 12, 19] Furthermore, a staphylococcus is recovered from the stools of only a minority of patients with pseudomembranous enterocolitis,[4] and ischemia produces specific lesions which we have already discussed.

From the histologic appearances, it seems that pseudomembranous colitis is due to a soluble toxin which diminishes in intensity as it penetrates the bowel wall. Where it is most concentrated at the mucosal surface, it causes necrosis; in lesser concentration it stimulates the crypt epithelium to excess mucus secretion; in the submucosa it causes increased permeability and edema. In all probability, the changes of pseudomembranous colitis can be elicited by a variety of toxins present in the lumen when the bowel is rendered susceptible by obstruction, chronic cardiorenal disease, or other debilitating disorders.

Necrotizing Enterocolitis

In 1947, Jeckeln[17] in Germany reported a necrotizing enteritis which he called *Darmbrand,* literally "gut burn" and analogous to "heart burn." This was later shown by Zeissler and Rassfield-Sternberg[43] and by Fick and Wolken[11] to be due to the beta toxin of *Clostridium welchii* Type F (now recommended to be included in Type C[38]). A similar disorder, described by Murrell and Roth,[30] affects the jejunum of New Guinea natives and is due to pork infected with *C. welchii* Type C.[8]

Involvement of the colon by the same type of necrotizing process has also been reported by Killingback and Williams,[18] Duncan,[7] Renwick, McGovern, and Spence.[36] Case 6 of Renwick, et al. points to the likelihood of *C. welchii* being responsible in these cases also. This was the case of a 55-year-old man with acute myeloblastic leukemia who was admitted to hospital with obvious clinical septicemia, abdominal pain, and absent bowel sounds. *C. welchii* of undetermined type was grown from his blood. The patient died 12 hours after admission, and at autopsy there was typical necrotizing colitis.

Clinically, necrotizing colitis presents with acute onset of abdominal pain which suggests an intra-abdominal emergency requiring immediate surgery.

PATHOLOGY. The entire colon may be affected or the process may be restricted to a small segment; in either case, the small intestine may be involved in some part. The affected bowel is dilated and has patchy greenish-brown foci of necrosis along its length. These may be plainly visible on opening the peritoneal cavity, but the extent of the disease is usually greater on the mucosal than the serosal surface. Microscopically, there is coagulative necrosis of the mucosa and, to a certain extent, of the submucosa also. There may be an infiltrate of polymorphonuclear neutrophil leucocytes at the junction of the necrotic and nonnecrotic zones, but at a later stage leucocytes infiltrate the necrotic tissue also. Killingback and Williams[18] stress the finding of gram-positive bacilli in the necrotic tissue. The significance of this is doubtful, as bacteria tend to invade any necrotic intestinal mucosa. Ulcers are formed when necrotic mucosal tissue is discarded; there is then the danger of perforation.

The histologic diagnosis of necrotizing enterocolitis depends upon finding necrosis of the mucosa with none of the characteristics of ischemic disease or other specific forms of colitis. The gross specimen, together with its characteristic clostridial odor, usually presents an obvious diagnosis.

Staphylococcal Enterocolitis

It is well known that certain strains of *Staphylococcus pyogenes* produce an enterotoxin which causes diarrhea and that many of the patients who have diarrhea under tetracycline therapy are in fact suffering from staphylococcal enteritis. This diarrhea, however, subsides with the administration of antibiotics to which the staphylococcus is sensitive.[5, 15]

Apart from simple staphylococcal diarrhea, there is always the possibility that the staphylococcus may invade established lesions of ulcerative colitis, Crohn's disease, or ischemic enterocolitis. This, however, seems to happen very rarely.

Ulcerative lesions of the intestinal tract due to staphylococcus are rare; Powell,[33] in an analysis of 40 autopsy cases in which there had been staphylococcal septicemia, found none. In 22 autopsies in which death had been due to staphylococcal septicemia, the writer found none with enterocolitis. Nevertheless, the staphylococcus should not be dismissed as a possible pathogen for the colon. In a certain proportion of patients with pseudomembranous colitis, *S. pyogenes* has been recovered from the stool as the dominant organism, and staphylococcal enterotoxin may well be one of the toxic agents which produce this reaction.[4] This is difficult to prove, and attempts to reproduce the changes of pseudomembranous enterocolitis in experimental animals by using *S. pyogenes* have not been successful. Inflammations of the alimentary tract have been induced and have been called pseudomembranous enterocolitis, but the illustrations and histologic descriptions have been those of non-specific inflammation with leucocytic infiltration through all coats of the intestinal wall, [1, 37, 39, 40] whereas in pseudomembranous enterocolitis, there is usually no leucocytic infiltration of the bowel wall.

One must conclude that apart from simple staphylococcal enteritis, ulcerative lesions of the intestine due to the staphylococcus are extremely rare.

Colitis Cystica Profunda

Colitis cystica profunda is not a separate entity. It can occur in any ulcerative lesion of the colon and is due to epithelialization of deep ulcers. It is found most frequently in the rectosigmoid region,[9] and there is a danger that it may be mistaken in sigmoidoscopic biopsies for carcinoma. Epstein, et al.[9] were not able to establish the etiology in their four cases, but we have encountered the condition in Crohn's disease, in ulcerative colitis, and in ischemic colitis (Fig. 31).

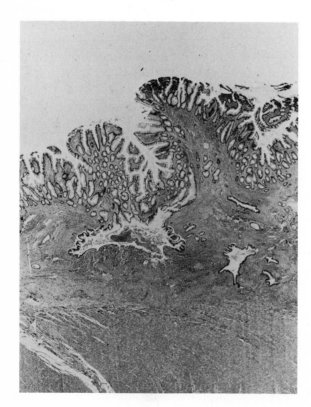

Fig. 31. Downgrowth of epithelium during healing of deep ulcers in ulcerative colitis has produced an appearance that could be mistaken for carcinomatous invasion in a small sigmoidoscopic biopsy. H&E. X60.

Obstructive Colitis

"Colitis and antecedent carcinoma" is the title given by Millar[27] to a condition in which there is a carcinoma of the sigmoid or descending colon associated with a segmental colitis proximal to it. The length of the affected segment varies from a few centimeters to about 25 centimeters. Between the segment of bowel exhibiting the colitis and the carcinoma, there is a zone of normal bowel mucosa varying in length from a few centimeters to about 20 centimeters or longer. This condition may simulate acute ulcerative colitis both clinically and radiologically, and the carcinoma may not be recognized. One of Millar's cases and one of the three cases seen in Royal Prince Alfred Hospital presented in this way (Fig. 32).

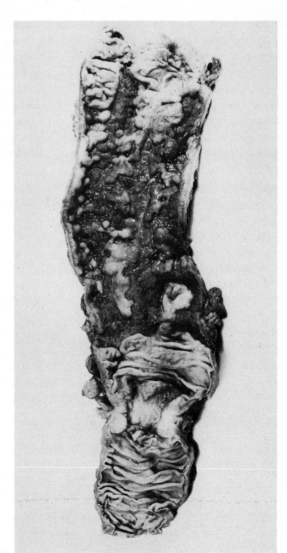

Fig. 32. Carcinoma of the sigmoid colon with deep ulceration of the bowel proximally. There is a short segment of normal mucosa between the carcinoma and the ulceration.

Macroscopically, there is linear ulceration overlying the *taeniae coli,* while between the ulcers the mucosa appears normal. Microscopically, the bases of the ulcers are lined by granulation tissue, and, although occasional vessels appear to have been occluded by organized thrombus, the pathogenesis of the condition is obscure. Between the ulcers the mucosa appears normal.

Summary

In *ulcerative colitis,* the diagnostic feature is inflammation of the mucosa with degeneration of crypt epithelium beginning at any level of the crypt. The mucosa adjacent to an ulcer is never normal.

The main lesion in *Crohn's disease* is lymphocytic aggregates together with fibrosis of the submucosa. Destruction of crypt epithelium always begins at the crypt base, and the mucosa adjacent to an ulcer is usually normal.

Ischemic colitis is characterized by hemorrhage in the mucosa and fibrin thrombi in mucosal vessels often extending into submucosal vessels. Hemosiderin granules are found in the cicatricial tissue of the chronic lesion.

Pseudomembranous colitis starts with necrosis of the surface epithelium and increased mucus production in the crypts. The fibrinous exudate and mucus coalesce with the necrotic surface epithelium in the form of plaques.

The diagnostic criteria outlined in this essay should enable most cases of colitis to be categorized without much difficulty. Even so, cases will arise from time to time in which the features are not sufficiently explicit for classification.

References

1. Bennett, I.L. Jr., Wood, J.S. Jr., and Yardley, J.H. Staphylococcal pseudomembranous enterocolitis in chinchillas; a clinico-pathologic study. Trans. Ass. Amer. Physicians, 69:116, 1956.
2. Bloomfield, D.A., and Walters, M.N.I. Pseudo-membranous enterocolitis. Med. J. Aust., 2:854, 1960.
3. Crohn, B.B., and Berg, A.A. Right-sided (regional) colitis. J.A.M.A., 110:32, 1938.
4. Dearing, W.H., Baggenstoss, A.H., and Weed, L.A. Studies on the relationship of *Staphylococcus aureus* to pseudomembranous enteritis and to post-antibiotic enteritis. Gastroenterology, 38:441, 1960.
5. ——— and Heilman, F.R. Micrococcic (staphylococcic) enteritis as a complication of antibiotic therapy: Its response to erythromycin. Proc. Mayo Clin., 28:121, 1953.
6. Deutsch, S. Physiology of the splanchnic circulation and its alteration by general anesthesia and hemorrhage in man. Amer. J. Surg., 114:353, 1967.
7. Duncan, T. Necrotising colitis: Case report. Amer. J. Surg., 108:885, 1964.
8. Egerton, J., and Walker, P. Isolation of *Clostridium perfringens* type C from necrotic enteritis of man in New Guinea. J. Path. Bact., 88:275, 1964.
9. Epstein, S.E., Ascari, W.Q., Ablow, R.C., Seaman, W.B., and Lattes, R. Colitis cystic profunda. Amer. J. Clin. Path., 45:186, 1966.
10. Ferrer, M.I., Bradley, S.E., Wheeler, H.O., Enson, Y., Preisig, R., and Harvey, R.M. The effect of digoxin in the splanchnic circulation in ventricular failure. Circulation, 32:524, 1965.

11. Fick, K., and Wolken, A. Necrotic jejunitis. Lancet, 1:519, 1949.
12. Goulston, S.J.M., and McGovern, V.J. Pseudomembranous colitis. Gut, 6:207, 1965.
13. Gray, G.K., Lockhart-Mummery, H.E., and Morson, B.C. Crohn's disease of the anal region. Gut, 6:515, 1965.
14. Hardaway, R.M., and McKay, D.G. Pseudomembranous enterocolitis. Arch. Surg., 78:446, 1959.
15. Jackson, G.G., Haight, T.H., Kass, E.H., Womack, C.R., Gocke, T.M., and Finland, M. Terramycin therapy of pneumonia: Clinical and bacteriologic studies in 91 cases. Ann. Intern. Med., 35:1175, 1951.
16. Jaffe, R.H., and Laing, D. Changes of digestive tract in uremia; pathologic anatomic study. Arch. Intern. Med., 53:851, 1934.
17. Jeckeln, E. Enteritis necroticans. Deutsch. Med. Wschr., 73:172, 1948.
18. Killingback, M., and Williams, K.L. Necrotising colitis. Brit. J. Surg., 9:175, 1961.
19. Kleckner, M.S., Bargen, J.A., and Baggenstoss, A.H. Pseudomembranous enterocolitis: Clinicopathologic study of 14 cases in which the disease was not preceded by an operation. Gastroenterology, 21:211, 1952.
20. Lockhart-Mummery, H.E., and Morson, B.C. Crohn's disease (regional enteritis) of the large intestine and its distinction from ulcerative colitis. Gut, 1:87, 1960.
21. ——— and Morson, B.C. Crohn's disease of the large intestine. Gut, 5:493, 1964.
22. McGovern, V.J., and Archer, G.T. The pathogenesis of ulcerative colitis. Aust. Ann. Med., 6:68, 1957.
23. ——— and Goulston, S.J.M. Ischaemic enterocolitis. Gut, 6:213, 1965.
24. ——— and Goulston, S.J.M. Crohn's disease of the colon. Gut, 9:164, 1968.
25. Marston, A. The bowel in shock. Lancet, 2:365, 1962.
26 ——— Pheils, M.T., Thomas, M.L., and Morson, B.C. Ischemic colitis. Gut, 7:1, 1966.
27. Millar, D.M. Colitis and antecedent carcinoma. Dis. Colon Rectum, 8:243, 1965.
28. Morson, B.C., and Lockhart-Mummery, H.E. Anal lesions in Crohn's disease. Lancet, 2:1122, 1959.
29. ——— and Pang, L.S.C. Rectal biopsy as an aid to cancer control in ulcerative colitis. Gut, 8:423, 1967.
30. Murrell, T., and Roth, L. Necrotizing jejunitis: A newly discovered disease in the highlands of New Guinea. Med. J. Aust., 1:61, 1963.
31. Penner, A., and Bernheim, A. Acute post-operative enterocolitis. Arch. Path., 27:966, 1939.
32. Pettet, J.D., Baggenstoss, A.H., Dearing, W.H., and Judd, E.S. Postoperative pseudomembranous enterocolitis. Surg. Gynec. Obstet., 98:546, 1954.
33. Powell, D.E.B. Non-suppurative lesions in staphylococcal septicaemia. J. Path. Bact., 82:141, 1961.
34. Reiner, L. Mesenteric vascular occlusion studied by post mortem injection of the mesenteric arterial circulation. In Pathology Annual 1966, Sommers, S.C., ed. New York, Appleton-Century-Crofts, 1966, Vol. 1, p. 193.
35. ——— Schlesinger, J.J., and Miller, G.M. Pseudomembranous colitis following aureomycin and chloramphenicol. Arch. Path., 54:39, 1952.
36. Renwick, S.B., McGovern, V.J., and Spence, J. Necrotizing enterocolitis: A report of six cases. Med. J. Aust., 2:413, 1966.
37. Speare, G.M. Staphylococcus pseudomembranous enterocolitis; a complication of antibiotic therapy. Amer. J. Surg., 88:523, 1954.
38. Sterne, M., and Warrock, G.H. The types of *Clostridium perfringens*. J. Path. Bact., 88:279, 1964.
39. Tan, T.L., Drake, C.T., Jacobson, M.J., and Van Prohaska, J. The experimental development of pseudomembranous enterocolitis. Surg. Gynec. Obstet., 108:415, 1959.
40. Van Prohaska, J. Pseudo-membranous (staphylococcal) enterocolitis. Arch. Surg., 79:197, 1959.

41. Wilson, G.S., and Miles, A.A. Topley and Wilson's Principles of Bacteriology and
     Immunity, 5th ed. London, Edward Arnold Ltd., 1964, p. 1240.
42. Wilson, R., and Qualheim, R.E. A form of acute haemorrhagic enterocolitis afflict-
     ing chronically ill individuals. Gastroenterology, 27:431, 1954.
43. Zeissler, J., and Rassfeld-Sternberg, L. Enteritis necroticans due to *Clostridium
     welchii* type F. Brit. Med. J., 1:267, 1949.

EXTRANODAL MALIGNANT LYMPHOMAS AND PSEUDOLYMPHOMAS

SIDNEY L SALTZSTEIN*

Extranodal malignant lymphomas differ in their clinical behavior from those malignant lymphomas arising in the more usual sites. The prognosis, usually better than either that of malignant lymphomas in general or that of carcinomas of the particular organ, is related to cell type and to regional lymph node involvement. Treatment primarily is surgical; late deaths are uncommon.

The reported prognosis of extranodal lymphomas is further improved by the inclusion in many series of cases of benign "pseudolymphomas." These lesions, reactive in nature, must be separated by the pathologist from malignant lymphomas so that patients are not subjected unnecessarily to radical surgical procedures, radiotherapy, or chemotherapy. Counterbalancing this, many series of extranodal lymphomas contain examples of disseminated malignant lymphomas of the usual type, in which the first or most prominent clinical findings are related to some extranodal site. These too must be separated from the extranodal malignant lymphomas because of their poorer prognosis and because of the differences in appropriate therapy.

Definitions

An extranodal malignant lymphoma is defined as a malignant lymphoma of any cell type (lymphocytic, reticulum cell, or Hodgkin's) involving primarily an organ other than the lymph nodes, liver, spleen, bone marrows, thymus, or Waldeyer's ring.

* The assistance of Mr. Cramer Lewis, Department of Ilustration, Washington University School of Medicine, St. Louis, Missouri, and of Mr. Edward J. Peterson, Office of Learning Resources, UCSD School of Medicine, San Diego, California, in the preparation of the illustrations is gratefully acknowledged.

There must be no evidence of dissemination in that only the organ (or the organ and its immediately adjacent lymph nodes) is involved by the malignant lymphoma and the bone marrow and peripheral blood are free of the neoplasm. To exclude those cases of malignant lymphoma of the usual type in which dissemination already has occurred but is not apparent at the time of diagnosis, there must be no evidence of dissemination for at least three months after diagnosis. Also excluded will be cases in which the diagnosis of an extranodal lymphoma was made at autopsy only. Burkitt's lymphoma will not be included in this discussion.

A pseudolymphoma is a benign reactive process of known or unknown cause, usually forming a tumor, with sufficient proliferation of reticuloendothelial elements to be confused with a malignant lymphoma. In essence, a pseudolymphoma is the extranodal counterpart of a reactive lymph node.

Two terms will be avoided in this presentation as they have various conflicting meanings. The first of these is "lymphosarcoma" which, depending upon the author, can mean all malignant lymphomas, malignant lymphomas of both lymphocytic types, malignant lymphomas of the well-differentiated lymphocytic type, or even all lymphoid lesions including pseudolymphomas. The other term which will not be used is "follicle," as this can mean either nodules of tumor or lymphoid germinal centers. The words "nodule" and "germinal center" will be used instead.

Malignant lymphomas will be classified according to the system Rappaport[52] devised for lymph nodes, but for simplification, only the well-differentiated and poorly-differentiated lymphocytic types, the reticulum cell type, and the Hodgkin's type will be used (Table 1).

Table 1. Classification: Malignant Lymphoma*

Malignant Lymphoma, Lymphocytic Type, Well Differentiated
Malignant Lymphoma, Lymphocytic Type, Poorly Differentiated
Malignant Lymphoma, Reticulum Cell Type
Malignant Lymphoma, Hodgkin's Type

* Modified after Rappaport, H., Winter, W.J., and Hicks, E.B. *Cancer*, 9:792, 1956.

Extranodal malignant lymphomas and pseudolymphomas have been described in virtually every organ of the human body. The most frequent sites are the lungs, stomach, small intestine, and large intestine. Extranodal malignant lymphomas and pseudolymphomas of these four sites will be discussed in detail separately. As a generalization, the observations pertaining to these lesions of these four sites can be extrapolated to the rest of the body.

Lung

Primary malignant lymphomas and pseudolymphomas of the lung are rare. As of 1963, only 102 reported cases were available for study.[56] A few scattered reports have appeared since.[16, 17, 26, 29, 31, 48, 51] Obviously, not all cases are reported; this writer has seen many in consultation since 1963. Compared to the estimate of 61,000 new cases of cancer of the lung in the United States alone each year,[3] malignant lymphomas and pseudolymphomas make up only an infinitesimal portion of primary lung tumors. Extrapolating from the American Cancer Society figures,[3] there must be at least 18,000 new cases of malignant lymphoma of all sites in the United States each year. Here again, malignant lymphomas which are primary in the lung represent only a very small fraction of all malignant lymphomas.

Presenting Symptoms. These tumors generally cause no symptoms and are detected on routine roentgenograms of the chest. Patients who do have symptoms complain of chills, fever, cough, chest pain, weakness, fatigue, and weight loss. Patients with malignant lymphomas of the reticulum cell type tend to be younger than those with malignant lymphomas of the lymphocytic type.

Radiologic Appearance. The radiologic picture is equally nonspecific; these lesions may present as large masses involving an entire lung, as small coin lesions, or as anything in between. The pseudolymphomas often demonstrate air bronchograms and only rarely show pleural effusion or lymphadenopathy.[31]

Gross Appearance. Operative findings reflect the gross appearance of these tumors. They may be firm masses occupying an entire lobe or lung, or they may be only a few centimeters in diameter. The tumors usually abut on the pleural surface. On section they are pink-white, fairly well demarcated, but not encapsulated (Figs. 1, 2). Pseudolymphomas and malignant lymphomas of the lymphocytic type are solid; malignant lymphomas of the reticulum and Hodgkin's types frequently are cystic (Fig. 2). Lymph nodes may be enlarged, but this does not invariably indicate involvement by tumor.

Microscopic Appearance. As seen under the microscope, the lesions are composed of masses of reticuloendothelial elements and remnants of the preexisting lung structure (Fig. 3). The pseudolymphomas and the lymphocytic type of malignant lymphoma tend to grow intraseptally about the periphery (Fig. 4); the reticulum cell and Hodgkin's types of malignant lymphoma tend to be more circumscribed. Necrosis is common in the reticulum cell type and accounts for the cystic gross appearance; pseudolymphomas and malignant lymphomas of the lymphocytic type show little, if any, necrosis. Growth beneath intact bronchial epithelium is frequent (Fig. 5). Vessel "invasion" can be found.

Differential Diagnosis. The diagnosis of a malignant lymphoma of the reticulum cell type is not difficult to establish if the characteristics of this neoplasm as it appears in lymph nodes are kept in mind. This tumor is composed of solid sheets of large, moderately pleomorphic cells without any suggestion of glandular or other differentiation. The individual cells have large, oval or bean-shaped nuclei with large nucleoli (Fig. 6). Large cell undifferentiated bronchogenic carcinoma, metastatic unpigmented malignant melanoma, metastatic renal adenocarcinoma, and metastatic seminoma are about the only sources of confusion. Eosinophilic granuloma of the lung conceivably could cause confusion.

Similarly, the diagnosis of malignant lymphoma, Hodgkin's type, is based on the finding of Reed-Sternberg cells, as it would be elsewhere in the body (Fig. 7). If one is strict in what he accepts as Reed-Sternberg cells and diligent in his search for them, he should neither overdiagnose or underdiagnose malignant lymphoma of the Hodgkin's type. This writer has not seen an example of this tumor arising in the lung in his personal experience but has had the opportunity to review the sections of four cases reported by Kern, et al.[38]

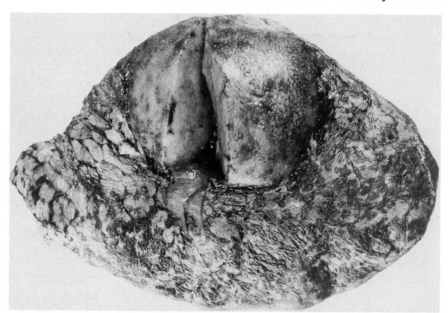

Fig. 1.   This pulmonary malignant lymphoma of the lymphocytic type abuts on the pleura.
The solid, well-demarcated nature of the lesion is seen. The gross appearance of a pseudolymphoma would be identical. W. U. III. #62-2534. (Reprinted from Saltzstein, S. L. *Cancer*,
16:928, 1963, with permission.)

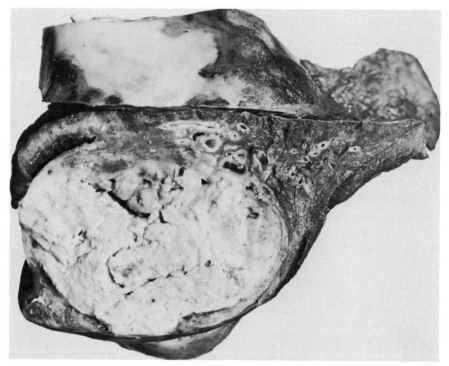

Fig. 2.   Gross photograph of a malignant lymphoma, reticulum cell type, of the lung,
showing the central necrosis and cyst formation. The lesion appears well demarcated. W. U.
III. #55-3939. (Reprinted from Saltzstein, S. L. *Cancer*, 16:928, 1963, with permission.)

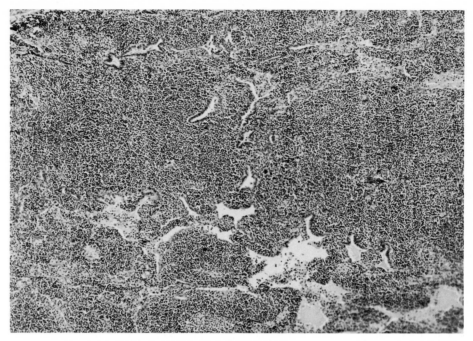

Fig. 3.   The central portion of both malignant lymphomas and pseudolymphomas shows a dense infiltrate replacing the pulmonary parenchyma. A few remaining bronchioles and vessels can be identified. W. U. III. #61-1763. H&E. X93.

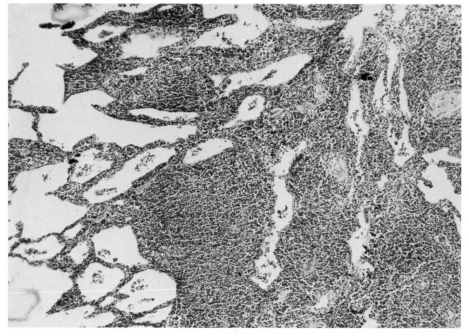

Fig. 4.   Photomicrograph of the periphery of a pseudolymphoma showing the intraseptal growth seen in both malignant lymphomas of the lymphocytic type and pseudolymphomas. Other areas of this lesion showed many well-defined germinal centers. W. U. III. #62-224. H&E. X55.

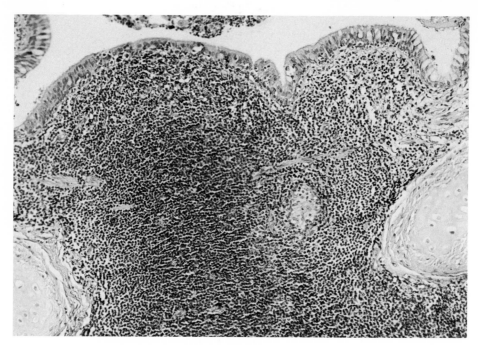

Fig. 5. Prominent endobronchial growth may be seen in either a malignant lymphoma or a pseudolymphoma. W. U. III. #61-1764. H&E. X170.

Malignant lymphomas of the lymphocytic type must be differentiated from "oat cell" carcinoma of the lung, on one hand, and from pseudolymphomas on the other. "Oat cell" carcinomas are large endobronchial tumors composed of pleomorphic, dark cells which are slightly larger than lymphocytes. These cells often are spindle-shaped and mitotic figures are seen frequently. Confusion between "oat cell" carcinoma and malignant lymphoma of the lymphocytic type has occurred in the cytologic evaluation of sputum specimens.

More germane to this discussion is the separation of a malignant lymphoma of the lymphocytic type from a pseudolymphoma. If one extends to the lung the criteria established by Rappaport, et al.[52] for distinguishing malignant lymphomas from reactive hyperplasia in lymph nodes, one usually can separate malignant lymphomas from pseudolymphomas (Table 2). Favoring pseudolymphoma are lym-

Table 2. Differential Diagnosis

	PSEUDOLYMPHOMA	MALIGNANT LYMPHOMA
Germinal Centers	Usually Present	Absent
Infiltrate	Mixed, Mature	Uniform, Immature
Nodes	Never Involved	Often Involved

phoid germinal centers and a mixed cellular infiltrate of various inflammatory cells (Fig. 8). A uniform infiltrate of mature or immature lymphocytes without germinal centers rules for a diagnosis of malignant lymphoma; tumor in the regional lymph nodes obviously establishes the diagnosis of malignant lymphoma. Pleural seeding

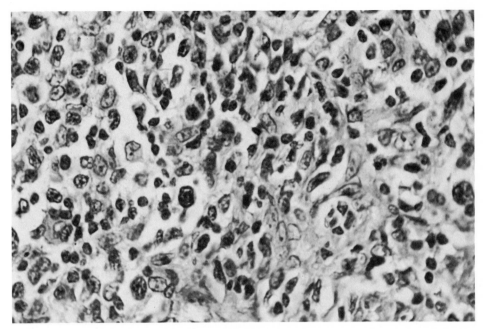

Fig. 6.   The characteristic large cells with bean-shaped nuclei and prominent nucleoli of a malignant lymphoma, reticulum cell type, are seen in this pulmonary tumor. W. U. III. #62-3562. H&E. X600. (Reprinted from Saltzstein, S. L. *Cancer*, 16:928, 1963, with permission.)

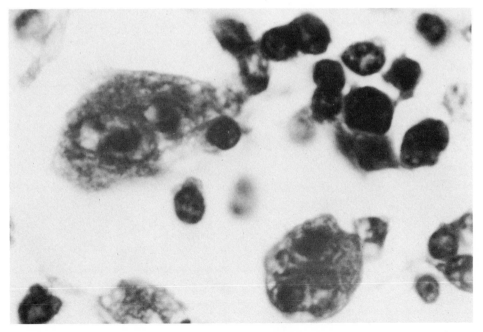

Fig. 7.   Classical Reed-Sternberg cells are seen in this example of a malignant lymphoma of the Hodgkin's type arising in the lung. UCSD OLR. H&E. X400. (Original section obtained through the courtesy of Dr. William Kern and Dr. Jules Kernen, Los Angeles.)

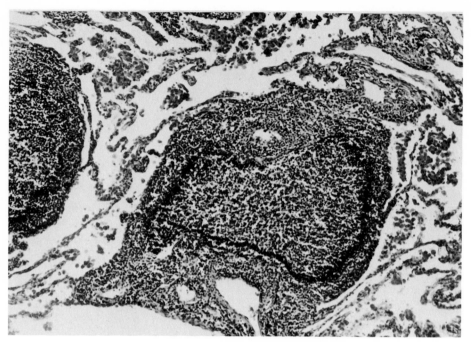

Fig. 8.   Prominent germinal centers are seen in the intraseptal growth of this pulmonary pseudolymphoma. UCSD OLR. H&E. X25.

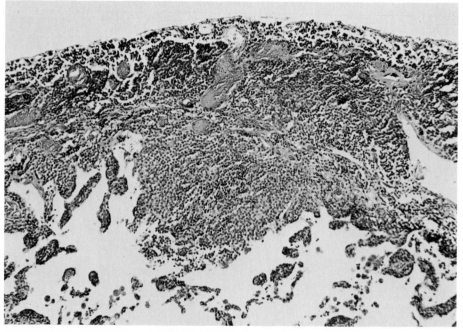

Fig. 9.   Pleural seeding of the tumor, as seen here, favors a diagnosis of malignant lymphoma. W. U. Ill. #62-3560. H&E. X130.

strongly favors a diagnosis of malignancy (Fig. 9). As in the case with lymph nodes, occasionally one will be unable to separate pseudolymphoma from malignant lymphoma of the lymphocytic type.

Another non-neoplastic disease which may be difficult or even impossible to separate from malignant lymphomas arising in the lung is the lymphomatoid variant of the limited form of Wegener's granuloma.[40] In both there is diffuse proliferation of immature reticuloendothelial cells. Favoring the diagnosis of Wegener's granuloma are vasculitis, necrosis, and "plasmacytoid" cells in the infiltrate. Special stains for elastic tissue to demonstrate the destruction of vessels resulting from the vasculitis can be very helpful in separating these entities. The vascular changes may be easier to evaluate in the portions of the sections containing less of the reticuloendothelial cell infiltrate.

Treatment. Complete surgical excision (lobectomy or even pneumonectomy) is the treatment of choice as it establishes the diagnosis, removes nonfunctioning lung tissue, and much of the time is sufficient to cure the patient. Radiotherapy should be reserved for those patients with involvement of regional lymph nodes or with evidence of recurrence. Very obviously, patients with pseudolymphomas do not require radiotherapy.

Prognosis. If it is to happen, recurrence of the malignant lymphoma with progression to death occurs very rapidly. Virtually all patients who die from this condition died within 2½ years, although recurrences leading to the death of the patient have been reported at 5½ and 6¼ years.[17, 48] Nonfatal recurrences may occur later but respond well to radiotherapy or to surgical excision. Most of the reported nonfatal recurrences are very poorly documented; in only one instance was tissue excised and examined.

It is difficult to establish the prognosis of patients with malignant lymphomas of the lymphocytic type because of the admixture of cases of pseudolymphoma in all reports. Combining these two lesions, a relative five-year survival rate of 70 percent is reported. In an attempt to separate the mortality resulting from the lymphocytic type of malignant lymphoma from this combined group, it can be shown that only 20 percent of the patients in this combined group died of malignant lymphoma. The influence of nodal involvement is apparent: only one of 42 patients whose nodes were known to be free of tumor died of lymphoma, while almost 40 percent of the others died of lymphoma.

The five-year relative survival rate of patients with reticulum cell type of malignant lymphoma is only 53 percent. Here again, of six patients known to have no involvement of regional nodes by tumor, only one died of lymphoma, while over half of the other patients died of lymphoma.

The prognosis of malignant lymphoma, Hodgkin's type, of the lung is not known exactly but must be very poor. The total English language experience is only 23 cases.* Of these, only one[12] is reported to have lived more than five years and

---

* In addition to the cases cited and reported by Kern, et al.[38] in 1961, this author would add the one reported by Bass and Reibstein,[6] the second case of Robins,[53] Starkey's sixth and seventh cases,[66] Snyder's case,[64] and the first case of Meese, et al.,[43] Monahan's case,[45] Gregory, et al.'s first case,[24] and Joseph's first and fourth cases.[36] Contrary to Kern, et al., I would not accept the cases of Rubenfeld and Clark[54] and of Rubinovich,[55] as in both cases,

a second as long as three years.[21] Interestingly, one of the two had involvement of the regional lymph nodes and the other invasion of the pericardium.

Stomach

Gastric lymphomas are the commonest extranodal malignant lymphomas. Most series state that from 1 to 5 percent of all gastric cancers are malignant lymphomas.[42, 67, 69] Thus, the annual incidence of these tumors should be from 200 to 1,000 in the United States alone.[3] It is obvious that the great majority of gastric malignant lymphomas are not reported. Sperling summarized 17 series reported from 1939 to 1965 which included only 852 patients.[65] Many series include cases of malignant lymphoma not truly originating in the stomach, as well as many examples of pseudo-lymphoma, further diluting the data pertinent to primary malignant lymphomas of the stomach.

The stomach is also a common site of pseudolymphomas. Of the lymphoid tumors of the stomach, between one-fourth and one-half have been found to be pseudolymphomas.[7, 18, 33, 63] This undoubtedly is a reflection of the commonness of peptic ulcer, which is at least one cause of gastric pseudolymphomas (Fig. 10).[18] In spite of the histologic and clinical evidence that many gastric lymphoid lesions are pseudolymphomas rather than malignant lymphomas, not all authors have accepted completely the concept of pseudolymphomas.[73]

Presenting Symptoms. Unlike malignant lymphomas and pesudolymphomas of the lung, those of the stomach usually produce symptoms. Pain, often like that of peptic ulcer, is the commonest symptom.[21, 35, 46, 62, 70] Weight loss with or without anorexia is almost as common. Bleeding, nausea, and vomiting are described less often. The only physical sign of significance is a mass in the epigastrium; this is present in less than half of the patients. Laboratory studies may show an anemia if there has been sufficient blood loss. Achlorhydria is noted in only one-fourth of the patients.

Radiologic Appearance. Roentgenographic studies will establish the presence of a gastric lesion, but rarely will a specific diagnosis of lymphoma be offerred.[35, 62, 70, 73] Signs favoring malignant lymphoma over carcinoma of the stomach include a large superficial ulcer often on the posterior wall or lesser curvature, enlarged rugae close to a polypoid mass or ulcer, a thick, nonpliable wall, a large tumor with little change in the capacity and contour of the stomach, a smooth mucosal surface, and multiple polypoid masses or ulcers.[62] On the other hand, the findings noted with pseudolymphomas include ulcerating tumors, constricting or infiltrating lesions, isolated ulcer craters, and, least often, enlarged rugae.[50]

Gross Appearance. When the lesion is first seen, either by the surgeon or by

---

the histologic diagnosis was made at autopsy only. More recent cases to be excluded are Samuels, et al.'s third, fourth, and sixth,[59] Meese, et al.'s second, third, and fourth,[43] Joseph's third and fifth,[36] and both those reported by Gonpnathan and Sataline.[23] In all of these cases, the diagnosis of malignant lymphoma, Hodgkin's type, was made on nodal tissue. Although a "suggestive" diagnosis was made from tissue removed at bronchoscopy in Joseph's second case,[36] a supraclavicular lymph node excised only "a little later" showed malignant lymphoma, Hodgkin's type. The second and third cases of Gregory, et al.[24] arose in the thymus.

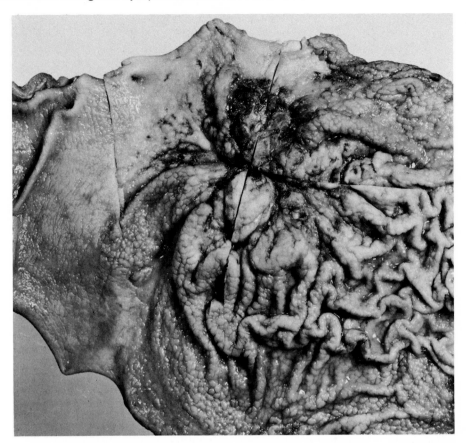

Fig. 10. Gross photograph of a gastric pseudolymphoma showing both an ulceration and a mass. The rugae are only slightly more prominent than normal. W. U. III. #55-4180. (Reprinted from Faris, T. D., and Saltzstein, S. L. *Cancer*, 17:207, 1964, with permission.)

the pathologist, the usual impression is that it is carcinoma. About one-half of the malignant lymphomas, as well as the pseudolymphomas, are ulcerated. Many others have one or more polypoid masses of tumor. Intramural growth is common. The frequently described large, brain-like rugae are seen only rarely and even then are not specific to lymphoma. Any combination of these various patterns may be present (Fig. 11).

Microscopic Appearance and Differential Diagnosis. The distinction between malignant lymphoma, pseudolymphoma, and carcinoma can be made only by thorough histologic examination. Whether this will entail biopsy of the tumor or of a lymph node, excision of an ulcerated lesion, or subtotal gastrectomy as an "excisional biopsy" will depend on the particular situation. Frozen section may be useful. Most carcinomas can be separated readily from the lymphomas, but an occasional carcinoma of the linitis plastica type may require demonstration of intracellular mucin production.

All of the malignant lymphomas and pseudolymphomas are characterized by a dense infiltrate composed of reticuloendothelial cells (Fig. 11). This may be

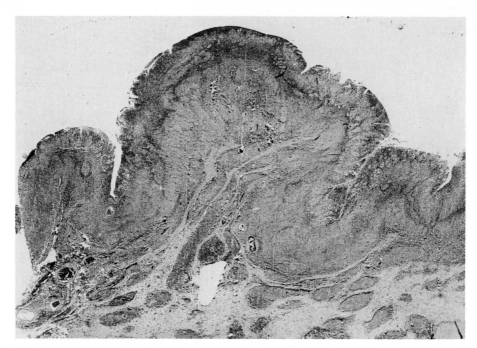

Fig. 11.   Low-power photomicrograph of a gastric pseudolymphoma showing the proliferation of reticuloendothelial elements to form a mass. W. U. III. #63-4328. H&E. X15. (Reprinted from Faris, T. D., and Saltzstein, S. L. *Cancer*, 17:207, 1964, with permission.)

limited to the mucosa, or may penetrate through the entire gastric wall (Figs. 12, 14, 15). As elsewhere, the diagnosis of malignant lymphoma of the reticulum cell and Hodgkin's types can be made if one is careful (Figs. 16, 17). Again, it is the distinction between malignant lymphoma of the well-differentiated lymphocytic type and pseudolymphoma that may be difficult and, at times, impossible.[37] Favoring the diagnosis of pseudolymphoma are a mixed infiltrate of various inflammatory cells, lymphoid germinal centers, and obviously, regional lymph nodes free of malignant lymphoma (Figs. 12, 13; Table 2). The opposite of each of these militates for a diagnosis of malignant lymphoma, i.e., a uniform monotonous infiltrate often of less-than-mature lymphocytes, no germinal centers in the lesion, and nodal involvement by malignant lymphoma (Figs. 14, 15).

   Treatment.   Virtually every author recommends surgical resection of gastric lymphomas if this can be done. This should include the regional lymph nodes in a manner analogous to procedures carried out for gastric carcinoma. The margins of grossly normal tissue about the primary tumor should be greater for a lymphoma than for a carcinoma because of the propensity of lymphomas to be large and to have multiple areas of tumor in the stomach.[42, 62] Although many five-year survivals are reported among those treated by surgical extirpation alone, most authors employ radiotherapy in the postoperative period. Long-term survivors, including some patients with unresectable tumors, are reported among the patients treated by radiotherapy alone. The placing of metal clips in the area of the tumor at operation to aid the radiotherapist is well worthwhile.

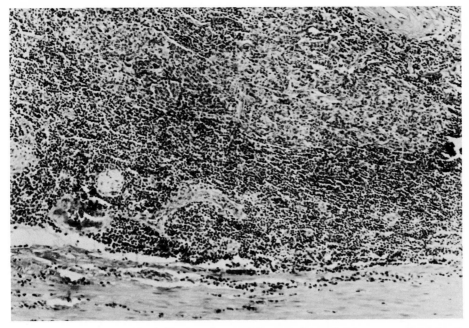

Fig. 12.   The pleomorphic infiltrate of a gastric pseudolymphoma may extend to the muscular wall, as seen here, or even deeper. The depth of infiltration is no guide to the distinction between a malignant lymphoma and a pseudolymphoma. UCSD OLR. H&E. X25.

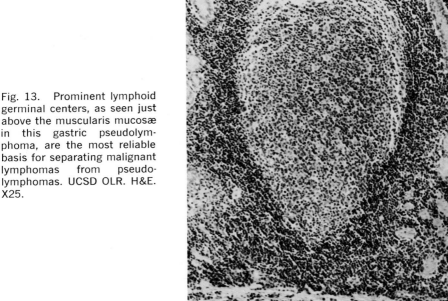

Fig. 13.   Prominent lymphoid germinal centers, as seen just above the muscularis mucosæ in this gastric pseudolymphoma, are the most reliable basis for separating malignant lymphomas from pseudolymphomas. UCSD OLR. H&E. X25.

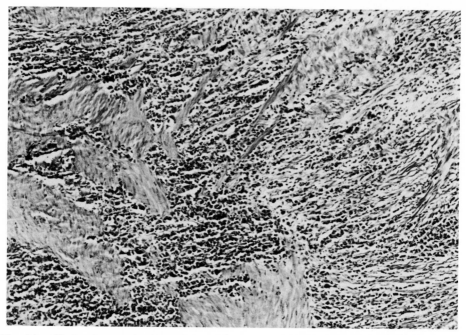

Fig. 14. Photomicrograph showing infiltration into the muscular wall of the stomach in a malignant lymphoma of the reticulum cell type. The distinction from a pseudolymphoma is made on the characteristics of the cells rather than on the depth of the infiltrate. UCSD OLR. H&E. X25.

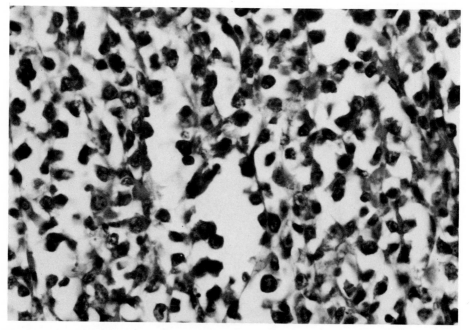

Fig. 15. A solid sheet of immature lymphocytes, with no other cellular elements, establishes the diagnosis of malignant lymphoma, lymphocytic type, poorly differentiated in this gastric lesion. UCSD OLR. H&E. X160.

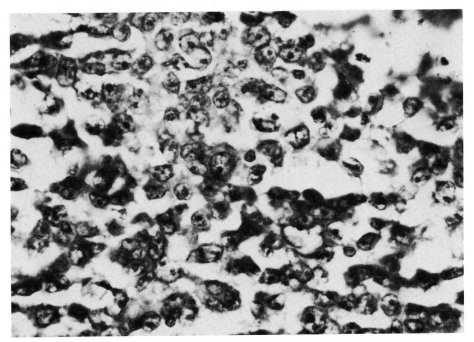

Fig. 16.   In the stomach as elsewhere, malignant lymphomas of the reticulum cell type are recognized by large cells with large, bean-shaped nuclei and prominent nucleoli. UCSD OLR. H&E. X160.

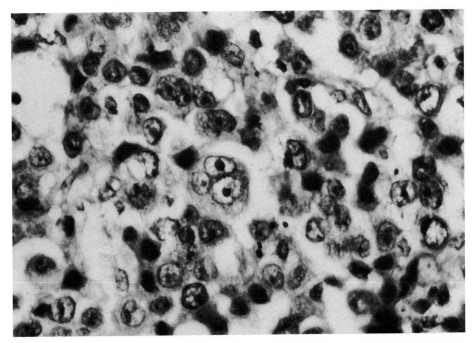

Fig. 17.   A typical Reed-Sternberg cell is seen in the center of this photomicrograph of a gastric malignant lymphoma of the Hodgkin's type. UCSD OLR. H&E. X160.

Prognosis. The five-year survival of all patients with malignant lymphomas of the stomach is about 34 percent.[65] This figure probably is inaccurate because many of the series included in Sperling's review mix together primary malignant lymphomas of the stomach, generalized malignant lymphomas secondarily involving the stomach, and pseudolymphomas. In the four series in which pseudolymphomas are separated out, the five-year survival of the remaining patients with primary malignant lymphomas of the stomach ranges from 7 to 70 percent.[7, 18, 33, 63] Three of these series are very small; in the fourth, 88 (67 percent) of 131 patients with primary gastric malignant lymphomas lived five years or more.

In contradistinction to primary pulmonary malignant lymphomas, late recurrences are reasonably common in gastric lymphomas. For this reason, ten-year survival figures may be more meaningful.

The influence of cell type on survival is well demonstrated. The five-year survival in patients with malignant lymphomas of the reticulum cell type ranges from 36 to 50 percent. In the same three series, the corresponding figures for patients with malignant lymphomas of the lymphocytic type range from 83 to 100 percent.[35, 43, 67] The ten-year survival rates are 30 percent and 77 percent, respectively. Most series do not contain many examples of malignant lymphomas of the Hodgkin's type arising in the stomach; Cornes reports 32 percent five-year and 5 percent ten-year survival rates in a group of 22 patients.[12] My personal experience exactly parallels the cited series.[57]

Nodal involvement by the malignant lymphoma cuts the five-year survival to about half of that in patients without nodal involvement.[2, 21, 35, 67] Larger tumors also carry poorer prognosis, as do those which invade deeply into the gastric wall.[35] A nodular pattern appears to improve the prognosis, similar to the situation in malignant lymphomas originating in lymph nodes.[35, 52, 77]

Small Intestine

In the small intestine, malignant lymphomas are relatively common. In various series, malignant lymphomas make up from one-sixth to one-third of all cancers of the small intestine.[34, 47, 60, 79] One author states that malignant lymphoma is the commonest malignant tumor of the small intestine.[1] This relative commonness of malignant lymphoma undoubtedly is only a reflection of the rarity of malignant tumors arising in the small intestine; the total number of reported malignant lymphomas of both the small and large intestine is less than 200.[15]

Pseudolymphomas are correspondingly rare in the small intestine. Weaver and Batsakis reported only three cases and were unable to find any earlier reports in the literature.[75] Over approximately the same time interval they reported ten malignant lymphomas of the small intestine.[74] Lymphoid hyperplasia of the terminal ileum as seen in children also warrants inclusion in the group of pseudolymphomas.[1, 68]

Presenting Symptoms. Symptoms of malignant lymphoma and pseudolymphoma in the small intestine, as elsewhere, do not allow distinction between the two. Abdominal pain, symptoms of intestinal obstruction, and changes in bowel habits are the commonest complaints.[8, 15, 19, 32, 44, 68, 74, 75, 76] A spruelike syndrome is being reported more and more frequently.[65] On examination, a palpable abdominal mass and evidence of weight loss are frequently noted. Occult blood may be present in the stool. Evidence of intestinal perforation is seen with some frequency. Other malignant tumors of the gastrointestinal tract have been reported in association with malignant lymphomas.[11]

Radiologic Appearance. Roentgenograms may show a discrete tumor, multiple tumors, thickened mucosal folds, or ulceration in addition to the findings of obstruction.[65] The separation from regional enteritis may be difficult.

Gross Appearance. Operative and gross pathologic findings are fundamentally those of a tumor arising in the submucosa of the small intestine. These tumors are variously described as annular, nodular, polypoid, ulcerative, or some combination of these.[8, 15, 19, 74] Lesions may be multiple;[9, 17] perforation is noted on occasion.[8] Involvement of regional lymph nodes is very common,[2, 8, 19, 20, 74] but enlargement of these nodes does not guarantee their involvement by tumor.[15] The tumors have the grey to pink appearance of lymphoid tumors elsewhere. They are more common in the ileum than elsewhere in the small intestine.

Microscopic Appearance and Differential Diagnosis. As in the other sites discussed, the distinction between malignant lymphoma and pseudolymphoma is made on histologic examination. Malignant lymphomas of the reticulum cell and Hodgkin's types should present no real diagnostic difficulties, although metastatic amelanotic malignant melanoma may be confused with the former. The features distinguishing pseudolymphomas from malignant lymphomas of the lymphocytic type again are the mixed infiltrate of mature cells, active phagocytosis (as might be seen in a germinal center), germinal centers, and regional lymph nodes free of tumor (Fig. 18; Table 2).[68, 75, 76]

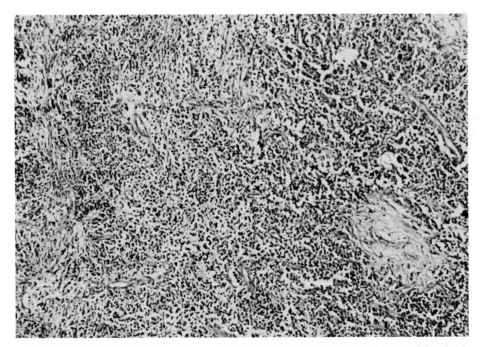

Fig. 18. In this malignant lymphoma, lymphocytic type, well-differentiated, arising in the jejunum, solid sheets of small lymphocytes can be seen infiltrating the outer portion of the intestinal wall. UCSD OLR. H&E. X25.

Treatment.   Surgical excision with wide margins of normal intestine and inclusion of regional lymph nodes is the standard treatment when feasible. Radiotherapy is generally given in addition, but it can be the only means of therapy.[10, 15]

Prognosis.   For several reasons, it is most difficult to estimate accurately the
prognosis of malignant lymphomas of the small intestine. Most series are quite small.
Many series contain a mixture of primary malignant lymphomas of the small intestine
along with disseminated disease involving the small intestine.[44] In other reports,
primary malignant lymphomas are well separated from other malignant lymphomas,
but small and large intestine are lumped together.[15, 78] Five-year survival rates range
from 10 to 50 percent, depending on the particular tumor and therapy.[2, 4, 8, 10, 15,
19, 20, 74] A 33 percent average seems reasonable.[34] The influence of cell type and
pattern is shown in that the survival for nodular malignant lymphoma is about 50
percent, while that of the diffuse lymphocytic type is 25 percent and that of the
reticulum cell type is only 10 to 11 percent.[15, 74] Cornes had no five-year survivors
with malignant lymphomas of the Hodgkin's type originating in the small intestine.[12]
There is some indication that lymph node involvement decreases the prognosis;
however, this is not as clear-cut as in the stomach or lung.[15, 20, 74] Certainly nodal
involvement does not preclude long-term survival.[15] The poor prognosis in children
reported by Mestel was not born out by Weaver and Batsakis.[44, 74] This probably
reflects Mestel's inclusion of many cases not truly primary in the small intestine,
as evidenced by death from dissemination in less than three months.

While a few recurrences have been noted in the period between five and ten
years, none have been reported after ten years. Most patients who are to die from
this condition will do so in the first two years.[15]

Large Intestine

The large intestine is the least common site in the gastrointestinal tract of
malignant lymphomas. Woodruff and Skorneck estimate that only 0.5 percent of
colonic malignancies are malignant lymphomas.[80] Glick and Soule in 1966 could
find only 38 reported cases of primary appendiceal or colonic lymphomas, to which
they, and later Wychulis, et al., added 50 more.[22, 82]

Pseudolymphomas, however, especially of the rectum, are very common. Individual series of 70 or 100 cases are not unusual.[13, 28] Of all of the pseudolymphomas
of the gastrointestinal tract, the average pathologist has the most experience with
those of the large intestine.[27, 30, 76]

Presenting Symptoms.   Patients with malignant lymphomas of the large intestine complain of abdominal pain, weight loss, rectal bleeding, and changes in
bowel habits.[22, 81, 82] There is an association with long-standing chronic ulcerative
colitis.[15, 82] A mass is found on abdominal or rectal examination in at least two-
thirds of these patients. Abdominal tenderness is almost as common. Lesions in the
rectum can be visualized and may be polypoid.

Radiologic Appearance.   Radiologic examination usually demonstrates either
a filling defect or a mass; only rarely is no abnormality seen.[81] The specific diagnosis
of malignant lymphoma usually is not made on roentgenographic study. Features
favoring malignant lymphoma over carcinoma are a longer involved segment, a wide

transition zone between the tumor and the normal intestine, a defect which is not annular, a mass out of proportion to the filling defect, dilation of the lesion, and flattening and obscuring of the mucosal changes by the contrast medium.[80, 81]

Gross Appearance. Malignant lymphomas most often occur in the area about the cecum, to a lesser extent in the rectosigmoid area, and least often in the mid-portion of the large intestine.[22, 80, 82] The tumors usually are circumscribed, but diffuse involvement has been reported. The circumscribed tumors may project into the lumen or may form large intramural and extracolonic masses. Lesions may be multiple. Annular lesions are quite rare.[22, 82]

Pseudolymphomas of the colon present somewhat differently. Bleeding is the usual symptom, but prolapse, the presence of a mass, or abdominal pain also may occur.[13, 28, 30] Examination shows one or many polypoid lesions ranging in size from 2 mm to 5 cm. These "lymphoid polyps" usually are sessile but may be pedunculated. At times, the polypoid lesions may be so numerous as to mimic multiple polyposis; this variant has been named "pseudoleukemia."[14]

Microscopic Appearance and Differential Diagnosis. Again, the final distinction between malignant lymphoma and pseudolymphoma is based on the histologic appearance. The diagnosis of malignant lymphoma of the reticulum cell and Hodgkin's types should not be any more troublesome here than elsewhere. Pseudo-lymphoma differs from malignant lymphoma of the lymphocytic type in the characteristic presence of germinal centers, a mixed cellular infiltrate, and relatively little involvement of the attenuated overlying colonic epithelium (Figs. 19, 20, 21; Table 2).[13, 28] Only rarely does a pseudolymphoma involve the circular muscle of the colon.[13]

Treatment. The usual treatment of a malignant lymphoma is surgical excision, as with a carcinoma. This may entail a segmental resection, a hemicolectomy, or even a total colectomy.[81] While some survivors have not received irradiation after operation, most patients have, and inclusion of this modality usually is recommended. This is true especially if there has been nodal involvement or extension to other organs.[82] Cook and Corbett reported two five-year survivors in ten patients with malignant lymphomas of the large intestine treated by irradiation alone.[10]

Prognosis. Only from the recent reports from the Mayo Clinic may any conclusions regarding prognosis be made.[22, 82] The five-year survival is 55 percent or better; the ten-year figure is 50 percent. Almost all of these patients had involvement of pericolic fat, and half had involvement of regional lymph nodes. Thus, the 55 percent five-year survival rate for malignant lymphoma exceeds the 50 percent five-year survival rate which could be expected with a similar group of colonic carcinomas (one-half Dukes' "B" and one-half Dukes' "C").[30] The data are inconclusive, but it appears that patients with lymphocytic type have a better chance of survival than those with the reticulum cell type. Only a few cases of the Hodgkin's type of malignant lymphoma originating in the large intestine have been reported. No meaningful estimate of prognosis can be made.[49, 61, 82]

As elsewhere, lymph node involvement worsens the prognosis. Wychulis, et al.[82] reported that 71 percent of their patients who died of recurrent malignant lymphoma had regional lymph node involvement originally, while only 32 percent of the survivors did. Extension beyond the colon also has an ominous significance.[82]

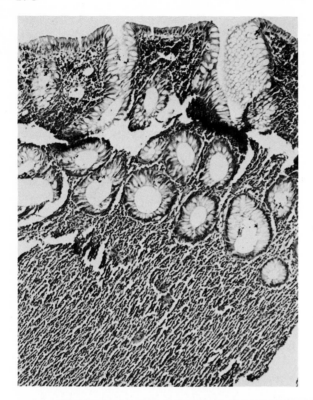

Fig. 19. This particular area seen in a malignant lymphoma, lymphocytic type, well-differentiated, arising in the rectum, would not allow distinction from a pseudolymphoma. A relatively small area of lymphocytes is not, in itself, a sufficient basis for a diagnosis of malignant lymphoma. See also Figures 20, 21. UCSD OLR. H&E. X25.

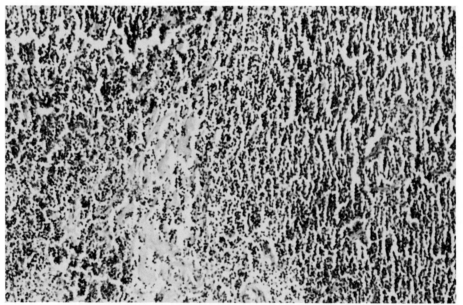

Fig. 20.   In another area of the same tumor as illustrated in Figure 19, the monotonous infiltrate of small lymphocytes is seen again. Multiple areas like this, with no germinal centers, allow one to make a diagnosis of malignant lymphoma. See also Figures 19, 21. UCSD OLR. H&E. X25.

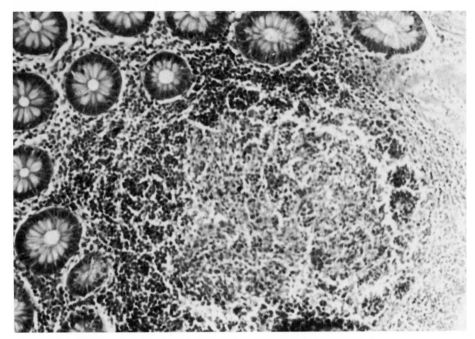

Fig. 21.   In this pseudolymphoma of the rectum ("lymphoid polyp"), prominent germinal centers allow separation from malignant lymphoma. Other areas were composed almost entirely of lymphocytes. Compare Figures 19, 20. UCSD OLR. H&E. X40.

Late recurrences are uncommon and apparently can be treated successfully by irradiation.[22, 82] Association with chronic ulcerative colitis indicates a poorer prognosis.[15, 82]

Discussion

The existence of both extranodal malignant lymphomas and pseudolymphomas is well established. The origin, etiology, and significance of these conditions merit further discussion.

The abundant lymphoid tissue in the submucosa of the gastrointestinal tract is the point of origin of malignant lymphomas in the stomach, small intestine, and large intestine. The lymphoid tissue which occurs regularly in the bronchial mucosa and in the fibrous tissue around the bronchial cartilages[41] can well explain the origin of malignant lymphomas in the lung. Primitive totipotential mesenchymal cells exist in the loose connective tissue everywhere, especially about blood vessels,[41] and can explain the development of malignant lymphomas anywhere in the body.

The etiology of extranodal malignant lymphomas is, like that of the usual malignant lymphomas, completely unknown. Only further study will determine if it is the same in all locations. It is of interest that chronic ulcerative colitis is associated with primary malignant lymphoma of the colon as well as with adenocarcinoma.[15, 82]

Extranodal malignant lymphomas have significance, and their separation from the usual malignant lymphoma is important because of their generally better prognosis and different therapy. For the first reason, separation from carcinoma also is important.

Pseudolymphomas are reactive lesions and, like other inflammatory lesions, can occur anywhere in the body. At times, every pathologist has seen dense lymphoid infiltrates, often with germinal centers, in almost every organ. In a sense, a pseudolymphoma is simply an extension of this and represents the extranodal counterpart of a reactive lymph node.

In the lungs, pseudolymphomas probably represent a form of chronic pneumonia in which lymphocytes predominate.[56] Pulmonary fibrous, xanthomatous, and plasma cell pseudotumors have been described as have lymphoid pseudotumors of the mediastinum.[9, 71, 72] The relationship to lymphoid interstitial pneumonia warrants intensive study.[40]

Gastric pseudolymphomas are generally part of the reaction to peptic ulcer (Fig. 22).[18] There is no reason why chronic gastritis alone could not lead to such a pseudolymphoma also.

Many of the pseudolymphomas of the small intestine are associated with regional enteritis and indeed may be only an extreme expression of that disease.[75] The pseudolymphomas of the very terminal ileum seen in young children are part of the generalized lymphoid hyperplasia characteristic of that age group.[1]

No specific factor can explain all of the colonic pseudolymphomas, but there

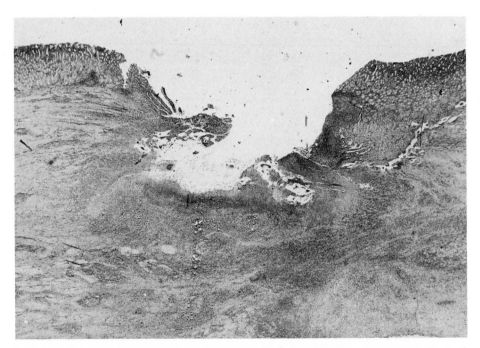

Fig. 22.   Photomicrograph showing a dense lymphocytic infiltration about a gastric peptic ulcer. This is felt to be one origin of gastric pseudolymphomas. W. U. III. #63-4326. H&E. X15. (Reprinted from Faris, T.D., and Saltzstein, S. L. *Cancer*, 17:207, 1964, with permission.)

is general agreement that they are of inflammatory origin.[13, 28] We have seen one of the cecum resulting from anticonvulsant drug therapy.[57]

The significance of pseudolymphomas is obvious: they are benign lesions and do not require the extensive surgery, radiotherapy, or chemotherapy that true malignant lymphomas require. Similarly, the emotional impact of a diagnosis of cancer on a patient and his family can be avoided.

Endoscopic biopsy and exfoliative cytology are of little use in the differentiation of extranodal malignant lymphomas, especially of the lymphocytic types, from pseudolymphomas because in both lesions there may be large areas composed mainly of lymphocytes (Figs. 19, 20, 21). A piece of tissue is necessary, large enough to study the structure and to have a reasonable chance to find germinal centers. This often will mean excision of the entire lesion. The diagnosis of malignant lymphoma of the reticulum cell type can be made at times on gastric cytologic material,[39] and Reed-Sternberg cells can be identified in material from endoscopic biopsies. As pseudolymphomas of the rectum usually are small, excisional biopsy should be performed.

Summary

Malignant lymphomas of any cell type can originate in organs other than the lymph nodes, liver, spleen, bone marrow, thymus, or Waldeyer's ring. In these extranodal locations, the malignant lymphomas have a better prognosis than the usual malignant lymphomas or other malignant tumors of the specific organ.

Cell type and nodal involvement affect the prognosis. Surgical excision is the treatment of choice. Late recurrences and late deaths are uncommon.

In these same sites, benign reactive pseudolymphomas also can occur. These can be separated from malignant lymphomas by their mixed cellular infiltrate, the presence of lymphoid germinal centers, and the absence of involvement of lymph nodes.

References

1. Ackerman, L.V. Surgical Pathology, 3rd ed. St. Louis, C. V. Mosby Co., 1964, pp. 413-414, 418.
2. Allen, A.W., Donaldson, G., Sniffen, R.C., and Goodale, F. Primary malignant lymphoma of the gastrointestinal tract. Ann. Surg., 140:428, 1954.
3. Statistics on cancer. CA, 18:13, 1968.
4. Azzopardi, J.G., and Menzies, T. Primary malignant lymphoma of the alimentary tract. Brit. J. Surg., 47:358, 1960.
5. Barba, W.P. Benign lymphoid hyperplasia of the rectum. J. Pediat., 41:328, 1952.
6. Bass, H.E., and Reibstein, H.B. Hodgkin's disease of the lung. New York J. Med., 50:345, 1950.
7. Berry, G.R., and Mathews, W.H. Gastric lymphosarcoma and pseudolymphoma. Canad. Med. Ass. J., 96:1312, 1967.
8. Burman, S.O., and van Wyk, F.A.K. Lymphomas of small intestine and cecum. Ann. Surg., 143:349, 1956.
9. Castleman, B., Iverson, L., and Mendendez, V.P. Localized mediastinal lymph node hyperplasia resembling thymoma. Cancer, 9:822, 1956.

10. Cook, J.C., and Corbett, D.P. Roentgen therapy of primary gastrointestinal lymphoma. Radiology, 78:562, 1962.
11. Cornes, J.S. Multiple primary cancers: Primary malignant lymphomas and carcinomas of the intestinal tract in the same patient. J. Clin. Path., 13:483, 1960.
12 ────── Hodgkin's disease of the gastrointestinal tract. Proc. Roy. Soc. Med., 60: 732, 1967.
13. ────── Wallace, M.H., and Morson, B.C. Benign lymphomas of the rectum and anal canal: A study of 100 cases. J. Path. Bact., 82:371, 1961.
14. Cosens, G.S. Gastrointestinal pseudoleukemia: A case report. Ann. Surg., 148:129, 1958.
15. Dawson, J.M.P., Cornes, J.S., and Morson, B.C. Primary malignant lymphoid tumours of the intestinal tract. Brit. J. Surg., 49:80, 1961.
16. Ehrenstein, F. Primary puimonary lymphoma. J. Thorac. Cardiovasc. Surg., 52:31, 1966.
17. Ellison, R.G., Bailey, A.W., Yeh, T.J., Corpe, R.F., Liang, J., and Stergus, I. Primary lymphosarcoma of the lung. Amer. Surg., 30:737, 1964.
18. Faris, T.D., and Saltzstein, S.L. Gastric lymphoid hyperplasia: A lesion confused with lymphosarcoma. Cancer, 17:207, 1964.
19. Faulkner, J.W., and Dockerty, M.B. Lymphosarcoma of the small intestine. Surg. Gynec. Obstet., 95:76, 1952.
20. Frazer, J.W. Malignant lymphomas of the gastrointestinal tract. Surg. Gynec. Obstet., 108:182, 1959.
21. Friedman, A.I. Primary lymphosarcoma of the stomach: A clinical study of 75 cases. Amer. J. Med., 26:783, 1959.
22. Glick, D.D., and Soule, E.H. Primary malignant lymphoma of colon or appendix. Arch. Surg., 92:144, 1966.
23. Gonpnathan, H., and Sataline, L.R. Pulmonary Hodgkin's disease with cavitary lesion. Ohio Med. J., 62:238, 1966.
24. Gregory, J.J., Ribaudo, C.A., and Grace, W.J. Endobronchial Hodgkin's disease: Report of three cases. Ann. Intern. Med., 62:579, 1965.
25. Grismer, J.T., Raab, D.E., Dornbach, R., and Krafft, W. Primary lymphosarcoma: An interesting solitary lesion of the lung. Minn. Med., 49:242, 1966.
26. Havard, C.W.H., Nichols, J.B., and Stansfeld, A.G. Primary lymphosarcoma of the lung. Thorax, 17:190, 1962.
27. Hayes, H.T., Burr, H.B., and Pruit, L.T. Lymphoid tumors of the colon and rectum: Report of a case of simple lymphoma of rectum. Surgery, 7:540, 1940.
28. Helwig, E.B., and Hansen, J. Lymphoid polyps (benign lymphoma) and malignant lymphoma of the rectum and anus. Surg. Gynec. Obstet., 92:233, 1951.
29. Hilbun, B.M., and Chavez, C.M. Lymphoma of the lung. J. Thorac. Cardiovasc. Surg., 53:721, 1967.
30. Holtz, F., and Schmidt, L.A. Lymphoid polyps (benign lymphoma) of the rectum and anus. Surg. Gynec. Obstet., 106:639, 1958.
31. Hutchinson, W.B., Friedenberg, M.J., and Saltzstein, S. Primary pulmonary pseudo-lymphoma. Radiology, 82:48, 1964.
32. Jackson, P.P., and Coady, C.J. Primary lymphomas of the GI tract. Arch. Surg., 78:458, 1959.
33. Jacobs, D.S. Primary gastric malignant lymphoma and pseudolymphoma. Amer. J. Clin. Path., 40:379, 1963.
34. James, A.G. Cancer Prognosis Manual, 2nd ed. New York, American Cancer Society, 1966, pp. 51, 53.
35. Joseph, J.I., and Lattes, R. Gastric lymphosarcoma: Clinicopathologic analysis of 71 cases and its relation to disseminated lymphosarcoma. Amer. J. Clin. Path., 45:653, 1966.
36. Joseph, M. Hodgkin's disease of the lungs. Med. J. Aust., 1:795, 1965.
37. Kay, S. Lymphoid tumors of the stomach. Surg. Gynec. Obstet., 118:1059, 1964.

38. Kern, W.H., Crepeau, A.G., and Jones, J.C. Primary Hodgkin's disease of the lung: Report of four cases and review of the literature. Cancer, 14:1151, 1961.
39. Kernen, J.A., and Bales, C. Cytologic diagnosis of gastric cancer. Calif. Med., 108: 104, 1968.
40. Liebow, A.A. Personal communication, 1968.
41. Maximow, A.A., and Bloom, W. A Textbook of Histology, 7th ed. Philadelphia, W. B. Saunders Co., 1957, pp. 68-70, 437.
42. McNeer, G., and Berg, J. The clinical behavior and management of primary malignant lymphoma of the stomach. Surgery, 46:829, 1959.
43. Meese, E.H., Doohen, D.J., Elliott, R.C., and Timmes, J.J. Primary organ involvement in intrathoracic Hodgkin's disease. Dis. Chest., 46:699, 1964.
44. Mestel, A.L. Lymphosarcoma of the small intestine in infancy and childhood. Ann. Surg., 149:87, 1959.
45. Monahan, D.T. Hodgkin's disease of the lung. J. Thorac. Cardiovasc. Surg., 49:173, 1965.
46. Nicoloff, D.M., Haynes, L.B., and Wangensteen, O.H. Primary lymphosarcoma of the gastrointestinal tract. Surg. Gynec. Obstet., 117:433, 1963.
47. Pagtalunan, R.J.G., Mayo, C.W., and Dockerty, M.B. Primary malignant tumors of the small intestine. Amer. J. Surg., 108:13, 1964.
48. Papaionnou, A.N., and Watson, W.L. Primary lymphoma of the lung. An appraisal of its natural history and a comparison with other localized lymphomas. J. Thorac. Cardiovasc. Surg., 49:373, 1965.
49. Parkhurst, G.F., and MacMillan, S.F. Longevity in lymphomas of the lower intestinal tract. J.A.M.A. 179:351, 1967.
50. Perez, C.A., and Dorfman, R.F. Benign lymphoid hyperplasia of the stomach and duodenum. Radiology, 87:505, 1966.
51. Rabiah, F.A. Primary lymphocytic lymphoma (lymphosarcoma) of the lung. Amer. Surg., 34:275, 1968.
52. Rappaport, H., Winter, W.J., and Hicks, E.B. Follicular lymphoma. Cancer, 9:792, 1956.
53. Robbins, L.L. Roentgenological appearance of parenchymal involvement of lung by malignant lymphoma. Cancer, 6:80, 1953.
54. Rubenfeld, S., and Clark, E. An unusual case of Hodgkin's disease of lung. Radiology, 28:614, 1937.
55. Rubinovich, A.Z. A case of pulmonary lymphogranulomatosis. Klin. Med. (Moskva), 35:144, 1957. Abstracted in Abstr. Sov. Med., B-2:908, 1958.
56. Saltzstein, S.L. Pulmonary malignant lymphomas and pseudolymphomas: Classification, therapy, and prognosis. Cancer, 16:928, 1963.
57. ――― Unpublished data, Barnes Hospital, 1963.
58. ――― and Ackerman, L.V. Lymphadenopathy induced by anticonvulsant drugs and mimicking clinically and pathologically malignant lymphomas. Cancer, 12:164, 1959.
59. Samuels, M.L., Howe, C.D., Dodd, G.D., Jr., Fuller, L.M., Shullenberger, C.C., and Leary, W.L. Endobronchial malignant lymphoma: Report of five cases in adults. Amer. J. Roentgen., 85:87, 1961.
60. Schmutzer, K.J., Holleran, W.M., and Regan, J.F. Tumors of the small bowel. Amer. J. Surg., 108:270, 1964.
61. Shapiro, H.A. Primary Hodgkin's disease of the rectum. Arch. Intern. Med., 107: 270, 1961.
62. Sherrick, D.W., Hodgson, J.R., and Dockerty, M.B. The roentgenologic diagnosis of primary gastric lymphoma. Radiology, 84:925, 1965.
63. Smith, J.L., and Helwig, E.B. Malignant lymphoma of the stomach: Its diagnosis, distinction, and biologic behavior. Amer. J. Path., 34:553, 1958.
64. Snyder, J.M. Discussion. J. Thorac. Surg., 31:44, 1956.

65. Sperling, L. Malignant lymphoma of the gastrointestinal tract. Progr. Clin. Cancer, 2:338, 1966.
66. Starkey, G.W.B. Discussion. J. Thorac. Surg., 31:43, 1956.
67. Stobbe, J.A., Dockerty, M.B., and Bernatz, P.E. Primary gastric lymphoma and its grades of malignancy. Amer. J. Surg., 112:10, 1966.
68. Swartley, R.N., and Stayman, J.W. Lymphoid hyperplasia of the intestinal tract requiring surgical intervention. Ann. Surg., 155:238, 1962.
69. Thorbjarnson, B., Beal, J.M., and Pearce, J.M. Primary malignant lymphoid tumors of the stomach. Cancer, 9:712, 1956.
70. ———— Pearce, J.M. and Beal, J.M. Sarcoma of the stomach. Amer. J. Surg., 97:36, 1959.
71. Titus, J.L., Harrison, E.G., Clagett, O.T., Anderson, M.W., and Knaff, L.J. Xanthomatous and inflammatory pseudotumors of the lung. Cancer, 15:522, 1962.
72. Umiker, W.O., and Iverson, L. Postinflammatory "tumors" of the lung: Report of four cases simulating xanthoma, fibroma, or plasma cell tumor. J. Thorac. Surg., 28:55, 1954.
73. Valdes-Dapena, A., Affolter, H., and Vilardell, F. The gradient of malignancy in lymphoid lesions of the stomach. Gastroenterology, 50:382, 1966.
74. Weaver, D.K., and Batsakis, J.G. Primary lymphomas of the small intestine. Amer. J. Gastroenterol., 42:620, 1964.
75. ———— and Batsakis, J.G. Pseudolymphomas of the small intestine. Amer. J. Gastroenterol., 44:374, 1965.
76. ———— and Batsakis, J.G. Primary lymphomas and related benign lesions of the intestines. Amer. J. Proctol., 17:229, 1966.
77. Welborn, J.K., Ponka, J.L., and Rebuck, J.W. Lymphoma of the stomach: A diagnostic and therapeutic problem. Arch. Surg., 90:480, 1965.
78. ———— Rebuck, J.W., and Ponka, J.L. Intestinal lymphosarcoma. Arch. Surg., 94:717, 1967.
79. Wheelock, M.C., Atkinson, A.J., and Pizzo, A. Lymphosarcoma of the ileum. Gastroenterology, 15:158, 1950.
80. Wolf, B.S., and Marshak, R.H. Roentgen features of diffuse lymphosarcoma of the colon. Radiology, 75:733, 1960.
81. Woodruff, J.H., Jr., and Skorneck, A.B. Malignant lymphoma of the colon and rectum: Roentgen diagnosis. Calif. Med., 96:181, 1962.
82. Wychulis, A.R., Beahrs, O.H., and Woolner, L.B. Malignant lymphoma of the colon. Arch. Surg., 93:215, 1966.

IN SITU CARCINOMA OF THE BREAST

MAURICE M. BLACK
ADA B. CHABON

Part I: Numerical Grading of Type and Extent

Invasive mammary carcinoma is commonly associated with a variety of proliferative changes in the mammary ducts, viz., benign appearing hyperplasia, atypical hyperplasia, in situ carcinoma, and diverse varieties of fibrocystic disease. This association between proliferative lesions and invasive carcinoma has been the stimulus for numerous attempts to define the precancerous potentialities of such lesions.[1, 2, 3] As a rule, investigators have approached the problem by comparing the incidence of histologic changes, such as adenosis (florid, sclerosing, blunt duct), papillomatosis, papillary hyperplasia, atypia, carcinoma in situ, apocrine metaplasia, etc., in breasts with and without invasive carcinoma. In our experience, this approach has been of limited value in that, except for in situ malignant changes, proliferative changes of the aforementioned types are found with almost the same frequency in benign and malignant breast lesions.

Nevertheless, our observations are in accord with others in suggesting that invasive breast cancer is associated with a greater degree of progressive and atypical proliferative alterations. We also had the impression that such changes commonly occurred in numerous segments of the same branching duct. Accordingly, we attempted to develop a grading system which might better define the degree of atypical proliferations occurring in different segments of the mammary duct system.

This paper describes a numerical grading system and its use in the classification of consecutive and selected samples of breast tissue. The grading system clearly differentiates between the proliferative changes in control and cancerous breasts, and it demonstrates that most breast cancers are associated with recognizable progressive changes in multiple portions of the duct system. These changes include lesions conventionally termed in situ carcinoma as well as lesser degrees of atypical proliferation. Such a spectrum of atypical changes occurring simultaneously in different segments of the branching ducts seems to constitute a biologic entity for which we have suggested the term "incipient carcinoma."

In the course of prior studies of breast tissue, we were impressed by the presence of lymphocytes in and among mammary ductular epithelial cells. The presence of lymphocytes within intestinal epithelium was reported a century ago.[4, 5] Scattered reports have also described a similar relationship between lymphocytes and other types of epithelial surfaces,[6] and, in a 1958 review, Trowell devoted a section to the subject of lymphocytes inside other cells (emperipolesis).[7] It appeared to us that intraepithelial lymphocyte accumulation (ILA) was diminished or absent in cancerous ducts. Therefore, we have included observations on the relationship between ILA and progressive atypical changes. It will be shown that ILA is routinely found in normal and hyperplastic ducts but is consistently depressed in the atypical proliferations of incipient carcinoma.

Material and Methods

The present study utilized slides of consecutive and selected breast lesions from the Surgical Pathology files of the New York Medical College, Flower and Fifth Avenue Hospitals. As a preliminary to the definitive study, we selected a number of cases which had been previously diagnosed as in situ carcinoma, as well as some cases of invasive carcinoma. All the available slides were studied in an attempt to characterize particular features to be assessed in the consecutive series. On the basis of such preliminary observations, it appeared that the features of interest could be best defined in terms of a numerical grading of the degree of atypical proliferative changes occurring in different portions of the duct system. For this purpose we have considered the branching ducts, from the nipple to and including the alveolar structure in terms of 4 divisions which we designate as A, B, C, and D. Division A includes the primary ducts and major interlobular subdivisions which are characterized by luminal diameters decidedly greater than the thickness of the epithelial lining. Division B refers to the terminal interlobular ducts. The epithelial lining is in the form of an outer layer of myoepithelial cells and an inner layer of columnar secretory cells. The luminal diameter of B ducts is approximately equal to that of the epithelial lining. Division C refers to the preterminal intralobular ducts. The anatomical structure is similar to that of the B ducts, although the inner epithelial cells are more cuboidal than columnar, and the lumen is smaller. The branches of the intralobular C ductules form the so-called acinar structures or D ductules. The latter are composed of an outer myoepithelial and an inner cuboidal layer of cells around a small but distinct lumen. In some lobules the myoepithelial layer is poorly defined or absent.

Each of the divisions of the duct system was assigned a numerical grade from 1 to 5, representative of cellular changes suggesting the proliferative sequence: (1) control → (2) hyperplasia → (3, 4) atypia → (5) in situ carcinoma. The salient features of the various grades in the different divisions (A, B, C, D) are described below.

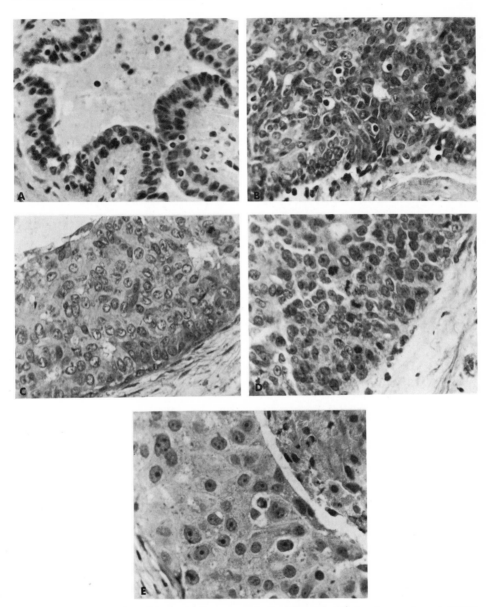

Fig. 1. A duct grading: (A) Control area, grade 1 of breast with in situ carcinoma (4723-62). Intraepithelial lymphocytes readily apparent. (B) Intraductal papillary hyperplasia, grade 2 in breast with in situ carcinoma (3598-66). Note ILA. (C) Grade 3 intraductal atypical hyperplasia, same case as in C (3598-66). Note monomorphic proliferation and lack of ILA. (D) Grade 4 intraductal atypical proliferations in breast with invasive carcinoma (4924-67). (E) Grade 5 intraductal atypical proliferation, in situ comedo carcinoma in breast with invasive carcinoma (688-67). Note lack of ILA.

A Ducts (Fig. 1). Hyperplasia (grade 2) is expressed as multilayering of the epithelium with or without intraductal papillations. The cellular proliferation includes both the myoepithelial and epithelial lining cells. The latter may often show

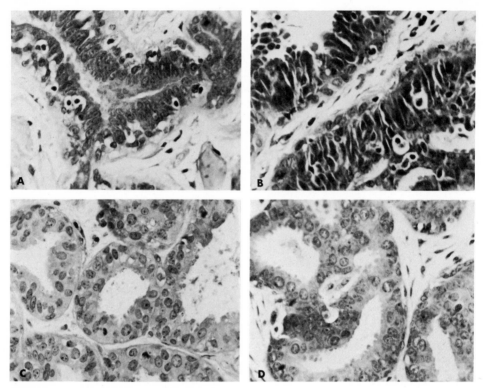

Fig. 2.   B duct grading: (A) Control area, grade 1 of breast with invasive carcinoma
(4938-67). ILA is readily seen despite the lack of periductal lymphoid cell infiltration. (B)
Ductular hyperplasia, grade 2 control area of breast with invasive carcinoma (134-67).
Note that polarity and ILA are maintained. (C) Grade 3 atypical ductular hyperplastic area
in breast with invasive carcinoma (1969-66). Note beginning loss of polarity, monomorphic
multilayering and lack of ILA. (D) Grade 4 atypical ductular proliferation in breast with
lobular in situ carcinoma. Same breast as depicted in Figure 1B and C (3598-66). Note
the lack of ILA.

prominent apical cytoplasmic blebs. Atypia (grade 3) is characterized by cellular
proliferations which are typically monomorphic. There is also some loss of polarity
of the cells and an increase in nuclear/cytoplasmic ratio. These changes become
more marked in grade 4 and eventuate in intraductular carcinoma of the papillary
or comedo variety (grade 5).

B Ducts (Fig. 2).   Hyperplasia (grade 2) is characterized by hypertrophy of
the inner columnar cells with increased basophilia of the cytoplasm. Atypia (grade
3) is recognized in the form of increased layering of the cells without accompanying
proliferation of myoepithelial cells. Irregular ductular proliferations may also be
seen, as well as increased nucleolar prominence. Progressive loss of cellular and
nuclear polarity occurs (grade 4) and eventuates in disorganized ductules containing
malignant appearing cells recognized as in situ ductular carcinoma (grade 5).

C Ducts (Fig. 3).   The proliferative changes in these intralobular ductules are
similar to those seen in B ductules. In the C ducts, however, the lumen is more commonly effaced by atypical and malignant transformations. In situ malignant changes

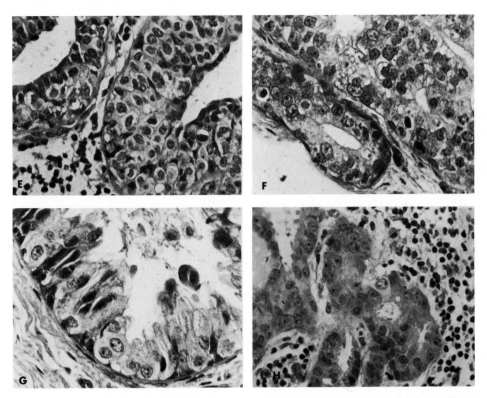

Fig. 2. (cont.)   B duct grading: (E) Another variant of in situ grade 4 atypia, in breast with invasive carcinoma (3866-67). Note the lack of ILA despite the accumulation of lymphoid cells in periductal stroma. (F) Grade 5 (intraductal carcinoma) in breast with invasive carcinoma. (G) Another variant of grade 5 malignant change in B ducts in breast with invasive carcinoma (688-67). (H) Invasive breast carcinoma (134-66) showing marked stromal lymphoid infiltrate but lack of intraepithelial lymphocytes in the cancerous ducts.

(grade 5) in C ducts are commonly but not always associated with analogous changes in their branches (D ducts). Nevertheless, atypia and malignant changes in C ducts may sometimes occur without analogous changes in D ducts.

D Ducts (Fig. 3).   Hyperplasia (grade 2) is characterized by cellular hypertrophy of both myoepithelial and epithelial cells. Atypia (grade 3) is associated with monomorphic proliferations which obliterate the lumen. Progressive loss of cell polarity occurs with increased nuclear prominence (grade 4) and in situ lobular carcinoma results (grade 5).

The grading system thus characterizes mammary parenchymal structures in terms of the degree of proliferative and atypical changes in different anatomical divisions of the duct system. Such changes are expressed as a profile of grades or summarized as the average of the duct grades.

We have also graded another structural variant, apocrine changes. It is well known that varying sized ducts or cysts in control and cancerous breasts may be lined by cells characterized by eosinophilic cytoplasm in place of the conventional type of epithelium. Such changes are usually referred to as apocrine metaplasia,

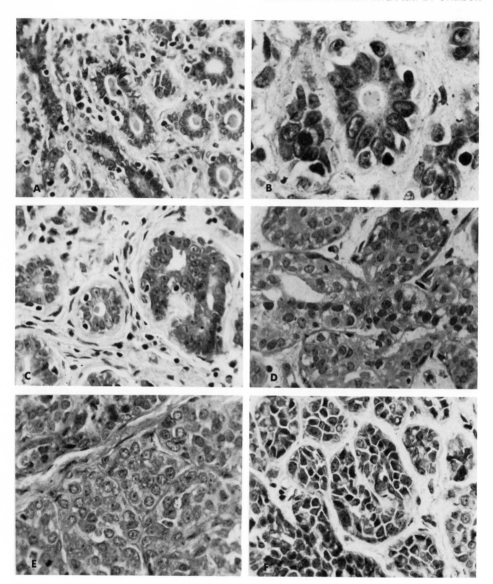

Fig. 3.   Intralobular duct (C and D) grading: (A) Control intralobular ducts, grade 1 from breast with in situ lobular carcinoma (5603-67). The intraepithelial lymphocytes are readily seen. (B) Higher magnification of A demonstrating the association between the epithelial cells and lymphocytes. (C) Lobular duct hyperplasia, grade 2, in breast with invasive carcinoma (134-67). (D) Atypical hyperplasia, grade 3 of lobular ducts in breast with invasive carcinoma (1969-66). Note the cellular enlargement, altered polarity, and loss of ILA. (E) Lobular in situ atypia, grade 4, in breast which also had in situ malignant changes in A and B ducts and grade 3 apocrine changes (4587-62). (F) Lobular in situ carcinoma, grade 5 in breast which also had grade 4 changes in B ducts and grade 3 apocrine changes (5603-65).

and malignant tumors composed of such cells are termed papillary apocrine adeno-carcinomas. In our preliminary survey and in the course of routine examination of

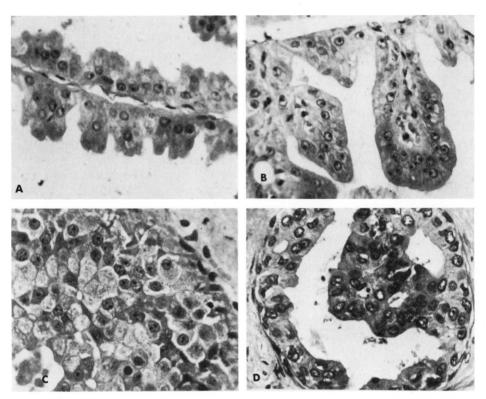

Fig. 4. Grading of apocrine metaplasia: (A) Apocrine grade 2, benign breast status (3129-68). (B) Apocrine grade 3 from breast with in situ lobular and ductular carcinoma (1045-68). (C) Apocrine grade 4 (L-69-73). (D) Apocrine grade 5. Intraductal papillary apocrine carcinoma (M-456-68).

surgical material, we had the impression that apocrine metaplasia with cell atypia was more frequent in cancerous breasts. In order to test this, we recorded the presence and degree of atypia of apocrine metaplasia. Note that this feature is independent of the anatomical division of the duct system, although it is more commonly seen in A and B ducts than in the intralobular C and D ductules.

Observations on apocrine epithelium were recorded under the designation Ap (Fig. 4). The normal status is presumed to be the absence of apocrine changes and is thus graded as 0. Where apocrine changes are found, they may show varying degrees of proliferative changes from a single layer of banal appearing cells (grade 1) to multilayered papillations made up of bizarre cells characteristic of papillary apocrine adenocarcinoma (grade 5). As used here, the designation of atypia (grade 3) implies multilayering and/or increased nuclear size with nucleolar prominence. Further loss of cell polarity, nuclear and nucleolar enlargement, and multinucleation are indicative of grade 4 changes. Note that the Ap parameter has a grading range from 0 through 5, while the specific duct gradings cover the range 1 through 5.

It should be noted that the grades assigned to the ducts and apocrine areas were the highest observed in the case. In almost all instances, lesser degrees of atypia were also seen, viz., grade 5 values were routinely accompanied by grades 3 and 4 in other areas.

Having defined the various features to be evaluated, we examined sections of 194 consecutive breast biopsies and/or mastectomies from the surgical pathology files. Since the consecutive series included only 4 cases of in situ carcinoma, we collected an additional 28 cases of in situ carcinoma from our own and other institutions. All sections pertaining to each case were examined and graded according to the above schema. Atypical changes were usually found in focalized areas, and in many instances different portions of the same branching duct were involved. This was true of breasts with in situ as well as invasive carcinoma. In contrast breast tissues peripheral to carcinomatous foci were usually indistinguishable from those of control breasts. As used below, such terms as multicentric, multifocal, and constellation of changes refer to alterations within different divisions of the same or neighboring ducts. While some instances of diffuse atypia were encountered, this was the exception rather than the rule.

As mentioned above, the various ducts were also examined for the presence of ILA. Since different areas of the same duct may show variations in the prominence of ILA, multiple areas were examined. ILA was considered to be present if the distribution was similar to that seen in control ducts. In cases of intraductal carcinoma, both the cancerous and control ducts were evaluated. There is little difficulty in broadly classifying ILA as normal or minimal (Figs. 1-4).

Results

Table 1 lists the diagnostic distribution of lesions encountered in the consecutive series of cases. The findings regarding the different parameters under consideration in the various groups are as follows:

Table 1.   Distribution of Diagnoses in Consecutive Series of Breast Lesions

DIAGNOSIS	NUMBER OF CASES
Non Cancer	
Fibroadenoma	38
Control*	97
Cancer	
In situ	4
Invasive	55
	194

* All nonfibroadenomatous and noncancerous lesions.

Fibroadenoma.   In many instances, the fibroadenoadenomas were "shelled out" by the surgeon without any appreciable amount of surrounding breast parenchyma. In 17 of the 38 cases, however, there was sufficient surrounding parenchyma to allow for grading. In all of these cases, the ductular system appeared essentially normal. None showed atypia of grades 3 or 4, and in only one was a significant degree of hyperplasia noted (C duct, grade 2).

Control (noncancer, nonfibroadenoma). This series included 97 samples of breast tissues removed because of nodularity, suspicious mammographic changes, or local tenderness. The histologic findings included all variants of so-called fibrocytic disease. Of these 97 cases only 12 showed duct and/or atypical apocrine metaplasia. The details of the findings in this subgroup of 12 cases are presented in Table 2. In

Table 2.   Duct Gradings in Noncancerous Breasts Having Atypia (Grade 3 or 4) in any Parameter*

CASE	AP	A	B	C	D	AVERAGE DUCTS		AGE
			DUCTS			DUCTS	DUCTS + AP	
2544-67	3	2	3	2	1	2.0	2.2	45
3731-67	3	1	2	2	2	1.8	2.0	51
3833-67	4	3	4	2	2	1.8	3.0	49
4258-67	0	3	1	1	1	1.5	1.2	43
5006-67	3	1	2	2	1	1.5	1.8	44
136-67	3	2	2	2	1	1.8	2.0	43
1542-67	3	3	3	3	3	3.0	3.0	50
1916-67	3	1	2	2	2	1.8	2.0	39
1987-67	3	1	2	2	2	1.8	2.0	50
2395-67	3	2	2	2	1	1.8	2.0	42
2460-67	3	3	2	2	2	2.3	2.4	42
1515-67	3	1	1	1	1	1.0	1.4	54
Average	2.9	1.9	2.2	1.9	1.6	1.9	2.1	44

* Exclusive of apocrine (Ap) features.

only one case was a grade of 4 observed in any of the ducts. This same case (3833-67) also showed grade 4 apocrine changes and a grade 3 atypia of A ducts. The average duct grading for this case, excluding the apocrine changes, was 2.8 and 3.0, including the apocrine changes. Note that an average duct grade > 2.0 were found in only three of the total series of 97 cases.

The ages of the patients with atypia vary from 39 to 54 years, with an average of 44 years. In the total series of 97 control cases, approximately 25 percent of the patients were less than 35 years of age while 10 percent were older than 54 years.

Cancer

IN SITU.   By definition and selection, this group has a grade of 5 in at least one of the duct divisions. In Table 3, we have listed the gradings in the individual cases. It is clearly evident that atypia and/or malignant changes occur in multiple segments of the ductular system. Note particularly that 17 of the 24 cases diagnosable as lobular in situ carcinoma on the basis of grade 5 in C and/or D ducts also had a grading of 5 in the extralobular ducts. The frequency of atypical apocrine changes in this series (64 percent) was greater than that in the control series (11 percent).

The average grade for the different parameters in this series clearly indicates the tendency toward atypical proliferation, while the average grade for each of the cases illustrates the tendency for such changes to occur in different subdivisions of the duct system. Thus, the average duct grade was greater than 2.0 in 30 out of 33 cases.

Table 3.   Duct Grading in 33 In Situ Carcinomas

| | | DUCTS | | | | AVERAGE | | |
CASE	AP	A	B	C	D	DUCTS	DUCTS + AP	AGE
M-1283-57	3	1	4	5	5	3.8	3.6	42
M-1402-67	3	5	1	1	1	2.0	2.2	62
M-125-67(L)*	4	4	5	5	5	4.7	4.6	50
M-125-67(R)*	4	4	5	5	5	4.7	4.6	50
M-3918-65	0	5	5	3	1	3.5	2.8	61
M-1379-51	0	5	5	5	5	5.0	4.0	50
M-1090-57	0	5	5	1	1	3.0	2.4	57
M-1388-49	5	1	1	1	1	1.0	1.8	—
1354-67	3	5	5	5	5	5.0	4.6	36
2289-67	4	5	5	5	3	4.5	4.4	53
2822-67	0	5	1	1	1	2.0	1.6	38
1479-67	5	5	5	5	4	4.7	4.8	43
2756-65	0	3	4	5	5	4.3	3.4	31
4723-62	0	1	3	5	5	3.5	2.8	62
361-68	0	5	1	5	5	4.0	3.2	36
7260-68	3	5	3	1	1	2.5	2.6	65
6197-60	0	5	5	5	5	5.0	4.0	49
5028-61	0	1	5	5	4	3.8	3.0	61
5603-65	3	1	4	4	5	3.5	3.4	41
75-59	3	5	5	5	5	5.0	4.6	50
4289-65*	4	2	3	4	4	3.3	3.4	57
4287-62	3	5	5	5	5	5.0	4.6	45
A-34087	3	4	4	5	5	4.5	4.2	—
A-35841	3	2	5	5	5	4.3	4.0	—
A-26535	5	5	5	5	5	5.0	5.0	—
A-25687	3	3	5	5	5	4.5	4.2	—
1045-68	3	4	4	3	5	4.0	3.8	42
3598-66*	5	5	4	5	5	4.7	4.8	51
2260-68	3	5	3	1	1	2.5	2.6	75
2480-66(L)*	0	5	4	4	5	4.5	3.6	44
2948-68(R)	0	1	1	1	1	4.8	4.8	43
1963-68(L)	0	1	5	5	1	3.0	2.4	67
2155-68*	3	4	4	5	5	4.5	4.2	—
Average	2.5	3.9	4.0	4.1	3.8	3.8	3.8	51

* Comments. M-125-67: bilateral, simultaneous carcinoma in situ. 4289-65: developed local recurrence in operative site two years later and axillary lymph node metastases three years after original mastectomy. 3598-66: had prior mastectomy of other breast for invasive carcinoma one year before. 2480-66: developed invasive carcinoma of opposite breast two years later. 2155-68: in situ carcinoma, right breast and simultaneous invasive carcinoma, left breast.

Of the 27 patients with in situ carcinoma for whom ages were available, the range was from 31 to 75 years with a mean value of 51 years. In six cases, the in situ malignant changes did not involve the intralobular ducts. Five of these six patients were more than 56 years of age, and the average age of the group was 60 years. However, in the group of 21 patients with lobular in situ changes, only four were older than 56 years, and the mean age was 48 years.

INVASIVE CARCINOMA.   Areas of in situ carcinoma were found in 31 of the 55 cases (56 percent) of invasive carcinoma, while an additional 11 cases had grade 3 or 4 changes in their ducts. Thus 77 percent of the breasts with invasive carcinoma also had atypia and/or in situ carcinoma. Apocrine metaplasia of an atypical type was also common in cancerous breasts. Eleven of the 55 cases had apocrine metaplasia grades 4 or 5, while an additional 13 cases had an Ap grading of 3. It should be noted that invasive carcinoma may overgrow adjacent areas of in situ carcinoma and thus obscure the relationship between in situ and invasive carcinoma. The true percentage of association between in situ and invasive carcinoma probably exceeds the values cited above.

Table 4.   Percent Distributions of Duct Grades in Control,
In Situ, and Invasive Carcinoma

PARAMETER	GRADE	PERCENT CONTROL (97 CASES)	PERCENT IN SITU (32 CASES)	PERCENT INVASIVE (55 CASES)
Apocrine	< 3	89	36	54
	3	10	40	25
	> 3	1	24	21
A ducts	< 3	96	27	33
	3	4	6	13
	> 3	—	67	54
B ducts	< 3	97	15	50
	3	2	12	6
	> 3	1	73	44
C ducts	< 3	99	21	56
	3	1	6	4
	> 3	—	73	40
D ducts	< 3	99	27	65
	3	1	3	4
	> 3	—	70	31
Average (A-D)	2.1	96	9	38
	2.1-3.0	3	9	19
	> 3.0	—	82	42

In Table 4 we have indicated the distribution of grades in the invasive cancer series as well as the equivalent values for the in situ carcinoma and the control series. It is apparent from these data that atypia and/or in situ malignant changes were commonly seen in multiple areas of the duct system of cancerous breasts but were rare in noncancerous breasts. Figure 5 depicts the diversity of intraductal atypia associated with invasive carcinoma.

The age distribution of the patients with invasive carcinoma ranged from 26 to 90 years with a mean value of 53 years. However, in those cases having foci of in situ lobular carcinoma (C and D ducts ≥ 4), the distribution shifted toward a younger age. The median age of the latter group is 48 years and the mean age is 47 years, values almost identical to those of the noninvasive, in situ lobular carcinoma group. This age distribution differs from that of patients with the invasive cancers without lobular in situ changes. The latter may be divided into a group of eight cases having nonlobular in situ malignant changes and a group of 24 cases without evidence of in situ carcinoma. The ages in the former group ranged from 43 to 90 years with a mean of 58 years. In the latter group, the age range was from

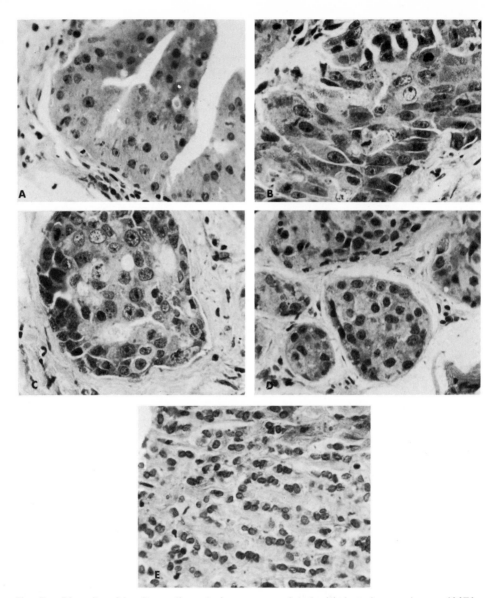

Fig. 5.   Diversity of in situ malignant changes associated with invasive carcinoma (4471-64). (A) Apocrine atypia, grade 3. (B) A duct, grade 5. (C) B duct, grade 5. (D) C and D ducts, grade 5. (E) Invasive carcinoma. Note that the invading cancer cells resemble the in situ lobular cancer cells more closely than the more anaplastic apocrine cells in the A and B ducts.

26 to 74 years with a mean of 57 years. It appears that the age distribution in the total invasive cancer series may be divided into two different distributions on the basis of the presence or absence of associated in situ lobular cancer. The age distribution of the invasive cancer group with in situ lobular carcinoma is similar to that of the lobular in situ carcinoma without invasion group. The age distribution

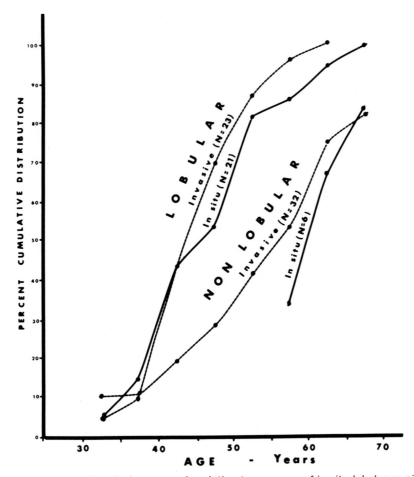

Fig. 6.   Cumulative distribution curves in relation to presence of in situ lobular carcinoma.

of the invasive cancer group without lobular in situ carcinoma is similar to that of the nonlobular in situ carcinoma group. The separation of the age distribution in relation to the presence of in situ lobular cancer is clearly demonstrated in the cumulative distribution curves (Fig. 6).

INTRAEPITHELIAL LYMPHOCYTE ACCUMULATION.   Representations of ILA in control, hyperplastic, and cancerous ducts are depicted in Figures 1 through 5. The findings in the series as a whole may be summarized as follows:

1. Scattered intraepithelial lymphocytes are found in all divisions of the mammary duct system, although they are usually more easily noted in intralobular ducts.

2. ILA is not correlated with the presence or absence of periductular stromal lymphoid cell infiltrations.

3. ILA is not diminished in ductular hyperplasia, papillary or nonpapillary, or in fibroadenomatous changes.

4. ILA is markedly reduced in foci of intraductular malignant changes (grade

5) and in grades 3 and 4 atypia. In none of the areas of in situ carcinoma did ILA approximate that seen in the control ducts of the same case.

5. ILA in control ducts (grades 1 and 2) of cancerous breasts is similar to that in homologous ducts of noncancerous breasts.

Comments

A grading system has been devised which permits numerical classification of atypical proliferative changes in different portions of the mammary duct system. Cases may thus be characterized by a profile of grades, while the overall findings in the case may be summarized in terms of the average of the duct grades. This approach clearly demonstrates that the great majority of invasive breast cancers are associated with a variety of atypical ductular changes. Such changes range from grade 3 (atypical hyperplasia) to well-defined in situ carcinoma (grade 5), which tend to occur simultaneously in different divisions of the duct system. Simultaneous involvement of different duct segments is also observed in breasts with in situ carcinomas lacking invasion. Eighty-five percent of the noninvasive in situ carcinomas and 87 percent of invasive carcinomas with foci of in situ changes had average duct grades $\geqslant 3.0$. In noncancerous breasts, grade 3 atypia of any single duct area is infrequent (<5 percent), and multiple areas of duct involvement are rarely seen.

Atypical apocrine metaplasia is also more commonly seen in association with invasive and in situ carcinomas. Thus, Ap grade $\geqslant 3$ was found in 21 of 27 in situ carcinomas (64 percent) and in 26 of 55 cases of invasive carcinoma (48 percent). This frequency is much greater than was observed in the control noncancer cases: 11 of 97 noncancerous, nonfibroadenoma breast biopsies, and 0 of 17 samples of breast tissues removed with a fibroadenoma.

In 26 of the invasive breast cancer cases, we were unable to find associated grade 5 lesions (in situ carcinoma). Nevertheless, three of the 26 cases had average duct grades between 3.0 and 4.0; nine had an Ap grade of 3 or 4, while duct grades of 3 or 4 were found in A ducts (ten cases), B ducts (six cases), C ducts (four cases), and D ducts (two cases). Two or more duct divisions were grade 3 or 4 in six cases, while six cases had both apocrine atypia and at least one duct grade of 3. A biologic relationship between atypia (grades 3 and 4) and in situ carcinoma (grade 5) is also suggested by the finding that ILA is diminished in both. It would appear that the lymphocytes are acting as an indicator of subtle change in the epithelial cells which precede the development of cytologic characteristics recognized as in situ carcinoma.

It appears that lesions which are conventionally termed in situ carcinoma are part of a more general biologic entity for which we would suggest the term *incipient carcinoma*. Conceptually, the term encompasses the gamut of atypical intraductal changes (grades 3 to 5); it also connotes the synchronous presence of such changes in different subdivisions of the branching ducts. However, as indicated below, it does not imply knowledge of the invasive potentialities of any particular forms of atypical proliferation. From an operational standpoint, we would apply the term to breast lesions having average duct grades $\geqslant 3.0$ and/or foci which would be conventionally termed in situ carcinoma. Actually, breast biopsies having two or more grade 3 values in ducts and/or apocrine foci would seem to be highly suspicious, even in the absence of any grade 5 areas. Such findings should alert the pathologist and the surgeon to the need for additional studies and careful follow-up of the patient. We would emphasize the need for the collection and follow-up of such cases. Ultimately, this is the sine qua non for defining the biologic significance of the various grades of change described above.

There seems to be little doubt that incipient carcinomas are related in some fashion to invasive carcinomas. From a structural standpoint, it is tempting to presume a sequential progression from incipient to invasive carcinoma or to consider the relationship between incipient and invasive carcinoma to be analogous to the initiation and promotion phases described in experimental carcinogenesis.[8] However, one cannot readily predict the invasion of the various synchronous in situ "malignant" changes. Thus, areas of lobular carcinoma in situ are commonly seen in association with invasive breast carcinoma, yet only rarely does the invasive cancer seem to arise from such foci (Fig. 5). Of the 32 patients with in situ carcinoma (see footnote to Table 3), one had simultaneous bilateral in situ carcinomas, one had simultaneous invasive carcinoma of the opposite breast, one had prior resection (one year) for invasive carcinoma of the other breast, one developed invasive carcinoma of the other breast within two years, and one patient had local recurrences of invasive carcinoma with axillary metastases two and three years respectively after a modified simple mastectomy for in situ carcinoma. These data indicate that incipient carcinomas have the features of a precancerous change, a preinvasive carcinoma, or a favored coincidental occurrence. The findings also raise the question whether extramammary host factors, viz., hormonal and immunologic, might not influence the ultimate biologic behavior of incipient carcinoma.

At first glance, the age distribution data for in situ and invasive cancers suggest that the former precedes the latter temporally. However, the situation is seen to be more complex when the cases are divided in terms of the presence or absence of in situ lobular carcinoma. As mentioned above, the mean age of the patients with in situ lobular carcinoma was essentially the same as the mean age of patients with invasive breast cancer having areas of lobular in situ changes (47 years). Furthermore, as indicated in Figure 6, the cumulative incidence with age is also similar in both groups. In contrast, an entirely different age distribution relationship was found for cases of nonlobular intraductal carcinoma (comedo, papillary, Paget's disease) and for invasive cancer without in situ lobular changes. The mean ages were some 10 years older than the mean age values of the lobular in situ groups, and the cumulative distribution curves differed sharply.

It appears that, in terms of development, breast cancer includes two different populations. If this proves to be the case in more extended studies, it would offer some explanations of the characteristic menopausal plateau in the incidence of breast cancer. According to this view, the plateau would reflect the almost complete occurrence of these breast cancers with in situ lobular changes. The secondary rise would be due to the increasing yield of carcinomas without in situ lobular carcinoma. It is noteworthy that Lilienfeld and Lewis[9] have suggested that the plateau reflects the existence of two linear curves consisting of those prior to and those after the 40 to 45 year age group. Their data and ours raise questions as to differences in hormonal influences on the development and behavior of the two groups.

More direct insight into the relationship between incipient and invasive cancer might be obtained by a comparative study of breast tissues of patients from geographical areas having differing incidence rates of cancer, viz., Japan and the United States or Great Britain. In the light of our observations, it would be of particular interest to know if the low incidence of breast cancer in Japan is associated with a low incidence of incipient carcinoma.

Finally, we should comment on the phenomenon of ILA in control and cancerous ducts. Although the intimate relationship between lymphocytes and epithelial cells has long been recognized by anatomists, pathologists have largely ignored the phenomenon and have made no contributions regarding pathologic variations. To the best of our knowledge, the diminution in ILA in association with malignant transformation of the epithelium has not been previously reported. The observation that incipient carcinoma exhibits a marked reduction in ILA further emphasizes the need to define the modus vivendi and biologic significance of the phenomenon. We are currently ignorant of the function of intraepithelial lymphocytes and do not know whether such cells are functioning immunologically. We have been unable to demonstrate IgG, IgA, or IgM immunocytochemically in intraepithelial lymphocytes. Nevertheless, the lack of ILA in foci of in situ carcinoma suggests that interactions between cancer cells and the lymphoreticuloendothelial (L-RE) system may precede the invasive phase of carcinogenesis. This possibility has prompted us to investigate the reactivity of lymph nodes draining in situ carcinomas. Such studies demonstrate that preinvasive carcinomas do indeed incite L-RE reactivity (see Part II, pp. 201-209).

Despite its prevalence and innumerable investigations, breast carcinoma continues to pose major problems. The newer diagnostic techniques of mammography and thermography, combined with the increasing use of mammotrophic hormones are presenting pathologists with additional numbers of unusual proliferative changes. It is hoped that the classification schema described above will aid the pathologist in the characterization of breast lesions. An enhanced precision in classification would not only be of practical value diagnostically but is requisite for the acquisition of more adequate knowledge of the biologic and biochemical changes associated with the development of breast cancer.

At the present time, there is a growing research interest in so-called "minimal deviation" neoplasms. Farber[10] has properly stated that the criteria for selection of a "minimal deviation system" for biochemical analysis must be biologic rather than biochemical. He notes that any neoplasm showing invasion and metastasis may be too advanced to be considered minimally deviated. Our data suggest that incipient carcinoma of the breast might well qualify as a minimal deviation neoplasm and provide particularly favorable material for both biologic and biochemical investigations of carcinogenesis. The research potential of human surgical pathologic specimens has by no means been exhausted. It remains a most necessary reference source of the realities regarding the development and behavior of spontaneous cancer.

Part II: Lymph Node Reactivity

In the course of a study of proliferative lesions of the breast, we observed that lymphocytes are characteristically found within the epithelium of normal and hyperplastic mammary ducts (see Part I, pp. 185-200). In contrast, such intraepithelial lymphocyte accumulation (ILA) was markedly reduced in invading cancerous ducts and in foci of in situ breast carcinoma. The latter observation suggested that tumor-lymphoreticuloendothelial (L-RE) interactions might be initiated in the preinvasive stage of carcinogenesis. This possibility is also supported by the frequent occurrence of stromal lymphoid infiltrates in the region of developing carcinomas of various types, viz., cervix uteri, melanoma, breast, or skin.[11] If the host L-RE system is indeed capable of recognizing and responding to preinvasive cancer, then some structural representation of such response should be found in the draining lymph nodes.

The occurrence of structural changes in axillary lymph nodes draining invasive breast cancer has been amply documented in numerous reports from this and other laboratories.[11-19] Furthermore, the data suggest that the biologic behavior of breast cancer reflects a tumor-host interaction wherein the tumor-antagonistic influence of the host may be correlated with histologic changes in the draining lymph nodes. Most particularly, a favorable prognostic influence is associated with a distinctive type of intrasinusoidal histiocytic proliferation, sinus histiocytosis (SH).

However, only a minority of patients with invasive breast cancer show SH reactivity in their resected axillary lymph nodes. Instead, many of them show a variety of degenerative changes in their sinusoidal histiocytes, viz., vacuolization, hyalinization, and fibrosis. Such degenerative changes are routinely found in the axillary lymph nodes of patients who have died of cancer or who succumb to the disease after limited postoperative survivals. In fact, the appearance of the lymph nodes of many breast cancer patients is reminiscent of lymph nodes exposed to overstimulation by antigen.[19] This is not unexpected, since, at the time of diagnosis, most invasive breast cancers are actually far advanced lesions in a biologic sense.

Farber has recently emphasized the need to utilize biologically early lesions, so-called minimal deviation tumors, in studies of the biochemistry of carcinogenesis.[20] The same caveat would apply to investigations of tumor-host interactions. Since in situ carcinomas constitute the minimal changes consistent with a diagnosis of malignancy, the lymph nodes draining such lesions should provide particularly favorable material for an investigation of the response of the L-RE system to biologically early cancer.

This paper reports on the characteristics of lymph nodes draining in situ breast carcinomas and compares the findings with those of lymph nodes draining invasive breast cancer. It will be shown that similar types of lymph node responses are associated with in situ and invasive carcinoma. It therefore appears that tumor-L-RE interactions precede the invasive phase of carcinogenesis. However, the in situ cancer series is distinguished by a higher incidence of prognostically favorable patterns of lymph node reactivity.

Materials and Methods

The present study is based on a collected series of 33 cases of in situ breast carcinoma with at least partial axillary lymphadenectomy.* The number of lymph nodes per case varied from two to 20 with an average of 11. For comparison, we have included observations on lymph nodes from 23 consecutive cases of invasive breast cancer with axillary metastases (Class II) and 32 cases of invasive breast cancer without axillary metastases (Class I). Each lymph node of the in situ and the invasive series was examined for SH, syncytial histiocytosis (Syn H), follicular prominence, and degenerative changes (degenerative SH, atrophy, hyalinization), as described previously.[13,18] The SH reactivity was graded from 0 to 5 plus, a zero reading being given to those lymph nodes which were extensively invaded by metastases. Lymph nodes which lacked an SH response despite minimal or no metastatic involvement were graded 1 plus. An SH grade of 5 was applied to lymph nodes showing prominent sinusoids distended by compactly arranged histiocytes. Such lymph nodes were also characterized by a hyperplastic pulp, minimal secondary follicles and inconspicuous plasma cells. Intermediate degrees of such reactivity were assigned progressive values from 2 to 4.

Syncytial histiocytosis (Syn H) refers to a reactive pattern which is similar to SH except that moderately prominent secondary follicles are seen in the cortex and plasma cell transformations are seen in the medullary cords. In addition, the sinusoidal histiocytes tend to have larger and more chromatic nuclei, and the cytoplasm is less distinct and less eosinophilic than is seen in SH. The Syn H pattern has also been found in previous studies to be prognostically favorable. In the present study, Syn H was classified for each lymph node as present or absent.

On the basis of the above observations, individual cases could be characterized according to the maximal SH grade (SH_{max}) of any of their lymph nodes and as positive or negative in regard to Syn H. The SH and Syn H reactions were also combined in an adjusted value by considering a positive Syn H reading as equivalent to a 4 plus SH. The adjusted SH_{max} values represent the highest value observed in any of the lymph nodes in terms of SH and Syn H reactivity. The degree of such reactivity, in the total lymph node sample of a particular patient or series of patients, was recorded in terms of the average value (SH_{av}) and the relative frequency of particular degrees of adjusted SH reactivity in the total lymph node population, viz., number of nodes having adjusted SH ≥ 2 over the total number of nodes examined.

As used in this paper, the designation "in situ carcinoma" refers to atypical proliferations of ductular epithelium which are conventionally recognized by pathologists as indicative of malignancy. No areas of extraductal invasion or lymph node metastases were present in any of these cases.

---

* Fifteen of the 33 cases were obtained from the Surgical Pathology files of the Flower and Fifth Avenue Hospitals. Eight cases were from a series previously studied through the courtesy of Dr. H. D. Moon, Professor and Chairman, Department of Pathology, School of Medicine, University of California. Seven cases were kindly provided by Dr. V. Palladino, Director of Laboratories, Meadowbrook Hospital. The remaining three cases were seen through the courtesy of Dr. S. C. Sommers, Director of Laboratories, Lenox Hill Hospital.

In keeping with our findings in a previous study, we have subdivided the in situ carcinoma cases into two subgroups, viz., lobular carcinoma in situ and non-lobular carcinoma in situ. *Lobular carcinoma in situ* includes those cases wherein malignant changes are found in the intralobular ducts. As a rule, the extralobular ducts also show varying degrees of atypia. *Nonlobular carcinoma in situ* includes those cases having in situ malignant changes in their extralobular ducts but which are lacking intralobular malignancy, as exemplified by comedo carcinoma, papillary adenocarcinoma, and Paget's disease. Further details regarding the structural features of in situ carcinoma may be found in Part I of this article (see pp. 185-200).

Results

Lymph nodes draining in situ carcinomas of the breast display all the structural changes which are observed in lymph nodes draining invasive breast carcinoma. In both series, it is only a small minority of cases which fail to show some alterations from the structural characteristics of control lymph nodes. In both the in situ and invasive cancer series, the most frequently observed changes are in the sinusoidal histiocytes. Such changes take the form of reactive changes (SH and/or Syn H) and degenerative changes (degenerative SH, sinus hyalinization, and fibrosis). In contrast, follicular hyperplasia and extensive plasma cell transformations are infrequent in both the in situ and invasive cancer cases.

Despite the similarity in the types of lymph node changes seen in the in situ and invasive series, the in situ cancer series shows a distinctly greater incidence of SH and Syn H reactivity. The detailed findings in the lymph nodes of patients with in situ carcinoma are presented in Tables 5 and 6, while Tables 7 and 8 summarize

Table 5.   Reactivity of Lymph Nodes Draining In Situ Lobular Carcinoma

CASE	SH_{max}	SYN H	ADJUSTED SH_{max}	ADJUSTED SH_{av}	ADJUSTED SH_{max} $\geqslant 2$/No.	$\geqslant 3$/No.
1045-68	2	—	2	1.2	1/5	0/5
1479-68	4	+	4	2.2	7/14	6/14
4188-65	3	—	3	2.7	4/6	4/6
M-1283-57	3	—	3	1.4	2/11	2/11
M-125-67	1	+	4	4.0	4/4	4/4
4289-65	5	—	5	4.7	4/4	4/4
2155-68	3	—	3	1.8	7/12	3/12
3598-68	4	+	4	3.7	11/11	10/11
C-214742	4	+	4	3.1	11/15	11/15
5028-61	2	—	2	2.0	2/2	2/2
6197-60	3	—	3	2.1	6/8	3/8
1354-67	4	—	4	1.6	6/13	2/13
2289-67	2	—	2	1.1	2/20	0/20
361-68	2	+	4	1.6	3/20	2/20
4689-62	5	—	5	2.3	11/17	8/17
M-1379-51	3	+	4	2.0	2/5	2/5
2480-66	1	+	4	1.6	2/10	2/10
Average	3.0	7/17	3.5	2.3	48%	37%

Table 6. Reactivity of Lymph Nodes Draining In Situ Nonlobular Carcinoma

CASE	SH$_{max}$	SYN H	ADJUSTED SH$_{max}$	ADJUSTED SH$_{av}$	ADJUSTED SH$_{max}$ ≥ 2/No.	ADJUSTED SH$_{max}$ ≥ 3/No.
2260-68	1	+	4	1.3	2/14	2/14
2822-67	1	—	1	1.0	0/13	0/13
M-1402-67	4	+	4	2.6	11/14	6/14
M-3918-65	1	+	4	2.9	5/8	5/8
M-1388-49	1	—	1	1.0	0/5	0/5
M-1090-57	1	—	1	1.0	0/14	0/14
L-4242-68	5	+	3	3.3	6/7	5/7
L-5897-67	2	+	4	1.5	7/18	1/18
L-153138	1	+	4	1.4	1/8	1/8
C-246028	3	—	3	1.2	2/17	1/17
C-203647	1	+	4	1.2	1/17	1/17
C-064513	1	—	1	1.0	0/9	0/9
C-108788	1	—	1	1.0	0/10	0/10
C-185779	4	—	4	1.7	5/10	1/10
C-145323	4	+	4	2.2	5/11	5/11
C-154877	1	—	1	1.0	0/12	0/12
Average	2.0	8/16	2.9	1.6	24%	15%

Table 7. Percent Distribution of Adjusted SH$_{max}$ Values in Axillary Lymph Nodes

Group	ADJUSTED SH$_{max}$* 1	2	3	≥ 4	MEAN	PERCENT NODES ≥ 2	≥ 3
In Situ (33)	18	9	15	58	3.2	36	26
Lobular (17)	—	17	24	59	3.5	48	37
Non Lobular (16)	38	—	6	56	2.9	24	15
Invasive (55)	49	11	13	27	2.2	15	6
Class I (32)	48	9	9	34	2.3	21	9
Class II (23) †	53	13	17	17	2.0	10	3

* As judged by Chi square procedure, the distribution in the in situ group differs significantly from that of the invasive group (p < 0.005). The differences between the lobular and nonlobular groups and the Class I versus Class II groups are not statistically significant with the sample size available.
† Reactivity of lymph nodes without metastatic replacement.

Table 8. Percent Distribution of Adjusted SH$_{av}$ Values in Axillary Lymph Nodes

Group	ADJUSTED SH$_{av}$* < 1.5	1.5-2.4	≥ 2.5	MEAN
In Situ (33)	40	36	24	2.0
Lobular (17)	18	53	29	2.3
Non Lobular (16)	62	19	19	1.6
Invasive (55)	77	21	2	1.3
Class I (32)	69	27	3	1.4
Class II (23) †	88	12	—	1.2

* As judged by the Chi square procedure, the distribution in the in situ group differs significantly from that of the invasive group (p < 0.001) as does the lobular from the non lobular group (p < 0.01). The differences between the Class I and Class II series are not significant (p < 0.20) for the sample size.
† Reactivity of lymph nodes without metastatic replacement.

the data and provide a comparison with the findings in the invasive cancer series. It is evident that the lymph nodes draining in situ carcinomas have a greater degree of SH reactivity than the nodes draining invasive breast cancers. Adjusted SH_{max} values ≥ 4 were found in 58 percent of the in situ series in contrast to 27 percent of the invasive cancer series. Conversely, 60 percent of the patients with invasive breast cancer had only minimal degrees of SH reactivity (< 3 plus) whereas only 27 percent of the patients with in situ carcinoma had similarly inadequate responses. The difference in SH reactivity is also reflected in the mean adjusted SH_{max} values and in the relative frequency of SH reactivity ≥ 2 plus and ≥ 3 plus among the total number of lymph nodes examined in the two series. The adjusted SH_{av} value, which provides an index of SH reactivity in the lymph node population, also discriminates between the in situ and invasive series. An adjusted SH_{av} value ≥ 2.5 was found in only 23 percent of the patients with invasive cancer but in 60 percent of the in situ cancer series.

Tables 7 and 8 also provide a comparison of the SH reactivity in the subgroups of the in situ and invasive cancer series. The data demonstrate that SH reactivity is greater in the lobular group of in situ carcinoma than in the nonlobular group and greater in the Class I invasive cases than in the Class II cases. Note that the SH reactivity indicated for the Class II cases was based on those lymph nodes without replacement by metastases. Inclusion of such involved nodes in the calculation of the adjusted SH_{av} value further depresses the mean value from 1.20 to 0.96. We would emphasize that, even in invasive breast cancer patients without axillary metastases, the SH reactivity was decidedly less than in the patients with in situ lobular carcinoma. The differences between the SH reactivity of the Class I series and the nonlobular carcinoma in situ series are in a similar direction but of a lesser degree.

A recent study suggested that carcinoma in one breast may provoke reactive changes in the heterolateral lymph nodes.[18] It is therefore pertinent to comment specifically on four of the patients with in situ carcinoma who also had malignant changes in the opposite breast (Table 9). While the small number of cases does not permit generalization, certain features are noteworthy. The SH reactivity in the lymph nodes draining the lobular in situ carcinoma was greater in a patient (M-

Table 9. Lymph Node Reactivity in Patients with In Situ Carcinoma in One Breast and a Second Carcinoma in the Opposite Breast

CASE	TUMOR	ADJUSTED SH_{max}	ADJUSTED SH_{av}	ADJUSTED SH$_{max}$ ≥ 2/No.	≥ 3/No.
M-125-67	Lobular in situ	4	4.0	4/4	4/4
M-125-67	Lobular in situ	No lymph nodes removed.			
2155-68	Lobular in situ	3	1.8	7/12	3/12
1963-68	Invasive, Cl. II plus lobular	3	0.6	1/38	1/38
2480-66	Mixed in situ	4	1.6	2/10	2/10
2948-68	Invasive, Cl. II	3	1.1	3/23	2/23
3598-66	Lobular in situ	4	3.7	11/11	10/11
———-65	Invasive cancer opposite breast one year before (slides unavailable for study).				

125-67) who had a simultaneous heterolateral lobular in situ carcinoma than in a patient (2155-68, 1963-68) who had a simultaneous invasive carcinoma in her opposite breast. The SH reactivity in the lymph nodes draining the in situ carcinomas was greater than that found in the heterolateral nodes which drained invasive carcinomas, which appeared simultaneously (2155-68, 1963-68), or subsequently (2480-66, 2948-68). In the patient with an in situ carcinoma (3598-66) detected one year after the resection of a heterolateral invasive carcinoma, the SH reactivity of the lymph nodes draining the in situ lesion was greater than the average for the invasive or in situ series. While we have been unable to obtain slides of the original tumor and lymph nodes which were resected elsewhere, it is known that this patient is clinically free of disease at this time (August, 1968).

Comments

The present study demonstrates that in situ carcinoma resembles invasive breast cancer in regard to the types of change induced in the draining axillary lymph nodes. As judged by such lymph node reactivity, tumor-L-RE interactions are initiated in the preinvasive phase of carcinogenesis. It is therefore pertinent to question whether the transition from in situ to invasive cancer might not be correlated with L-RE reactivity. In this connection, it is noteworthy that Carter and Gershon[21] have described a relationship between dissemination and lymph node reactivity in experimental transplantable lymphomas. Two similar-appearing lymphomas from a common source differed decisively in their ability to metastasize and in their effect on lymph node structure. One variant grew locally but did not establish metastatic foci, despite the presence of circulating tumor cells in blood and lymph. The other variant developed widespread metastases. The nonmetastasizing lymphoma was regularly associated with a distinctive proliferation of sinus histiocytes in the regional nodes, a reaction which was absent in the nodes of hamsters bearing the metastasizing tumor.

Anastassiades and Pryce[19] have suggested that many potential tumors may be killed immunologically in inceptio, a phenomenon which would depend on the development of antigenicity in preinvasive malignancies against which the L-RE system would react. It is therefore noteworthy that prognostically favorable lymph node reactions are less frequent in patients with invasive carcinoma than in patients with in situ carcinoma. In the lobular in situ carcinoma group, the adjusted SH_{av} was 2.3, and 83 percent of the cases showed an adjusted $SH_{max} \geq 3$ plus. These values are superior to those found in Class I cases of invasive carcinoma, viz., 1.3 and 40 percent, respectively. Such data are at least consistent with the possibility that L-RE reactivity may impede the transformation from in situ to invasive carcinoma.

However, if preinvasive carcinomas uniformly incite a tumor-antagonistic response in the host L-RE system, then whence the development of invasive carcinoma? In a recent editorial, Old and Boyse[22] have discussed mechanisms whereby the development of clinical cancer might occur despite antigenicity of the tumor cells. The most direct mechanism would be a tumor growth potential which exceeded the controlling capacity of the immune response. The other devices which they suggest involve either impairment of the immunologic responsiveness or alterations in the antigenicity of the cancer cells. Diminution in immunologic responsiveness may occur via nonspecific immunosuppression, immunologic tolerance, or immunologic enhancement, while altered antigenicity may occur by immunoselection or antigenic modulation. It is appropriate to consider the implication of some of these alternatives in terms of the lymph node patterns encountered in patients bearing in situ and invasive breast cancer.

An appreciable percentage of patients with advanced cancer do exhibit impairment of their ability to develop circulating antibodies and delayed hypersensitivity and also show depressed homograft rejection.[23] However, immunologic competence does not appear to be impaired in patients with more localized disease. Thus, there is no evidence that the transition from preinvasive to invasive carcinoma is dependent on a generalized loss of the host immunologic competence.

Immunologic tolerance presumes that the tumor antigen is treated as self by virtue of exposure of the host to the antigen before the development of immunologic competence. In such circumstances, the lymph nodes would be indifferent to the developing and progressively growing tumor. However, our observations and those of Anastassiades and Pryce[19] show that in only some 10 percent of breast cancer patients are the axillary lymph nodes devoid of reactive or degenerative changes. Such findings are inconsistent with a state of tolerance.

Immunologic enhancement refers to the experimental observation that the rejection of tumor transplants can be impaired by antisera against isoantigens of the tumor. Since this phenomenon depends on the production of circulating antibodies against the tumor antigens, there should be some reflection of such activity in the draining lymph nodes, viz., secondary follicles and plasma cell transformations. As indicated above, such patterns are uncommon in lymph nodes draining breast cancer except for the medullary cancers wherein the survival is better than average. As judged by axillary lymph node structure, it is highly improbable that either immunologic tolerance or enhancement are critically involved in the development of invasive carcinoma of the human breast.

The observed lymph node structure also limits the assumption that invasive cancer cells lack antigenicity. In theory, immunoselection would lead either to total elimination of antigenic cancer cells or to the survival of those cells having minimal antigenicity. If antigenicity were reduced to a minimal level, then minimal L-RE response would be expected, an expectation not found in fact. If, however, the residual antigenicity provoked L-RE responsiveness, then the phenomenon becomes a variant of the direct mechanism of tumor growth potential "breaking through" an immunologic barrier. It is noteworthy that only this mechanism leads to the expectation of reactive and degenerative lymph nodes and thus corresponds with the actual observations in both in situ and invasive breast cancer.

The spectrum of changes in lymph nodes draining in situ as well as invasive cancers suggests that SH reactivity becomes transformed with time to degenerative vacuolization, hyalinization, fibrosis, and lymphoid atrophy. This interpretation is favored by Anastassiades and Pryce[19] who point out the similarity between the degenerative changes in cancer-draining lymph nodes and antigenically overstimulated nodes. We are certainly in accord with such a possibility and have so stated in previous publications.[11, 17, 18] However, the present data also suggest the additional possibility that some tumor "antigens" might produce degenerative changes in draining lymph nodes in a more direct fashion than the transitional changes suggested above.

The designation "in situ or preinvasive carcinoma" includes a wide diversity of atypical proliferations in various divisions of the branching duct system. Furthermore, the intrinsic appearance of any particular focus is not per se readily correlated with its ability to invade. In recognition of the constellation of lobular and nonlobular intraductal changes and the uncertainty regarding their biologic behavior, we suggested the term "incipient carcinoma" (see p. 198). The present study demonstrates that the heterogeneity of ductular changes in incipient carcinoma is associated with heterogeneity of lymph node reactivity. Furthermore the data suggest some correlation between the type of ductular change and the lymph node response. Thus, the subgroup classified as in situ lobular carcinoma had a greater degree of SH reactivity than the nonlobular carcinoma group.

The differences between SH reactivity of lymph nodes draining in situ lobular carcinomas and those draining nonlobular in situ carcinomas deserves some additional comment. As defined above, the lobular in situ series includes all cases having malignant transformation of their intralobular ducts. It includes those cases wherein the malignant changes are predominantly found in the intralobular ducts (nine cases) as well as a mixed group having prominent malignant changes in the extralobular ducts (eight cases). It is thus possible to divide the in situ cancers into three subgroups, viz., nonlobular, mixed, and lobular. Table 10 provides a com-

Table 10. Reactivity of Lymph Nodes Draining Different Types of In Situ Carcinoma

| Group | Number | ADJUSTED | | PERCENT ADJUSTED SH_{max} | |
		SH_{max}	SH_{av}	$\geqslant 2/No.$	$\geqslant 3/No.$
Nonlobular	16	2.9	1.3	24	15
Mixed	8	3.5	1.8	35	22
Lobular	9	3.5	2.7	62	54

parison of the SH reactivity found in these three groups of in situ carcinoma. These data emphasize the difference between the nonlobular and the lobular group and demonstrate that the reactivity in the mixed group is intermediate between the lobular and nonlobular groups. It thus appears that different types of in situ malignancy differ in their effects on draining lymph nodes. It is not clear, however, whether the observed differences reflect differences in amount or type of tumor antigens.

While the various observations do not define the modus operandi of tumor-L-RE interactions, they do emphasize the reality and complexity of the phenomenon. More importantly, they suggest new directions for investigation. It would be of no small interest if one could isolate fractions from lobular carcinoma in situ which could induce SH reactivity in lymph nodes, or fractions from nonlobular in situ lesions which caused degenerative lymph node changes. Such data would be most pertinent to experimental attempts to control cancer immunologically. If invasive cancers contain fractions which have L-RE depressing activity, attempts to "immunize with antigen" derived from invasive breast cancer might depress rather than stimulate L-RE reactivity.

It also appears that antigenic stimulation of most breast cancer patients would be of limited therapeutic value in view of the frequency of degenerative changes in their lymph nodes. Such patients are probably already overstimulated. Nevertheless, the routine, so-called "prophylactic use of cytotoxic agents or ionizing irradiation," might constitute a hazard to the minority of patients where L-RE reactivity seems to exert a significant tumor-antagonistic influence.[24] However, it is also possible that appropriately dosed chemotherapy might be a particularly useful adjunct in some patients having host reactivity. Precedent for such expectation is found in regard to the favorable results of chemotherapy of choriocarcinoma of pregnancy and Burkitt's tumor. In any case, there is a need to collect clinical data on the relationship between chemical and radiation therapy and the lymph node reactivity.

While the available data seem to impose limitations on immunologic approaches to the control of breast cancer, they do not negate this possibility. Rather, they direct attention to the importance of a hitherto neglected aspect, the in situ phase. The application of modern immunologic techniques to the problem of the tumor-host relationship in preinvasive breast cancer might well yield practical as well as conceptual dividends. We would emphasize the importance of focusing attention on human breast cancer and monitoring such studies by detailed microscopic examinations of the primary tumor and regional lymph nodes. Immunologic studies of experimentally induced animal tumors or cancer cells growing in tissue culture may delineate biologic potentialities and aid the development of technical procedures. To that end such studies are of interest; however, it remains to be proven what relationship, if any, such studies have to human cancer. There is a present need to coordinate the disciplines of immunology, epidemiology, and biochemistry with pathology in a concerted investigation of the biologic behavior of *human* cancer.

In Part I we suggested that incipient carcinomas correspond to "minimal deviation" neoplasms and as such are worthy of detailed biologic and biochemical investigations. The present study indicates that incipient carcinomas of the breast may also be uniquely useful in providing information regarding the role of the L-RE system in the development and behavior of human cancer.

References

1. Foote, F.W., and Stewart, F.W. Comparative studies of cancerous versus non cancerous breasts. II. Ann. Surg., 121:196, 1945.
2. Karpas, C.M., Leis, H.P., Oppenheim, A., and Mersheimer, W. Relationship of fibrocystic disease to carcinoma of the breast. Ann. Surg., 162:1, 1965.
3. Stein, A.A. Carcinoma in situ of the breast. *In* Pathology Annual 1967, Sommers, S.C. ed. New York, Appleton-Century-Crofts, 1967, Vol. 2, pp. 47-75.
4. Arstein, C. Uber Becherzellen und ihre Beziehung zur Fetteresorption in Sekretion. Arch. Mikrosk. Anat., 39:527, 1847.
5. Andrew, W., and Collins, C.K. Lymphocytes within cells of intestinal epithelium in man. Anat. Rec., 96:445, 1946.
6. Humble, J.G., Jayne, W.H.W., and Pulvertaft, R.J.V. Biological interaction between lymphocytes and other cells. Brit. J. Haematol., 2:283, 1956.
7. Trowell, O.A. The lymphocyte. Internat. Rev. Cytol., 7:235, 1958.
8. Berenblum, I. The two stage mechanism of carcinogenesis as an analytical tool.

In Cellular Control Mechanisms and Cancer, Muhlbock, O., and Emmelot, P., eds. Amsterdam, Elsevier Press, Inc., 1964, pp. 259-267.

9. Lilienfeld, A.M., and Lewis, M.L. Some factors involved in the incidence of breast cancer. Proceedings of the Third National Cancer Conference. J.B. Lippincott Co., 1956, Philadelphia, pp. 105-112.

10. Farber, E. On the concept of minimal deviation in the study of the biochemistry of cancer. Cancer Res., 28:1210, 1968.

11. Black, M.M., and Speer, F.D. Immunology of cancer. Surg. Gynec. Obstet., 109:105, 1959.

12. ———— and Speer, F.D. Sinus histiocytosis of lymph nodes in cancer. Surg. Gynec. Obstet., 106:163, 1958.

13. ———— and Speer, F.D. Lymph node reactivity in cancer patients. Surg. Gynec. Obstet., 110:477, 1960.

14. Cutler, S.J., Black, M.M., and Goldenberg, I.S. Prognostic factors in cancer of the female breast. I. An investigation of some interrelations. Cancer, 16:1589, 1963.

15. ———— Black, M.M., Friedell, G.H., Vidone, R.A., and Goldenberg, I.S. Prognostic factors in cancer of the female breast. II. Reproducibility of histopathologic classification. Cancer, 19:75, 1966.

16. Masse, L., Masse, C., and Chassaigne, J.P. Le prognostic des cancers du sein en function de la surcharge en histiocytes des sinus des ganglions axillaires. Mem. Acad. Chir., 86:940, 1960.

17. Black, M.M. Reactivity of the lymphreticuloendothelial system in human cancer. Prog. Clin. Cancer. New York, Grune & Stratton, Inc. 1965, pp. 26-49.

18. ———— and Asire, A.J. Palpable axillary lymph nodes in breast cancer. Structural and biological considerations. Cancer, in press.

19. Anastassiades, O. Th., and Pryce, D.M. Immunological significance of the morphological changes in lymph nodes draining breast cancer. Brit. J. Cancer, 20:239, 1966.

20. Farber, E. On the concept of minimal deviation in the study of the biochemistry of cancer. Cancer Res., 28:1210, 1968.

21. Carter, R.L., and Gershon, R.R. Studies on transplantable lymphomas in hamsters. I. Histologic responses in lymphoid tissues and their relationship to metastases. Amer. J. Path., 49:637, 1960.

22. Old, L.L., and Boyse, E.A. Prospects for immunotherapy of human cancer. Ann. Intern. Med., 69:393, 1968.

23. Southam, C.M. Summary: Evaluation of immunologic capability of cancer patients. Cancer Res., 28:1455, 1968.

24. Schwartz, R.S. Are immunosuppressive anticancer drugs self-defeating? Cancer Res., 28:1452, 1968.

SOFT TISSUE TUMORS:
Aids in Differential Diagnosis

GERALD FINE
ROBERT C. HORN, JR.

Controversy concerning the classification of primary soft tissue tumors has existed for years and can perhaps be most simply stated as a division between two schools, the "splitters" and the "lumpers." The grossest sort of lumping—classifying sarcomas as of spindle or round or polymorphous cell type—is fortunately now almost extinct. This change, which has been slow to evolve, has resulted from the study of groups of soft tissue tumors correlating cytologic features and microscopic growth patterns with biologic behavior. Such studies have been invaluable in terms of limbs saved from amputation for chondromyxoid fibroma of bone, atypical myositis ossificans, chondroblastoma of bone, fibromatosis, etc. At the same time, they have brought out the need for aggressive surgical attack upon extraosseous osteogenic sarcoma, myxoid liposarcoma, and small, circumscribed synovial sarcoma, among others. Further, there are indications that the most refined classification may become essential as chemotherapy is further developed and prhaps becomes specific for tumor cell type.

Despite the advances made in the classification of sarcomas, difficulties continue and uncertain diagnoses are numerous. This is well exemplified by the variety of diagnoses that can be obtained from various expert consultants in problem cases. Rather than discourage further efforts, the difficulties and uncertainties should serve to stimulate continued thorough study, not only by conventional methods, but with the addition of histochemical and enzymatic procedures as well as examination at the ultrastructural level.

The following discussion centers upon some of the problems we have encountered in the microscopic diagnosis of soft tissue tumors, emphasizing particularly those morphologic features and special techniques which we have found helpful in differential diagnosis.

In attempting to classify soft tissue tumors, every conceivable diagnostic possibility must be considered, including not only primary mesenchymal tumors but also tumors of nerve and nerve sheath origin, as well as those epithelial tumors which may mimic sarcomas, e.g., hypernephroid tumors of the kidney, malignant melanoma, etc. Also, the importance of sampling many different areas of any given tumor cannot be overemphasized. Even with the greatest care, there will be instances where a tumor's classification may be found at a later date to have been incorrect. This occurs most often when study is limited to small biopsy fragments in which histogenetically different tumors may manifest histologic similarity but where the opportunity to search for telltale differences in other portions of the tumor is lacking.

A closely related problem centers about the biopsy diagnosis of malignant mesenchymoma—the soft part tumor composed of cells differentiating into two or more different tissues, or unrelated tumor types (exclusive of fibrosarcoma, since all the mesenchymal tumors may have a fibrosarcomatous component).[26] The recognition of a second (or third, etc.) type of sarcoma upon examination of a complete tumor, recurrence, or metastasis following biopsy diagnosis of a different type of sarcoma may indicate that the tumor in question is a mesenchymoma rather than that the initial classification was incorrect. Furthermore, many, and perhaps all, of the soft tissue sarcomas may be composed in part of cells so primitive that their destined direction of differentiation can only be surmised by finding more differentiated companion cells. It is perfectly conceivable that such primitive cells, in some tumors at least, are uncommitted, and have the potentiality of differentiating into multiple tumor forms.

Extraosseous Osteogenic Sarcoma

The microscopic variations of this group of tumors are similar to those of osteogenic sarcomas arising in bone. They range from the overtly bone or osteoid forming tumor to those corresponding to the cellular lytic variety of osteogenic sarcoma (Fig. 1). Problems in diagnosis are not with the former but with those at the opposite end of the spectrum, where osteoid formation may be very subtle. Here, its only indication may be the entrapment of round or polygonal cells within an intensely eosinophilic, poorly fibrillar tissue which may or may not have cells aligned at its periphery. The cellular areas may be purely spindle-celled with varying amounts of collagen and little or abundant eosin-staining cytoplasm, with extensions of varying length, or they may have a mixed population of spindle and polygonal cells. The latter may be gigantic—mononuclear or multinuclear—the multinucleated forms having uniform nuclei and appearing identical with osteoclasts (Fig. 2). These multinucleated cells have proven helpful in the differential diagnosis of soft tissue sarcomas, since we have not observed them in tumors other than osteogenic sarcoma, giant cell tumor, and fibrous xanthoma.

Among the malignant tumors from which the osteogenic sarcoma must be distinguished are fibrosarcoma, rhabdomyosarcoma, and mesenchymoma.[5, 10, 26] The

5. Fine, G., and Stout, A.P. Osteogenic sarcoma of the extraskeletal soft tissue. Cancer, 9:1027, 1956.
6. Fisher, E.R. Histochemical observations on an alveolar soft-part sarcoma with reference to histogenesis. Amer. J. Path., 32:721, 1956.
7. Gray, G.F., Jr., Gonzalez-Licea, A., Hartmann, W.H., and Woods, A.C., Jr. Angiosarcoma in lymphedema: An unusual case of Stewart-Treves syndrome. Bull. Hopkins Hosp., 119:117, 1966.
8. Hamperl, H., and Lattes, R. Study of argyrophilia of nonchromaffin paragangliomas and granular cell myoblastomas. Cancer, 10:408, 1957.
9. Hiramoto, R., Jurandowski, J., Bernecky, J., and Pressman, D. Immunochemical differentiation of rhabdomyosarcoma. Cancer Res., 21:383, 1961.
10. Horn, R.C., and Enterline, H.T. Rhabdomyosarcoma: A clinocopathological study and classification of 39 cases. Cancer, 11:181, 1958.
11. Hutter, R.V.P., Stewart, F.W., and Foote, F.W., Jr. Fasciitis. A report of 70 cases with follow-up proving the benignity of the lesion. Cancer, 15:992, 1962.
12. Kauffmann, S.L., and Stout, A.P. Histiocytic tumors (fibrous xanthoma and histiocytoma) in children. Cancer, 14:469, 1961.
13. Kroll, A.J., Kuwabara, T., and Howard, G.M. Electron microscopy of a rhabdomyosarcoma of the orbit. Assoc. of Research and Ophthalmology, Investigative Ophthalmology, 2:523, 1963.
14. Landers, J.W., Chason, J.L., Gonzalez, J.E., and Palutke, W. Morphology and enzymatic activity of rat cerebral capillaries. Lab. Invest., 11:1253, 1962.
15. Marshall, R.B., and Horn, R.C. Nonchromaffin paraganglioma. A comparative study. Cancer, 14:779, 1961.
16. Morales, A.R., and Fine G. Lymphangiosarcoma in postmastectomy lymphedema. An electron microscopic and histochemical study. In preparation.
17. Pineda, A. Electron microscopy of the lemmocyte in peripheral nerve tumors (neurolemmomas). J. Neurol., 25:35, 1966.
18. Price, E.B., Jr., Silliphant, W.M., and Shuman, R. Nodular fasciitis: A clinicopathologic analysis of 65 cases. Amer. J. Clin. Path., 35:122, 1961.
19. Shipkey, F.H., Liberman, P.H., Foote, F.W., Jr., and Stewart, F.W. Ultrastructure of alveolar soft part sarcoma. Cancer, 17:821, 1964.
20. Smetana, H.F., and Scott, W.F., Jr. Malignant tumors of nonchromaffin paraganglia. Milit. Surg., 109:330, 1951.
21. Soule, E.H. Proliferative (nodular) fasciitis. Arch. Path., 73:437, 1962.
22. Stewart, F.W., and Treves, N. Lymphangiosarcoma in postmastectomy lymphedema. A report of six cases in elephantiasis chirurgica. Cancer, 1:64, 1948.
23. Stobbe, G.D., and Dargeon, H.W. Embryonal rhabdomyosarcoma of head and neck in children and adolescents. Cancer, 31:826, 1950.
24. Stout, A.P. Hemangio-endothelioma: A tumor of blood vessels featuring vascular endothelial cells. Ann. Surg., 118:445, 1943.
25. ———— Liposarcoma—the malignant tumor of lipoblasts. Ann. Surg., 119:86, 1944.
26. ———— Mesenchymoma—the mixed tumor of mesenchymal derivations. Ann. Surg., 127:278, 1948.
27. ———— Myxoma—the tumor of primitive mesenchyme. Ann. Surg., 127:706, 1948.
28. ———— Hemangiopericytoma (a study of 25 new cases). Cancer, 2:1027, 1949.
29. ———— and Verner, E.W. Chondrosarcoma of the extraskeletal soft tissues. Cancer, 6:581, 1953.
30. Winslow, D.J., and Enzinger, F.M. Hyaluronidase-sensitive acid mucopolysaccharides in liposarcomas. Amer. J. Path., 37:497, 1960.

TUMORS OF THE EXTRAHEPATIC BILIARY SYSTEM

GEORGE F. GRAY, JR.
ROBERT W. McDIVITT

Tumors of the gallbladder and bile ducts present numerous problems to clinicians and pathologists. The close proximity of the biliary tract to the liver, pancreas, and ampulla and the nearly identical histology of cancers arising in these organs often makes identification of the source of tumors difficult. Furthermore, benign neoplasms and various tumor-like conditions may be confused with cancer. Finally, the difficulties in making early diagnoses and the limitations of present methods of therapy are reflected by high mortality rates of biliary carcinomas.

The biliary duct system, liver, and pancreas develop from the *hepatic diverticulum,* a ventral outgrowth of gut endoderm. Although anomalies of development are fairly common, the extrahepatic biliary system usually consists of a right and left hepatic duct which emerge from the liver, join, and form the *common hepatic duct.* The common hepatic duct is about 4 cm in length and 0.5 cm wide. The *gallbladder,* a sac 7 to 10 cm long, about 2.5 cm in greatest diameter, with a capacity of about 30 to 35 cc, is connected to the common hepatic duct by a narrow and somewhat tortuous 4 cm long *cystic duct.* The cystic and common hepatic ducts join to form the *common bile duct,* a structure 7 cm in length, which in turn empties into the duodenum. The distal common duct passes immediately posterior to the head of the pancreas and may be joined by the pancreatic ducts just proximal to the ampulla.

The epithelium of the entire biliary system is of tall columnar type, usually thrown into folds and ridges, particularly in the gallbladder (Fig. 1). These mucosal folds become accentuated by edema. A rather thin muscularis normally surrounds the ducts and gallbladder, but it may become markedly thickened in chronic inflammatory disorders or with calculi. A dense connective tissue layer forms an

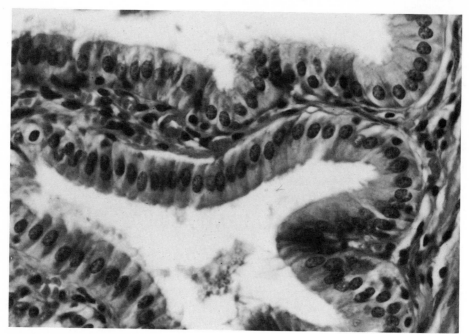

Fig. 1. Normal biliary mucosa. The epithelium is tall columnar with uniform basally located nuclei. H&E. X400.

adventitia external to the muscularis. Since the function of the biliary system is transport of bile from liver to duodenum, disturbance of this function by such abnormalities as tumor, calculus, or stricture may cause jaundice, pain, or alteration of alimentary function.

Cancer of the Gallbladder and Bile Ducts

INCIDENCE.   Most clinically significant tumors of the biliary tract are carcinomas. Biliary cancer is less common than carcinoma of the colon, stomach, esophagus, or pancreas, but it is more frequent than primary cancer of the small intestine or liver.[33] The incidence is more difficult to determine than that of tumors in many other sites because of the nonspecific morphology and difficulty of separation from cancers originating in the pancreas, ampulla, pylorus, or even other parts of the gastrointestinal tract; however, published reports include more than 4,000 biliary cancers.

From a group of 4,821 patients who had biliary operations, Thorbjarnarson and Glenn[69] reported 147 cancers, including 26 ampullary carcinomas and 90 (1.9 percent of cases) carcinomas of the gallbladder. Ochsner and Ochsner[49] found 20 gallbladder cancers in 1,523 cholecystectomies (1.3 percent of cases); Balagero[5] reported an identical incidence, 11 biliary tract cancers in 789 operations. Earlier, Strauch,[65] from reports by various authors, collected 482 gallbladder carcinomas in 34,242 biliary operations (1.4 percent of cases). Tumors may occur in all parts of the gallbladder but are most frequently in the largest part, the fundus.[69]

Bile duct carcinomas appear to be less frequent than gallbladder carcinomas. Thorbjarnarson and Glenn[69] found only 31 (0.6 percent of cases) in 4,821 biliary operations, as opposed to 90 gallbladder carcinomas. Salmon[57] found 83 cholecystic cancers, but only 60 duct cancers among 586 malignant tumors of the pancreas and biliary tree. While primary carcinomas occur throughout the duct system, there appears to be a slight predilection for the bifurcation of the right and left hepatic ducts and for the junction of the cystic, hepatic, and common bile ducts. In some instances, however, tumors do not appear to be well localized.[35] Thus, in 173 bile duct tumors, Braasch[10] and his associates found 57 in the hepatic ducts, 62 in the distal common bile duct, 27 at the junction of the cystic, hepatic, and common bile ducts, and 27 which were spread throughout the entire system. A similar distribution has been observed by others.[12] Tumors of the distal common duct are easily confused with tumors arising in the head of the pancreas or ampulla.

AGE.   About half the patients with gallbladder cancer are in the seventh decade.[69] Although gallbladder cancer has been reported in the third[40] and fourth decades, it is infrequent before age 50 and after age 80.[65] The age distribution of patients with bile duct carcinoma is similar. Pallette[51] found the average age for gallbladder cancer was 65.3 years, for duct cancer 67.5 years.

SEX.   Gallbladder carcinomas are three times more common in women than in men. For example, Strauch[65] found, in a review of 1,016 cases, 75.3 percent in women and only 24.7 percent in men. However, there is little sex difference in incidence of biliary duct carcinomas.[57, 66]

Clinical Presentation

The similarity in presentation of cancer and calculus has been repeatedly emphasized.[9, 10, 17, 33, 40, 65] Pain is the most frequent symptom of cholecystic carcinoma. Weight loss and jaundice are the next most common complaints, followed by symptoms of digestive dysfunction such as bloating, flatulence, anorexia, and food intolerance. Abdominal swelling or a mass is an uncommon initial symptom, but a palpable gallbladder or a right upper quadrant mass is frequently found with advanced tumors. Hydrops of the gallbladder may result from cystic duct tumors.[50] Mild icterus detected chemically is more frequent than marked jaundice.[69] Patients with gallbladder cancers, particularly those associated with gallstones, frequently have a long history of symptoms of cholecystic disease. Persistence of symptoms referable to the biliary tract following cholecystectomy may indicate bile duct or pancreatic cancer.[7, 18, 54] On the other hand, gallbladder carcinoma presented as acute cholecystitis[68] in 11 percent of 90 cases, presumably because of obstruction of the gallbladder neck or cystic duct. One cystic duct cancer presented as gallbladder perforation.[52] Rapid onset of jaundice is more commonly a symptom of bile duct carcinoma, since these ducts may be obstructed by relatively small tumors. Of 76 patients with duct cancers, 62 percent presented with jaundice and 58 percent complained of pain.[68] Radiographic changes diagnostic of carcinoma are infrequent, since in many cases the findings are indistinguishable from those of other forms of biliary tract disease.[16, 25, 44, 55] Gallbladders with calcification of the wall ("porcelain" gallbladder) are relatively frequent sites of carcinoma.[53]

Etiology and Pathogenesis

Calculus is frequently associated with biliary cancer, prompting speculation that stones may have a causative role in the development of cancer of the gallbladder and bile ducts. Stones are found much more consistently with cancers of the gallbladder than with carcinomas of the ducts, being associated with 72 to 90 percent of gallbladder cancers.[40, 65] Calculi tend to be found more frequently in females (90 percent) than in males (59 percent) with cholecystic cancer.[69] A study of 11,129 autopsies in Oslo,[70] 45 percent of the total deaths, revealed gallstone incidence of 19.5 percent—27.5 percent in women and 12.7 percent in men. In this group, there were 39 unequivocal and 7 probable cancers of gallbladder origin (0.4 percent of cases). Of the 39 definite cancers, 36 were in women and 34 had associated stones. Similar studies in the United States have suggested that a 45-year-old person with stones has a 1.4 percent chance of developing gallbladder cancer, and that a 65-year-old person with stones has a 0.44 percent chance.[47]

Although calculi are the most common disorder associated with bile duct carcinomas, they are found much less frequently than with gallbladder carcinoma. Although some[51] have found calculi in nearly half (46 percent) of duct cancers, others[71] have found them in as few as 18 percent. Since it is not always clear whether these stones were within the gallbladder or within the duct system, evidence of a possible etiologic relationship is slight.

There has been little attention given to the type of gallstones, i.e., bilirubin, cholesterol, mixed, etc., associated with cancer. Such a study might give clues to possible etiologic factors common to calculi and stones.

Carcinomas are reported to occur in approximately 2 percent of choledochal cysts.[4, 67] Although this cancer incidence is higher than in the general population, it is not so frequent as to suggest an etiologic relationship such as bile stasis.[42] No other disorders are regularly associated with biliary tract carcinoma. Liver disease may result from chronic obstruction but does not appear to predispose to the development of biliary tract cancer. Diabetes[71] was found in 10 percent of one group of patients with bile duct carcinoma, and cancers of other organs were present in 6 percent of one large group of patients with cholecystic carcinoma,[69] but these associations are not noted in other studies.

In India there is a higher incidence of biliary and hepatic cancers in the North than in the South; variations in diet have been suggested as the cause,[43] even though no specific agent has been implicated. Nutritional factors have also been suggested to explain the apparent rarity, not only of biliary cancer, but of biliary diseases among Negroes in Uganda, among whom only 22 cases of biliary tract disease including 6 cancers of the gallbladder (1 female, 5 males) were found in 61,000 hospital admissions.[60] Obviously, other social and economic factors besides diet could affect apparent differences in occurrence of biliary carcinoma in Africa, the United States, Norway, and various regions of India. We have not found evidence of racial or ethnic variations in biliary cancer in the United States; there is specifically no indication that formation of gallstones early in life in patients with hemolytic disorders, which are common in American Negroes, leads to either increased or early development of biliary cancer.

Experimental Carcinogenesis

Experimental induction of biliary cancers has chiefly resulted from application of known carcinogenic chemicals or implantation of gallstones into laboratory animals. Methylcholanthrene, which is carcinogenic in many sites in a variety of experimental animals, has caused carcinoma when implanted into the gallbladders of cats and dogs.[29, 30] The cats developed invasive carcinoma with metastases 23 to 32 months after implantation, and one of five dogs had papillary adenocarcinoma in multiple sites of the biliary tree after 58 months. Another dog which did not have frank cancer had a diffuse papillary hyperplasia of the biliary epithelium. Aramite, another experimental carcinogen, caused adenocarcinomas of the intrahepatic and extrahepatic bile ducts, gallbladder, and ampulla of Vater in 15 of 19 dogs given this material orally.[64] Carcinogenesis required 38 to 101 months. These dogs also developed cirrhosis but neither calculi nor hepatocellular carcinoma was observed.

Foreign bodies such as glass beads or cholesterol pellets failed to induce carcinoma when introduced into the gallbladders of guinea pigs; however, the guinea pig does not appear to be a particularly susceptible animal, since methylcholanthrene produced only moderate epithelial dysplasia but not carcinoma.[22]

Three of 186 cats that had gallstones from cancer patients implanted in the gallbladder eventually developed carcinoma. However, the lack of suitable controls and the rather low incidence of cancer make evaluation of these experiments difficult.[31, 32]

Pathology

Adenocarcinoma is the predominant histologic type, comprising 85 percent or more of gallbladder and duct carcinomas. Variant forms include epidermoid carcinomas, which make up to 10 percent in some reports, and anaplastic carcinomas. The typical adenocarcinoma is composed of acini or tubules, frequently with papillary processes, which are lined by columnar epithelium often closely resembling normal biliary tract mucosa (Figs. 2, 3). Varying degrees of nuclear atypia may be present (Figs. 4, 5), but most carcinomas are well differentiated and are not usually characterized by a predominance of bizarre cell forms or abundant mitotic figures. Less frequently, the glandular or tubular pattern is partially or completely lost and the tumor grows in solid sheets or strands (Fig. 6). Biliary tract carcinomas may have a mixture of glandular and epidermoid features, similar to the pattern frequently seen with bronchogenic carcinoma (Fig. 7). In our own material, a glandular pattern is seen in all instances, although some of the tumors have epidermoid foci. Intercellular bridges may be seen, but keratinization is uncommon in biliary carcinoma. Vascular and perineural involvement is common and, when present, is a useful diagnostic feature (Figs. 8, 9). Mucin is frequently seen in tumors but also may be prominent in cholecystitis (Fig. 10).

Although scarring and thickening of the wall with diminution of the lumen may be the only gross characteristics of gallbladder or bile duct carcinoma, some gallbladder cancers protrude into the lumen as a solid or papillary tumor. Rarely a papillary growth on the mucosal surface without evidence of gross infiltration of

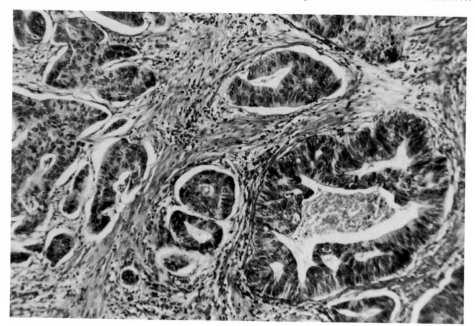

Fig. 2.   Adenocarcinoma. This is a typical well-differentiated adenocarcinoma of gallbladder. There is infiltration of the muscularis. H&E. X100.

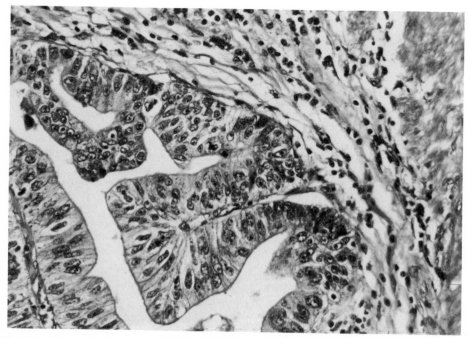

Fig. 3.   Cholecystic carcinoma. There is moderate pleomorphism and loss of basal orientation of nuclei. In the upper left is a papillary projection of epithelium without stroma.
H&E. X400.

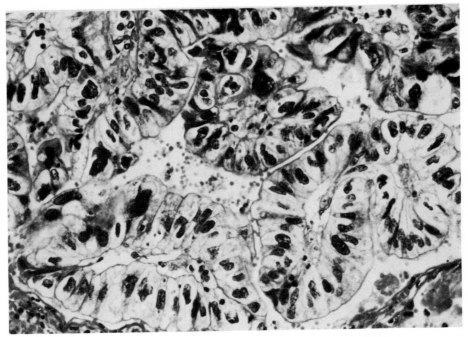

Fig. 4. Adenocarcinoma. The columnar cell shape persists despite rather marked nuclear pleomorphism. There is focal mucin production. H&E. X400.

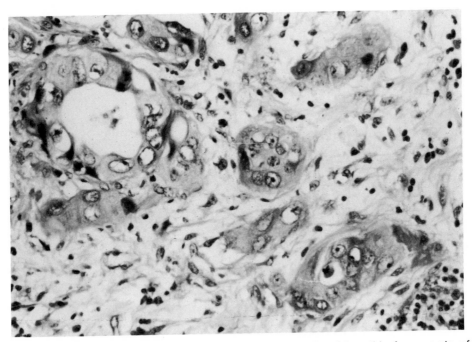

Fig. 5. Adenocarcinoma of bile duct. Definite atypia distinguishes this from crypts of normal epithelium (Fig. 12), but an acinar pattern remains. H&E. X250.

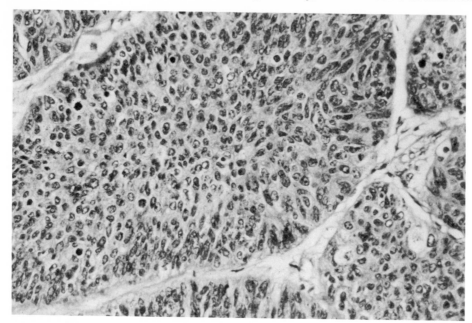

Fig. 6.   Epidermoid carcinoma. Cholecystic carcinoma metastatic to a pericholedochal lymph node grows in sheets without formation of acini. Keratinization in biliary epidermoid carcinomas is uncommon. H&E. X250.

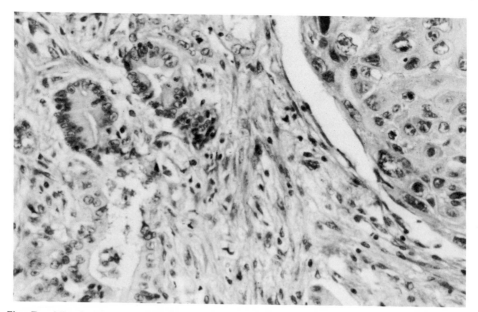

Fig. 7.   Mixed pattern in biliary cancer. In the upper right, a solid nest of epidermoid carcinoma has intercellular bridges ("prickle cells"). On the left, the tumor grows in a glandular pattern. This mixture of epidermoid and glandular elements is more common than pure epidermoid carcinoma of biliary origin. In the metastases, the epidermoid pattern may predominate (Fig. 6). Mucicarmine. X250.

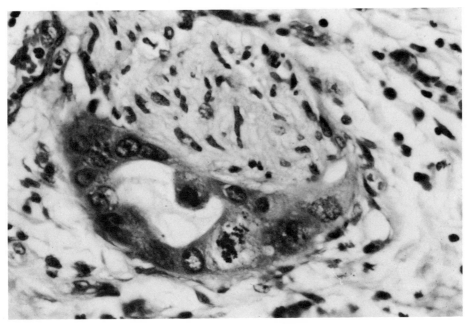

Fig. 8. Poorly differentiated adenocarcinoma. The large bizarre nuclei and prominent mitotic figures seen in this example are relatively infrequent in biliary carcinomas. A glandular pattern persists, and there is perineural infiltration. H&E. X400.

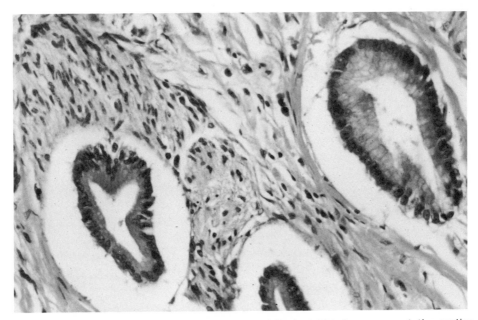

Fig. 9. Well-differentiated carcinoma of common bile duct. This is a representative section from the deep part of a scirrhous mass involving the distal half of the common bile duct and extending into the pancreas and ampulla. The tumor resembles normal epithelium (Fig. 1), but there is infiltration of perineural spaces. H&E. X250.

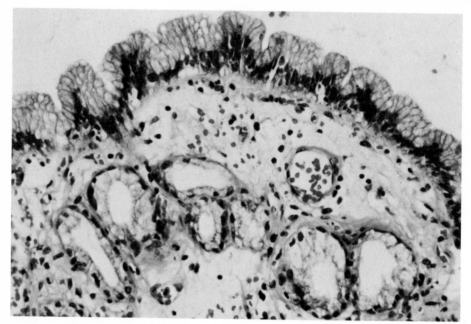

Fig. 10.   Mucin production in chronic cholecystitis. Mucin production may be markedly increased in inflammatory conditions. In this instance, there is mucin production in virtually all of the surface epithelium as well as in the small crypts below. H&E. X250.

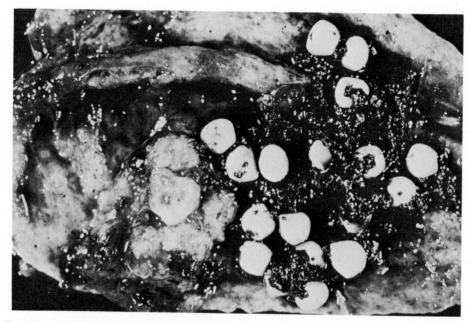

Fig. 11.   Papillary adenocarcinoma of gallbladder. A 78-year-old woman had a cholecystectomy for acute cholecystitis. In addition to calculi, a papillary tumor 3 cm in diameter was found in the fundus when the gallbladder was opened. There was superficial invasion of the muscularis by a well-differentiated adenocarcinoma, histologically identical to Figure 1.

the wall will prove to be superficial carcinoma, but there is no certain method to separate superficial carcinomas from adenomas by gross examination (Fig. 11).

Depth of tumor invasion is of greater prognostic significance than histologic variation. Discovery of cancer of the bile ducts in a preinvasive stage is most unlikely because symptomatic duct cancers are usually invasive, but in situ carcinoma of the gallbladder may be found incidentally after cholecystectomy for clinically benign disease. Approximately 3 percent of gallbladder cancers are reported as preinvasive.[2, 26, 69]

Most carcinomas have invaded the wall of the gallbladder or duct system, and more than half have metastasized or invaded adjacent structures by the time of diagnosis. Fahim[27] and associates found hepatic involvement in 34 percent of 151 patients with gallbladder cancer, mostly in the form of a local mass near the primary. Smaller but equal numbers had satellite nodules or disseminated liver metastases. One patient in four had metastasis to pericholedochal and pancreaticoduodenal lymph nodes but *not* to the lymph nodes of the hilum of the liver. Although local venous spread was found in 13 percent and perineural involvement in 24 percent of cases, these findings were not associated with apparent systemic disease. Direct peritoneal seeding was not found, and involvement of other abdominal organs was attributed to lymphatic spread. Extension along the duct system was identified in only 4 percent of cases, and it was a less frequent cause of jaundice than compression by metastases to periductal lymph nodes. Litwin[40] found a higher percentage of hepatic (63 percent) and lymph node (24 percent) involvement and also a higher incidence of omental (26 percent) and peritoneal (12 percent) involvement. Spread to the porta hepatis was observed in 12 percent, and 9 percent had lung metastasis. The apparent discrepancies between the findings of Litwin and Fahim, et al. are due to differences in the clinical stage of disease at examination.

Although no distant metastases were found in 60 percent of 22 cases of duct carcinoma studied by Coulter,[7] there were no survivors. Van Heerden[71] and associates found spread of disease beyond the primary site, but not necessarily distant metastases, in 71 percent of biliary cancers. The mode of spread of duct cancer is similar to that of cholecystic carcinoma except that the pancreas and ampulla are more likely to be involved by tumors of the distal common duct.

Differential Diagnosis

Adenomas may be distinguished from adenocarcinomas by lack of epithelial atypia and absence of invasion. Since careful orientation of tissue sections facilitates evaluation of invasion, a gallbladder with a suspected neoplasm should be carefully opened, gently washed free of bile and fixed for a few hours before taking sections. With the exception of extremely large lesions, which should be generously sampled, papillary lesions should be examined in their entirety to exclude invasion. Even with good tissue preparation, noninvasive carcinoma may be extremely difficult to distinguish from adenoma (Fig. 12). The histologic features of *nonneoplastic polyps* are quite different from carcinoma and should cause no confusion.

Chronic cholecystitis, particularly when associated with numerous stones, frequently results in thickening of muscularis with mucosal outpouchings deep into

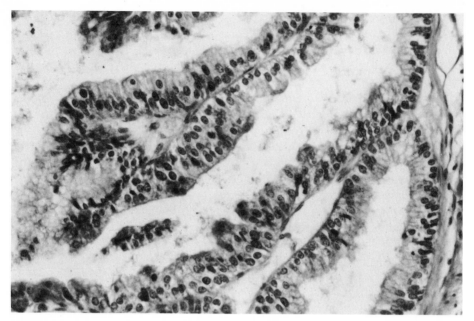

Fig. 12.   Adenoma versus noninvasive adenocarcinoma. This papillary tumor was discovered in the gallbladder of a 75-year-old woman after cholecystectomy for chronic cholecystitis and cholelithiasis. There was only slight nuclear atypia and no demonstrable invasion. The patient had no evidence of cancer three years postoperatively. This illustrates the difficulty in distinguishing adenomas from low-grade, noninfiltrating carcinomas. H&E. X250.

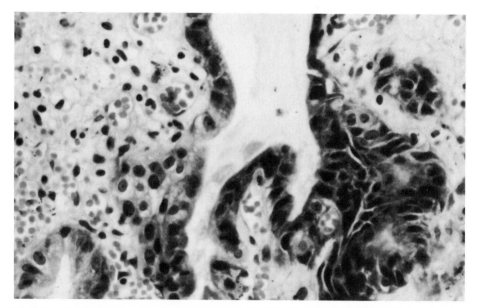

Fig. 13.   Atypia in chronic cholecystitis. The epithelial cells are flattened or cuboidal. The nuclei appear large and hyperchromatic. Atypia of this degree is frequently seen with mucosal erosion due to stones. There is no evidence that this type change progresses to malignancy. H&E. X400.

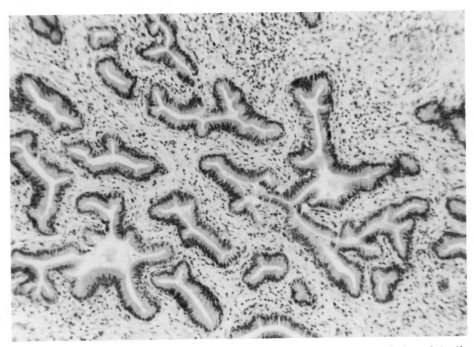

Fig. 14.   Mucosal crypts. Branching nests of normal epithelium extend deep into the wall. This is a normal finding in the neck of the gallbladder, the cystic duct and the distal common duct; it may be seen throughout the entire duct system with choledocholithiasis or following cholecystectomy. H&E. X100.

the wall (Rokitansky-Aschoff sinuses). These changes are usually diffuse but may be localized. Reactive epithelial atypia (Fig. 13) may be confused with cancer, particularly when it occurs in epithelial nests deep in the muscularis. Careful orientation of the specimen will help prevent error, and it must be remembered that epithelial crypts are common in the neck of the gallbladder and biliary ducts (Fig. 14).

Primary sclerosing cholangitis may be most difficult to distinguish from bile duct carcinoma, clinically and morphologically. Approximately 30 instances of this disorder have been recorded. Scarring with occlusion of the ducts following biliary tract surgery is far more common than primary sclerosis. The disease is characterized by either generalized or focal sclerosis of the extrahepatic biliary ducts with reduction or obliteration of the lumen. There is occasionally cholecystic involvement. A relationship to other sclerosing diseases, such as idiopathic retroperitoneal fibrosis or Riedel's struma, has been suggested,[6] but association with these disorders has been unusual. The symptoms, as with cancer, are usually those of chronic cholecystic disease. Jaundice is frequently the presenting complaint. At operation, a thickened sclerotic duct system which may closely resemble the gross appearance of duct cancer is found. Indeed, Altemeier[1] and associates believe that most patients who initially appear to have sclerosing cholangitis eventually will be shown to have scirrhous carcinoma of the bile ducts. The process may extend to the *intrahepatic duct;* in some instances, the bulk of the tumor may be within the liver and thus not recognized until autopsy. On the other hand, Glenn

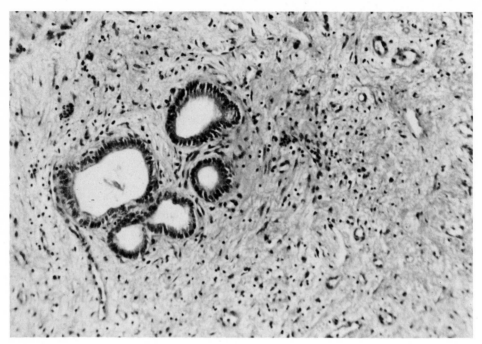

Fig. 15. Sclerosing cholangitis. Dense scar tissue replaces the wall of a bile duct. Only a few mucosal nests remain. At times it may be difficult to distinguish sclerosing cholangitis from well-differentiated adenocarcinoma (Fig. 9). H&E. X100.

and Whitsell[34] have reported seven instances of duct sclerosis with no antecedent biliary surgery and in which no tumor was found at biopsy. One of these patients was alive seven years after biliary diversion, a longer survival than would be expected with an unresected carcinoma. Autopsy follow-up in all proposed cases of this kind will ultimately determine whether this entity is different than sclerosing carcinoma. In the cases which have been accepted as sclerosing cholangitis, the most prominent histologic change has been scarring of the walls and ducts (Fig. 15). Since small islands of biliary mucosa may remain and focally resemble a well-differentiated biliary adenocarcinoma, it is imperative to examine as much tissue as can be obtained to get an overall picture of the disease process. Most surgeons understand that definitive diagnosis based on a single frozen section may not always be possible.

Other Malignant Tumors

A single *lymphoma* of the gallbladder was included in a group of 31 cancers.[48] The finding of lymphoma in the gallbladder should be regarded as evidence of systemic lymphoma until proven otherwise. *Malignant melanoma* in the biliary tract should also be regarded as metastatic until a careful search has excluded other primary sites. Six percent of patients with disseminated melanoma had involvement of the biliary tract,[19] but a few primary biliary melanomas have been reported, including one found at autopsy without tumor elsewhere.[56, 61] A few *leiomyosar-*

comas[10, 72] have been included in reports of gallbladder cancer. Since carcinoma may assume a spindly appearance, an erroneous diagnosis of sarcoma may result from inadequate examination. *Embryonal rhabdomyosarcoma*[20, 36] (sarcoma botryoides) has been recorded approximately a dozen times. All were in children ages 2 to 11, who presented with obstruction of the biliary system.

Prognosis

The poor prognosis of biliary carcinomas is exemplified by a follow-up study of 526 such patients. The five-year survival was 31 percent for ampullary cancer, 26 percent for pancreatic cancer, and zero for both gallbladder and bile duct cancer.[57] Nonetheless, an occasional patient with gallbladder cancer may be cured. Three of 90 (3.3 percent) patients of Thorbjarnarson and Glenn[69] lived seven years without disease; two of these, however, were not known to have carcinoma until the gallbladder was opened. Two of 76 (2.6 percent) patients of Van Heerden[71] and associates lived five years. The even higher five-year survival rate, 8 of 151 (5.9 percent), found by Fahim[26] and associates, was principally related to finding the tumors in an early stage, either in situ or with only superficial infiltration. In all eight instances, the discovery of the tumors was incidental to cholecystectomy for clinically benign disease. Although seven of the survivors had been treated by cholecystectomy alone, one also had wedge resection of the liver. The authors felt that radical surgery might have been beneficial to some of the 43 patients who had residual tumor following cholecystectomy. Appleman[2] and associates studied 21 long-term survivors of gallbladder cancer, and in all the diagnosis was unsuspected until the gallbladder was opened. Two solitary tumors were under 1.0 cm in diameter, 12 were multifocal, and 10 others were superficially invading the wall but not the liver. This histologic type of cancer among long-term survivors is the same as that seen in the fatal cases. The highest survival rates are reported from general hospitals where carcinomas are found in carefully examined gallbladders removed for clinically benign disease. Cancer hospitals treating patients referred for known or suspected cancer have fewer survivors.[63]

The prognosis of biliary duct cancer is even worse; only occasional long-term survivals are noted.[39, 45] Only 1 percent of 218 bile duct carcinomas reported by Den Besten and Leichty lived five years.[21] Other large studies include no long-term survivors.[57, 63]

Treatment

Long-term survival of biliary cancer has been associated only with complete surgical removal of localized disease. Although few gallbladder cancers are in situ when discovered, many more appear confined to the gallbladder and adjacent liver at the time of diagnosis. In this circumstance, right hepatic lobectomy has been proposed as a feasible method of treatment. One author estimated that as many as 15 percent of such patients might profit from this procedure.[15] The five-year cure of a patient with *invasive* carcinoma of the gallbladder treated by hepatic lobectomy[11] has stimulated interest in more radical surgery for this disease.

Palliation has been the primary goal in management of biliary duct cancers, since surgical resection of the tumor has been feasible only in rare instances; however, some believe that about 10 percent of patients with biliary cancer might benefit from more aggressive surgical procedures.[21, 39, 45] Radiation and chemotherapy usually have been used only for palliation. Cure of biliary carcinoma then depends on early, even fortuitous diagnosis, except in rare instances in which radical surgery has proved beneficial. The long history of biliary symptoms in many patients with carcinoma suggests that more cancers might have been found at a curative stage with earlier operation. Since carcinomas often cannot be distinguished from benign tumors by x-ray, any tumor demonstrated radiographically should be removed without delay. Furthermore, the relatively frequent association of carcinoma with acute cholecystitis suggests that when primary cholecystectomy is contraindicated, the gallbladder should be removed and the duct system explored as soon as is feasible to rule out carcinoma. Finally, since scirrhous carcinoma may masquerade as sclerosing cholangitis, resectable sclerotic lesions should be removed.

Benign Tumors of the Biliary Tract

The incidence of benign tumors of the biliary tract is difficult to determine because of inconsistent terminology in many reports; however, benign neoplasms seem to be rare, whereas non-neoplastic tumors are common. Small benign tumors of the gallbladder are likely to be asymptomatic and are frequently discovered only during surgery for cholelithiasis or at autopsy. Tiny tumors of the duct system may also be found only at autopsy, but even relatively small tumors may become symptomatic because of obstruction, especially when in the cystic duct.

Although radiographic studies may demonstrate tumors,[49] ordinarily they cannot be relied upon to distinguish the type. However, adenomas are more likely to be large, single and lobulated, whereas cholesterol polyps are usually small and multiple.[8] Of 52 polypoid lesions discovered on x-rays, 26 were cholesterolosis, 6 calculi, 4 inflammatory polyps, 8 Rokitansky-Aschoff sinuses (adenomyosis), and only 3 true adenomas.[48]

Inflammatory Lesions and Hyperplastic Conditions

Small focal mucosal or mural lesions are so frequent in gallbladders removed for stone or inflammation that little attention is given to these lesions. Most are of no clinical significance.

Cholesterol polyps result from focal subepithelial accumulation of cholesterol-containing macrophages, usually in association with diffuse cholesterolosis (Fig. 16). The polyps are usually multiple and small, only occasionally exceeding 5 mm in diameter. There is no constant relation to serum cholesterol levels or cholelithiasis.[58]

Inflammatory polyps are focal masses resulting from edema or granulation tissue and ordinarily are caused by local irritation by stones (Fig. 17).

Adenomyosis (adenomyomatosis)[28] is the proliferation of epithelium with outpouching of mucosa into or through a thickened muscularis. Some degree of

58. Seltzer, D.W., Dockerty, M.B., Stauffer, M.H., and Priestly, J.T. Papillomas (so-called) in the non-calculous gallbladder. Amer. J. Surg., 103:472, 1962.
59. Serpe, S.J., Todd, D., and Baruch, H. Cholecystitis due to granular cell myoblastoma of the cystic duct. Amer. J. Dig. Dis., 5:824, 1960.
60. Shaper, A.G. Diseases of the biliary tract in Africans in Uganda. E. African Med. J., 41:246, 1964.
61. Simard, C., George, P., Caulet, T., and Diebold, J. Les melanomes malins de la vesicule biliaire. Rapport de deux cas. J. Chir. (Paris), 92:51, 1966.
62. Smith, V.M., Feldman, M., Sr., and Warner, C.G. Neoplasms of the cystic and hepatic ducts, Amer. J. Dig. Dis., 7:804, 1962.
63. Statistical Report of End Results, 1949-1957. New York, Memorial Hospital for Cancer and Allied Diseases and the James Ewing Hospital of the City of New York, 1965.
64. Sternberg, S.S., Popper, H., Oser, B.L., and Oser, M. Gallbladder and bile duct carcinomas in dogs after long-term feeding of aramite. Cancer, 13:780, 1960.
65. Strauch, G.O. Primary carcinoma of the gallbladder: Presentation of 70 cases from the Rhode Island Hospital and a cumulative review of the last ten years of the American literature. Surgery, 47:368, 1960.
66. Strohl, E.L., Reed, W.H., Diffenbaugh, W.G., and Anderson, R.E. Carcinoma of the bile ducts. Arch. Surg., 87:567, 1963.
67. Thistlethwaite, J.R., and Horwitz, A. Choledochal cyst followed by carcinoma of the hepatic duct. Southern Med. J., 60:872, 1967.
68. Thorbjarnarson, B. Carcinoma of the gallbladder and acute cholecystitis. Ann. Surg., 151:241, 1960.
69. ——— and Glenn, F. Carcinoma of the gallbladder. Cancer, 12:1009, 1959.
70. Torvik, A., and Hoivik, B. Gallstones in an autopsy series. Incidence, complications and correlation with carcinoma of the gallbladder. Acta Chir. Scand., 120:168, 1960.
71. Van Heerden, J.A., Judd, E.S., and Dockerty, M.B. Carcinoma of the extrahepatic bile ducts: A clinicopathologic study. Amer. J. Surg., 113:49, 1967.
72. Whitcomb, F.F., Jr., Corley, G.J., Babigian, D.N., and Colcock, B.P. Leiomyosarcoma of the bile ducts. Gastroenterology, 52:94, 1967.

HUMAN RENAL VASCULAR LESIONS AND HYPERTENSION

LELAND D. STODDARD*
HOLDE PUCHTLER

This is an account of chronic hypertensive and malignant hypertensive renal vascular lesions in man. It is based on our personal experience. A discussion of the lesions is followed by an historical sketch of their recognition and significance. A technical appendix gives histochemical methods developed in our department.

Hypertension has been defined as an elevation of blood pressure above normal.[1] Normality, in general, has been called an ideal fiction. It is unprofitable to belabor the point that high blood pressure can be defined no better than the upper part of a distribution curve of blood pressure readings obtained from a large population. The medical importance of this distribution curve is not that it describes biologic variation but that it has pathologic significance, for the upper part includes persons subject to cardiac, vascular, renal, and other disturbances we call hypertensive disease.

Blood pressure varies, of course, and the cause and significance of an elevated reading is not always at once apparent. Ryle[47] gave credit to Sir Clifford Allbutt for the terms, "hyperpiesis" and "hyperpiesia," and went on to say:

"By hyperpiesis we understand the fact of raised blood-pressure; we know that it may be transient or persistent, and that it may accompany a variety of conditions, including arterial disease, chronic renal disease, lesions causing increased intracranial pressure, exophthalmic goitre, and so forth. By hyperpiesia we understand a peculiar and

* We thank Dr. Paul Kimmelstiel for valuable criticism and discussion and the editor for helpful comments. For support of research during the past ten years, we acknowledge the institutional budget, the Medical Research Foundation of Georgia, and grants from the National Institutes of Health and the Georgia Heart Association; and for support (in part) of research training, a departmental grant from the National Institutes of Health, GM-207.

interesting malady in which raised blood-pressure is the most constant and outstanding feature. Clifford Allbutt described it as a malady in which, at or towards middle life, the blood-pressure rises excessively—a malady having a course of its own, and deserving the name of a disease."

The terms hyperpiesis and hyperpiesia were not widely adopted, and the single noun, hypertension, ambiguously refers to "the fact of raised blood-pressure" and to hypertensive disease in which it is "the most constant and outstanding feature."

Hypertensive disease in man usually pursues a chronic course and the diastolic as well as the systolic blood pressure is elevated. Diastolic elevation represents increased peripheral resistance, and systolic elevation is the thrust to overcome it. The renal vascular lesions of chronic hypertensive disease are, however, also found in old persons who have only a systolic elevation and whose hearts are little, if at all, hypertrophied.

Malignant hypertension in man rarely occurs *de novo* but almost always is a new event in the course of chronic hypertensive disease. This is repeatedly verified when accurate medical histories are available, and it is attested to by cardiac hypertrophy found at autopsy. The renal vascular lesions of malignant hypertension, except rarely, are superimposed upon those of chronic hypertensive disease. However, in experimental animals, hypertension can be produced acutely by a variety of methods, and the animals develop in pure form lesions analogous to some which occur in human malignant hypertension.

The intrarenal vascular lesions associated with chronic hypertension in man are hyperplastic arteriosclerosis of larger arteries and hyaline sclerosis of preglomerular arterioles and their antecedent interlobular arteries. When hypertensive disease becomes malignant, formerly almost always fatal, the chronic lesions are complicated by a peculiar mucoid endarterial proliferation in larger arteries and by focal fibrinoid necrosis scattered along the vascular tree from larger arteries to glomeruli.

The Lesions

Hypertensive intrarenal vascular lesions can be conveniently described and discussed according to the following outline:
Arteriosclerosis
  Larger Arteries
    Hyperplastic arteriosclerosis of chronic hypertension.
    Mucoid endarterial fibrosis of malignant hypertension.
  Arterioles
    Hyaline arteriolosclerosis of chronic hypertension.
Fibrinoid Necrosis of Malignant Hypertension
  Arteries and arterioles
  Glomeruli

Arteriosclerosis

LARGER ARTERIES. *Hyperplastic arteriosclerosis* affects the interlobar and arcuate arteries and may extend to the interlobular arteries. It is an intimal proliferation of concentric lamellae of connective tissue which may in time be accompanied by atrophy of the media. Although the media in early lesions is normally thick, recent observations suggest that the muscle already begins to be replaced by collagen.[45] The proliferation fills part of the lumen but does not occlude the artery. (See illustration in Jackson, et al.[24]) A gradually developing, partially obstructive lesion, it produces cone-shaped[1] zones of atrophy having the same shape as infarcts caused by sudden, complete obstruction of corresponding arteries. These moderately coarse scars of arterionephrosclerosis are 3 to 5 mm across on the surface and can be traced in a radial section to the corticomedullary boundary where the sclerotic artery is at the vertex of the cone. In some cases, hyaline arteriolosclerosis is scarce, and for that reason Bell and Clawson[1] stated that arteriosclerosis precedes arteriolosclerosis. Often, however, both lesions occur together, which may mean that they usually develop concurrently.

Hyperplastic sclerosis is sometimes discussed as part of atherosclerosis, especially in older reports. The reason is difficult to understand, except that histologic sections were thick, and fat was sometimes demonstrated in Sudan-stained frozen sections. Hyperplastic sclerosis is not like atherosclerosis which begins with intimal lipid deposits or metamorphosed thrombi,[7] nor does it build up by aggregation of eccentric thrombotic masses accumulated in episodes. Finally, it does not become a necrotic, chalky gruel.

Hyperplastic arteriosclerosis is often called elastic hyperplastic sclerosis because the concentric lamellae of the intimal proliferation stain with resorcin-fuchsin of Weigert as does the internal elastica. Paradoxically, the proliferated lamellae, but not the internal elastica, also stain by a variety of techniques as collagen does.[24] The proliferated intimal lamellae are pseudoelastic, abnormal collagen that has some elastic physical properties.

Resorcin-fuchsin does not specifically stain elastic fibers in the chemical sense of the protein, elastin. It is thought that, "resorcin-fuchsin is bound by nonionic bonds, presumably hydrogen bonds, between a hydroxyl group of the resorcinal moiety of the dye and suitable bonding sites in tissues."[43] Bonding sites for the dye can be made available by several pretreatments of collagen and reticulum fibers which otherwise do not stain. For example, by immersion in hot water, inelastic tendon can be made to bind resorcin-fuchsin, and in addition to binding the dye, it also is more elastic than before. Immature collagen in infants also binds the dye.[27] It seems probable that collagen which binds resorcin-fuchsin is incompletely crosslinked and has free bonding sites for this dye.

The elastic intimal structure of muscular arteries, normal and abnormal, has some hemodynamic implications. The large elastic arteries absorb much of the pulsatile pressure. Muscular arteries leading off from them retain an internal and usually an external elastic lamella. A recent series of reinforcing histochemical, polarization, and fluorescence microscopic studies have shown that the structure of the internal elastica gradually changes in the ramifying intrarenal arterial tree.[46] In the sizable arteries (interlobar), the internal elastica is elastin. As the peripheral vessels become smaller, there is a gradual transition through a mixture of elastin and collagen to a basement membrane kind of matrix containing longitudinal collagen fibrils which terminate at the glomerular hilus and give way to the basement membrane of the glomerular capillaries. The internal elastica is stained throughout by resorcin-fuchsin because, where the membrane is collagenous, the collagen is the incompletely cross-linked, or immature, type. As noted, such collagen has some elasticity.

Some histochemical, physical, and biologic observations suggest that pseudo-elastic hyperplastic arteriosclerosis is an adaptation to rising blood pressure or perhaps a widened pulse pressure. The blood pressure rises during childhood, and intimal proliferation of pseudoelastic fibers begins in infancy.[26] The concentric lamellae of pseudoelastic collagen in hyperplastic arteriosclerosis are an exaggeration of the process. Such sclerosis is regularly found in old persons who have no diastolic hypertension or cardiac hypertrophy, but they do have less elastic aortas, some systolic elevation, and a widened pulse pressure. Hypertensive disease accelerates the lesion so that it appears at a younger age. Those who have studied the problem in the past agree fairly well that hyperplastic intrarenal arteriosclerosis is only more severe among those with hypertensive disease than among old persons, although Evans[13] has stated that the senile lesions were eccentric rather than concentric, a difference not generally commented upon.

To sum up, the concentric lamellae of connective tissue in hyperplastic arteriosclerosis are intimal proliferations of immature or incompletely cross-linked collagen. It has sites available for binding resorcin-fuchsin and presumably is more elastic than mature, fully cross-linked collagen. The lesion would better be called pseudoelastic, rather than elastic, hyperplastic sclerosis. A reasonable theory is that it is an anatomical adaptation to hemodynamic changes in blood pressure and pulsatile flow. Its presence in hypertensive disease may be less a consequence of elevated diastolic pressure than of systolic elevation and a widened pulse pressure.

Mucoid Endarterial Fibrosis in Malignant Hypertension. Pseudoelastic hyperplastic sclerosis often is described as a lesion of malignant hypertension. We think this designation is incorrect because the lesion is found in cases of benign hypertension and in elderly persons having no elevation of diastolic pressure or cardiac hypertrophy. In cases of malignant hypertension, hyperplastic sclerosis is a concomitant of antecedent chronic hypertension. But characteristic of malignant hypertension is a distinctive internal layer of mucoid endarterial fibrosis. It is found in arteries as large as interlobars and as small as interlobulars and is fairly widely distributed in the usual random histologic samples of the renal vascular tree. It may be sharply set off from or may merge with the concentric lamellae of pseudoelastic hyperplastic sclerosis. This inner band is usually wide enough to reduce the lumen appreciably. It has histologic features of young, recently proliferated connective tissue, such as one sometimes finds in granulation tissue, in arteries invaded by malignant tumors, or in organizing arterial thrombi. Nuclei are scattered in abundant basophilic ground substance, and widely separated young collagen sometimes stains deeply with resorcin-fuchsin. Its apparent age fits the course of the malignant phase of hypertension which lasts only weeks or a few months.

We had been struck by the frequency of this distinctive mucoid endarterial fibrosis in a large population of malignant hypertensive subjects autopsied at the Medical College of Georgia over the past fourteen years. Because many published accounts of malignant hypertension do not clearly describe this lesion or distinguish it from chronic pseudoelastic hyperplastic sclerosis, we wondered for a time whether it might have a geographical peculiarity, characterize malignant hypertension in blacks, or be related to administration of modern antipressor or other drugs. However, the lesion was clearly described and illustrated as early as 1931 by Klemperer and Otani.[32]

Brief mention should be made of obliterative endarterial fibrosis because it occurs in chronic pyelonephritis. Kimmelstiel, et al.[29] pointed out that arterial lesions augment the atrophy in chronic pyelonephritic scars. We find that such lesions, on the one hand, lack the distinctive concentric lamellae of chronic pseudoelastic hyperplastic sclerosis, and, on the other, their dense eosinophilic collagen contrasts with the mucoid endarterial fibrosis of malignant hypertension. The elevation of blood pressure in chronic pyelonephritis is not great, and the patients' hearts are, as a rule, not much hypertrophied. Even so, an interesting intrarenal vascular lesion occasionally found seems to recapitulate the development of chronic pyelonephritis, renal atrophy, and finally hypertension if it occurs. The lesion is a double layered intimal sclerosis: the outer layer is a dense fibrosis; the inner is a lamellated pseudoelastic hyperplastic sclerosis.

ARTERIOLES. *Hyaline sclerosis* of renal arterioles is the anatomical counterpart of chronic, clinical hypertensive disease, but if hypertension causes it there are also other causes, as we shall discuss later. The lesion is constant and most severe in preglomerular arterioles. It often extends to interlobular arteries but rarely into a glomerulus, except in diabetics. It is segmental and eccentric, but it can expand to circle the entire wall and narrow the lumen. (See illustrations in Moritz and Oldt.[39]) Small lesions cause no perceptible glomerular change, but as arteriolar sclerosis advances, the glomerulus atrophies. Tubular atrophy follows, and the atrophied nephron becomes a small, pitted scar. Atrophy of many nephrons leads to the familiar pits of arteriolonephrosclerosis, with the cortex of the contracted kidney thinner than its normal 7 mm and the pelvis surrounded by fat. In most cases, there also are slightly larger scars of arterionephrosclerosis caused by hyperplastic arteriosclerosis. Seldom does the kidney weigh less than 100 g. In advanced cases, it is easy to find pale, hypertrophied, surviving nephrons projecting above the dull red-gray scars. When death occurs early in the course of hypertensive disease, as, for example, in cases of ruptured bifurcational cerebral aneurysms, the kidneys are grossly normal and inconspicuous hyaline arteriolosclerosis must be searched for histologically.

Hyalin means no more than a glassy, homogeneous looking mass which stains well with eosin. Long ago, the smallest, and so presumably early, lesions were described beneath the endothelium of the intima. The higher resolution of electron microscopy added details. Small lesions seem to begin in spaces between the subendothelial and the smooth muscle basement membranes; the "elastic" fibers lie outside.[3] Larger lesions infiltrate the elastica and extend into interstitial spaces between smooth muscle cells of the media. However, the origin of hyaline sclerosis has been variously postulated from electron micrographs. To some, the lesions look distinct from all normal structures and seem best explained as infiltrations from the blood, between endothelial cells, and into the wall.[3, 16] Other observers see thickening of endothelial and muscle basement membranes as the initial lesion to which may be added components from degenerated muscle cells in advanced lesions.[38]

The chemical composition of vascular hyalin is not so homogeneous as its appearance. A number of substances have been demonstrated or suggested by histochemical and ultrastructural techniques.[16] Histochemical studies from our laboratory have led us to agree with the view that hematogenous infiltration best accounts for the composition of the lesion. Hyaline deposits reacted intensely with the dihydroxy-dinaphthyl-disulfide (DDD) reaction for sulfhydryl and disulfide groups and with the rosindole reaction for indoles and indole derivatives (tryptophane). Smooth muscle fibers were colored moderately by the DDD procedure and faintly by the rosindole reaction. Collagen, which does not contain tryptophane or cysteine/cystine, and the collagenous internal "elastic" membrane of arterioles remained unstained.[33] In model experiments with various fractions of plasma proteins, other proteins, and saccharides, the rosindole reaction colored only fibrinogen; fibrin; alpha, beta, and gamma globulin; elastase; and gliadin, a component of wheat flour.[49] The phosphotungstic acid-hematoxylin (PTAH) stain cannot be relied upon to demonstrate fibrin and other plasma proteins in hyaline deposits. Frequently, hyaline deposits which are colored deep blue by the rosindole reaction are stained red like collagen in adjacent sections treated with PTAH. In model experiments, no relation could be found between the chemical nature of the test substances and their coloration by PTAH.[49] Unfortunately, the rosindole reaction for demonstration of plasma proteins requires Carnoy fixation. The deposits also stain with the periodic-acid-Schiff (PAS) reaction. In our experience, Lillie's[34] allochrome procedure or its light-fast modification[50] are the methods of choice for formalin- or Zenker-fixed material; the bright red hyaline deposits contrast nicely with the yellow medial muscle cells and blue collagen. It is well known that Sudanophilic fat accumulates, but Fishberg[15] has stated it was not present in early lesions. None of these techniques serves to distinguish hyaline sclerosis from fibrinoid necrosis, which can complicate the lesion in malignant hypertension (see discussion on p. 259).

It is often said that hypertension precedes renal arteriolosclerosis. Failure to find it in renal biopsy samples taken early in the course of hypertensive disease is cited in evidence. However, the lesion is focal, as one can learn from following an arteriole in serial sections, and even in multiple, large autopsy blocks, one may have to search a while to find it if lesions are scarce and inconspicuous. It can be missed entirely in poorly prepared sections, especially from formalin-fixed blocks. We much prefer Zenker or Carnoy for satisfactory histologic preparations of kidneys. Goldblatt[18] found arteriolar necrosis after a few days of severe, acute hypertension in dogs but has repeatedly stated that no arteriolosclerosis can be found in animals that have been hypertensive for years.[19] There is no clear evidence in human beings or in experimental models that hyaline sclerosis is produced by chronic hypertension alone.

Hyaline arteriolosclerosis occurs in old age somewhat less regularly than hyperplastic renal arteriosclerosis. Except in diabetics, renal arteriolosclerosis before the age of 45 or 50 is a good indicator of hypertensive disease with elevated systolic and diastolic pressures. The amount of hyaline sclerosis of preglomerular arterioles rather parallels the duration of hypertension. At about 50 years of age, it begins to appear in persons who did not have a diastolic elevation or cardiac hypertrophy at autopsy, but they may have had systolic elevations and widened pulse pressures.

Fishberg's study[15] of the distribution of hyaline arteriolosclerosis in hypertensive subjects has been amply confirmed. It is most severe in the kidneys where its frequency approaches his invariably finding it. Following in frequency and severity are abdominal organs, notably adrenals, pancreas, and gut. Splenic arteriolosclerosis is unusually severe, but it is not a lesion of hypertension because it is found in almost all normotensive subjects by the age of 30.

Hyaline arteriosclerosis is most common in the vascular beds of four arteries that arise from a 5 cm length of the abdominal aorta—celiac, superior mesenteric, and renals—although it occurs elsewhere, as in the retinal arteries. The distribution of hyaline sclerosis might be clarified by accurate knowledge of pressure and wave propulsion in various parts of the arterial tree, but we think there is more to it than hemodynamics.

Bell and Clawson[1] noted severe hyaline sclerosis among diabetic hypertensive subjects. Since Kimmelstiel and Wilson's description,[31] hyaline arteriolosclerosis has been understood as a part of the complex of diabetic glomerulosclerosis. It can be found before hypertension develops in diabetics and uniquely involves the low-pressure efferent arteriole as well as the high-pressure afferent.

The distribution of hyaline sclerosis in the renal arterial tree is related to the structure of the internal elastic membranes.[42] We previously discussed histochemical differences in the internal "elastica" of arteries of different sizes. Hyaline sclerosis occurs only in the smaller vessels, especially arterioles, which have an internal membrane of collagen fibers embedded in a basement-membrane-like matrix. It is not found in larger arteries which have an internal membrane of elastin or elastin and collagen.

Moritz and Oldt[39] described other chronic hypertensive arteriolar lesions. Endothelial proliferation is beautifully illustrated in their paper. They found the lesion in renal vessels larger than afferent arterioles; it often was accompanied by medial thinning and collagen deposition. We have not been so impressed with it in chronic hypertension but have seen it dramatically in a few cases of malignant hypertension that developed without evidence of longstanding benign hypertension.

To sum up, hyaline arteriolosclerosis is most severe and constant in the kidneys of persons having chronic hypertension. In time, it causes atrophy of nephrons and arteriolonephrosclerosis. The lesion probably arises by infiltration of blood constituents but is chemically complex. Its etiology is not hypertension alone. It is unusually severe in diabetics. It develops in small vessels which have an internal "elastica" of collagen fibers embedded in a basement-membrane-like matrix, but this does not explain the earliest ultrastructural lesions which are subendothelial. Endothelial proliferation may also be found.

FIBRINOID NECROSIS OF MALIGNANT HYPERTENSION.   Necrosis of intrarenal arteries, arterioles, and glomeruli is the hallmark of malignant hypertension. Arterial necrosis occurs with unpredictable variation in other sites, too, notably, pancreas, gut, and retina. Some of the lesions usually cause small hemorrhages, and those in the kidney cause hematuria. The lesion is commonly called "fibrinoid necrosis" or sometimes, with less justification, "necrotizing arteritis" and "arteriolitis." It is important to understand that the lesions are focal and range from sparse to abundant and that they are superimposed on all the intrarenal vascular lesions already discussed; they are, indeed, necrotic because there is evidence of cell death.

What has just been stated indicates what to expect at autopsy and suggests some problems in needle biopsy sampling. A large or even normal size, swollen kidney covered with a rash of petechiae and hemorrhagic splotches is exceptional. Even in such a kidney, the fine scarring of arteriolonephrosclerosis can still be made out. Much more often, a moderately contracted, arteriolonephrosclerotic kidney is speckled with a few petechiae the size of a glomerulus and its adjacent proximal convoluted tubule. There may be as few as half a dozen red dots that have to be looked for over the stripped cortical surface of half a kidney. Specific lesions have to be selected for histologic study, and with a biopsy needle one would be lucky to find them. Fortunately, many covert lesions that have not yet caused glomerular bleeding are found for every one that has bled.

Related autopsy observations and the clinical course put one on the track of malignant hypertension. Chronic hypertension is reflected in a much hypertrophied, globular heart, but in malignant hypertension it is pallid and streaked with fat. Fibrinous pericarditis is found but not invariably and often inconspicuously. Hemorrhages in the pancreas, intestine, and retina are inconsistent. A typical clinical syndrome heralds these lesions: steadily rising blood pressure, progressive azotemia, fluctuating blood sodium and chloride, a mental state in and out of contact with reality, and retinal hemorrhages and hematuria. Before antipressor drugs were used, the course lasted only weeks or a few months and was fatal. Present day treatment can be life-saving.

Malignant hypertension is not often found with chronic renal lesions other than vascular nephrosclerosis. An unusual case of chronic glomerulonephritis ends with it, but the kidneys are small and greatly scarred and the heart less hypertrophied. If Kimmelstiel's criteria[29] are observed, chronic pyelonephritis will not be mistaken for nephrosclerosis and seldom will be found to end in malignant hypertension. Some cases of scleroderma (systemic sclerosis) end in malignant hypertension, and the intrarenal vascular lesions are indistinguishable.[14, 17]

Fibrinoid necrosis is found along with hyaline sclerosis—malignant hypertension in the wake of chronic hypertension—but the lesions can be distinguished in properly fixed and prepared material. Formalin fixation may be unsuitable and blurs the distinction. After Zenker or Carnoy, the bright, eosinophilic, smudgy focal lesions can be seen even in arterioles altered by hyaline sclerosis. Immunohistologic observations have demonstrated various plasma proteins in the lesions: fibrin or fibrinogen, albumin, gamma globulins, and even complement.[6, 14, 41] In more overt lesions, red blood cells in arterial walls show that the swelling is surely accounted for in part by seepage from the blood. Such intramural hemorrhage is easy to find in hyperplastic sclerotic arteries and, on occasion, can call attention to necrosis of a hyaline arteriole. Classic nuclear lesions, karyorrhexis and pyknosis, are seen by light microscopy in fibrinoid necrosis, but even a stray pyknotic nucleus is uncommon in hyaline sclerosis.

Glomerular lesions invariably accompany arterial necrosis in malignant hypertension, although they may not necessarily be caused by it. Klemperer and Otani[32] made serial section reconstructions to show that mucoid endarterial sclerosis of malignant hypertension obstructed the mouths of branches and infarcted glomeruli. Perhaps this is the explanation of a common nonhemorrhagic lesion: a large renal corpuscle with pale, dilated glomerular capillaries and much protein in Bowman's

space and the adjacent proximal tubule. (Surviving hyperplastic nephrons in contracted kidneys also contain extravasated protein, but it is denser, and the glomerulus
is not pallid.) Glomerular epithelium is swollen with protein droplets. A few red
blood cells in the filtered protein suggest an early stage of glomerular necrosis. In
other glomeruli, fibrinoid necrosis extends from the necrotic afferent arteriole; because all lobules are not always necrotic, it is difficult to think that the glomerulus
is infarcted either by fibrinoid necrosis of the arteriole or mucoid endarterial
fibrosis further upstream. Other glomerular lesions look quite like those in nephritis.
Epithelial proliferation and even leukocytes are found. Although Fahr[36] called
malignant nephrosclerosis a combination vascular and nephritic lesion, we find
necrotic lesions much commoner than inflammatory. The variety of glomerular
lesions in malignant hypertension is not easily explained by a single mechanism.

The cause of hypertensive vascular necrosis is disputed. Recourse is taken to
animal experiments. Hypertension of rats can be produced in a few weeks by reducing renal mass and giving salt, combined in most experiments with a third
maneuver such as administering a mineralocorticoid or inducing adrenal regeneration.[48] These animals develop fibrinoid necrosis in the renal vessels and in vessels
elsewhere.

Some years ago, one of us (LDS) had the chance to study Skelton's adrenal regeneration and related kinds of acute murine hypertensive lesions.[48] Except that
lesions of chronic hypertension were of course absent, their resemblance to the
necrotic lesions of human malignant hypertension was striking. There is, however, a
species difference: periarteritis of such arteries as the mesenteric is also found in the
hypertensive rats. A cellular inflammatory reaction (i.e., an arteritis) is most uncommon in human lesions, although we have occasionally encountered it, especially in
the interlobular renal arteries. Such cases were not mistaken instances of periarteritis or glomerulonephritis, for the renal glomerular lesions were scattered and
quite characteristic of malignant hypertension as were the other pathologic findings
and the clinical course.

We mentioned the demonstration of globulins and complement in some human
lesions (see p. 260). This suggests the possibility of an immune pathogenesis. Hypo-
thetical endothelial damage allowing infiltration of proteins might set the scene for
antigen-antibody reactions in some cases. It is tempting to think that more knowledge about variations at this stage of the process will lead to a better understanding
of species and individual variation in cellular inflammatory response.

Hypertension, itself, may cause fibrinoid necrosis in experimental animals.
Goldblatt[18] described and illustrated such lesions and said they were indistinguishable from lesions of human malignant hypertension. He produced the lesions in as
little as 48 to 72 hours by greatly constricting the renal arteries with his clamp. Interestingly, the lesions did not appear in the ischemic kidneys protected from the
elevated blood pressure. However, the pathogenesis is probably complex. The parts
played by pressure and ischemia have a new importance because of renal transplantation. Experiments testing extracorporeal perfusion and storage of kidneys are
directed toward maintaining human kidneys while a suitable recipient is found
among those awaiting renal transplantation.[2] Arterial and glomerular necrosis in a

few perfused canine kidneys we have studied seemed to be explained by a high perfusion pressure.[23]

To summarize, fibrinoid vascular necrosis can be experimentally produced by
acutely elevated blood pressure. In some experiments, the etiology was multifactorial
because salt was administered or, additionally, the endocrine state changed. An
immunopathogenesis has been suggested in some cases. In human malignant hypertension, the vascular necrosis is uncommonly complicated by arteritis and a cellular
infiltrate. A variety of glomerular lesions, necrotic, proliferative, and exudative, are
not easily accounted for by a single mechanism.

Historical Survey of Early Work

The relationship between hypertension and renal vascular lesions is customarily
traced back to Richard Bright's *Reports of Medical Cases* in 1827. Interested in
dropsy, Bright called attention to cases with albuminuria and organic change in the
structure of the kidney. Among the renal lesions, he illustrated by his own hand "a
hard contracted and granulated state of the kidney,"[5] and he noted that the left
ventricle was "particularly thick and firm" in a heart whose valves were normal.[4]
Hypertension, the connecting etiologic link, was not known at that time.

By 1872, Gull and Sutton[22] remarked that left ventricular hypertrophy was well
known in chronic Bright's disease with contracted kidneys. They attributed the
hypertrophy to vascular changes of "arterio-capillary fibrosis." In a curious way,
Gull and Sutton directed attention to the importance of vascular lesions by observations that were misinterpreted or even incorrect. They thought the scarring in the
kidney came from a primary periarteriolar and pericapillary fibrosis. Reminiscent
of the way "collagen disease" came to be extended in our time, they found "arterio-
capillary fibrosis" all over the body, a systemic malady.[21] Johnson[25] criticized their
observations and their interpretation at the time. He said the arterioles were thick
because of muscular hypertrophy. He thought that the heart and the arterioles both
hypertrophied to propel the blood through obstructed capillaries; later, he considered the hypertrophied arterioles themselves to be the peripheral obstruction.

As early as 1877, Mahomed[37] showed sphygmographic tracings of high arterial
tension, "the earliest and surest indication of this disease." He stated that the chronic
high arterial tension must inevitably lead to cardiac hypertrophy and thickening of
arteries, "in other words . . . to arterio-capillary fibrosis," of Gull and Sutton. Yet
Osler[40] did not list hypertension in the table of contents or the index of the first
edition of his textbook (1892); he mentioned it under "arterio-sclerosis," "chronic
interstitial nephritis," and "cardiac hypertrophy." In 1896, Riva-Rocci[44] described
the pressure cuff to measure blood pressure indirectly in man and, by the early
twentieth century, hypertensive disease was a clinical entity.

After vascular lesions were recognized in scarred, atrophied kidneys of hypertensive subjects, it was still some years before kidneys scarred because of vascular
sclerosis were separated from kidneys scarred because of antecedent nephritis, i.e.,
arterio-arteriolonephrosclerosis separated from chronic nephritis. Jores[28] is particularly credited with their clear separation in the first decade of the twentieth century.
Until then, what we know as vascular nephrosclerosis was generally considered

chronic interstitial nephritis. However, Cornil and Brault[10] in 1884 described vascular renal cirrhosis of arterial origin and set forth the features we recognize as hypertensive cardiovascular renal disease. One must have experience with "end-stage" kidneys to understand the difficulties: all scarred kidneys have some "inflammation," and chronic nephritis is complicated by hypertensive vascular lesions. As late as 1921, Evans[13] described intrarenal vascular sclerosis in detail and then explained at length why he thought both the vascular sclerosis and the parenchymal lesions resulted from renal inflammation. In the last edition of his textbook (1941), MacCallum[35] continued to discuss "arteriosclerotic nephritis" in the chapter on inflammation of the kidney, although he described the vascular lesions. He thought that not only interstitial inflammation but also glomerular lesions in this kind of renal disease were evidence of nephritis; he seemed not to separate chronic benign nephrosclerosis and malignant hypertension.

During this same period, it was learned that the vascular form of contracted kidneys usually ended in death by heart failure or cerebral apoplexy and, unlike chronic nephritis, seldom ended in renal failure. In other words, clinical hypertensive disease found its renal, cardiac, and vascular lesions. Further, hypertension secondary to nephritis was separated from hypertensive disease and vascular nephrosclerosis. By 1925, Fishberg[15] clearly stated, "The concept of essential hypertension includes those cases of chronic hypertension which neither clinically nor anatomically can be demonstrated to have evolved from antecedent inflammatory disease of the kidneys or from urinary obstruction." In the same paper, he gave an excellent account of hyaline arteriolosclerosis and its relation to hypertension. Hypertension-nephrosclerosis had been separated from hypertension secondary to other renal diseases.

In 1914, Volhard and Fahr[51] identified malignant hypertension among cases of primary hypertensive renal disease and related two groups of hypertensive disease to distinctive renal lesions. In their chronic benign form, renal insufficiency seldom occurred, and the kidneys were marked by arteriolosclerotic scarring. In malignant hypertension, death occurred in uremia; besides nephrosclerotic lesions, the kidneys had glomerular lesions like those in nephritis (combination form). The controversies stirred up by Volhard and Fahr's identification of malignant hypertension are tedious to trace through lengthy polemical German writing of that period. Later Fahr changed his views about the cause of the renal lesions in the malignant phase of hypertension and emphasized necrotizing arteritis rather than nephritis.[36] He also recognized a proliferative endarteritis. Clear expositions of malignant hypertension appeared in American publications by the late 1920's and early 1930's.[1, 30, 32] In last year's *Pathology Annual,* MacMahon[36] recounted this whole story at some length in the light of his own experience; this valuable paper also illustrates the lesions we have described in malignant hypertension (see Figs. 3, 5, 6, 7, 8, and 10[36]).

The search for a humoral vasopressor to link scarred kidneys to hypertension is a familiar story which continues to spin out connections of the renin-angiotensin mechanism with the juxtaglomerular apparatus and the adrenal cortex. The humoral etiology of renal hypertension gave new form to an old question about the primacy of vascular sclerosis or hypertension by limiting the argument to the kidney. Goldblatt had long been impressed by intrarenal vascular sclerosis in his autopsy studies

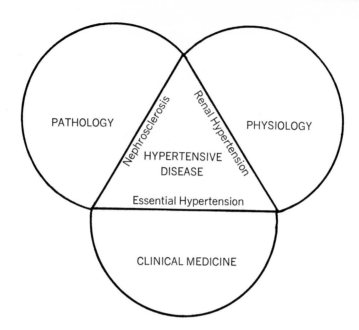

of hypertensive human beings, and he partially clamped the main renal artery as a way to produce renal ischemia only because he could think of no way to produce intrarenal arteriolosclerosis.[20] Since his famous experiments in the 1930's, he repeatedly contended that the intrarenal vascular sclerosis was the cause of renal hypertension. The opposite view is that elevated pressure causes the vascular lesions.

About a hundred years after Bright, the entity "hypertensive disease" emerged at the interfaces of pathology, clinical medicine, and physiology (see diagram). The entity served for more than a quarter century; then it began to be fragmented. As human counterparts of Goldblatt's clamp experiments were revealed by aortography and renal arteriography, cases of hypertension secondary to partial obstruction of the main renal artery were identified and surgically corrected. Another group, or perhaps several groups, of cases, are Conn's adrenal cortical hypertension with and without hypokalemia and with and without diabetes.[8, 9] Even more recently, cases having no increased peripheral resistance but hypertension as a consequence of sodium and water retention, increased blood volume, and increased cardiac output are being identified.[11, 12] It is unknown how large a group in the residue is triggered by vasomotor stress. As this process of fragmenting a scientific entity goes on, pathologists have an interesting opportunity to relate hypertensive renal vascular lesions to newly discovered mechanisms of disease. Out of all this will come new groupings of cases and probably overlapping new entities.

Technical Appendix

Carnoy Fixation

Investigations of the staining properties of fibrous proteins showed significant blocking of reactive groups by Zenker-formol and 10 percent formalin. In contrast, Carnoy's fluid does not cause irreversible chemical changes in the reactive groups and has therefore been recommended for histochemical studies of proteins and glycogen. This preservation of reactive groups made it possible to develop new staining methods on the basis of chemical, electron microscopic, and x-ray diffraction data, e.g., for incompletely cross-linked collagen,[60] basement membranes,[59] myoendothelial cells,[61] and muscle fibers. However, it is said that Carnoy's fluid causes considerable shrinkage and that the fixation procedure is too cumbersome for use in general hospital pathology. The fixation-embedding schedule described below overcomes these objections and has worked well for us for nine years.[65]

1. Cut tissue blocks 5 to 6 mm thick and place in Carnoy's solution (absolute alcohol-chloroform-glacial acetic acid 6:3:1). The ratio of fixative to tissue should be 20:1 to keep contamination of this nonaqueous fixative with tissue water within a few percent; this is important to prevent shrinkage. Let stand overnight at room temperature. During weekends and holidays tissues can be left in Carnoy's fluid up to 72 hours.

2. Transfer to absolute alcohol in the morning and wash in three changes of absolute alcohol for a total of 6 to 8 hours. Do not exceed this time limit; prolonged exposure to alcohol will cause shrinkage and hardening of tissues. During this time, blocks should be trimmed to a thickness of 2 to 3 mm and placed in receptacles.

3. Place in methyl benzoate overnight. Tissues can be stored in this fluid over weekends.

4. Transfer to an Autotechnicon in the morning; clear in xylene and xylene-paraffin mixture 1 hour each; infiltrate two to three changes of Paraplast for a total of 4 to 5 hours. The temperature of the paraffin bath should not exceed 60°C to avoid thermal shrinkage. Block as usual.

With this procedure, preservation of tissue structures is as good as in Zenker-fixed material and often considerably better than in formalin-fixed blocks from the same organ. Shrinkage artifacts described in the literature occur if one follows older procedures which recommend brief fixation for six hours or less and dehydration in absolute alcohol for 12 to 24 hours. This schedule does not permit stabilization of proteins by hydrogen-bond formation with the components of Carnoy's fluid, and the subsequent prolonged treatment with alcohol then causes collapse of protein structures. Therefore, tissues should be fixed for 15 hours and exposure to alcohol must be limited to less than eight hours.

Carnoy-fixation was found suitable for conventional stains (H&E, phosphotungstic acid-hematoxylin, allochrome, trichrome methods) and for histochemical demonstration of polysaccharides (PAS reaction) and proteins (amino, carboxyl, sulfhydryl and disulfide groups, tryptophane). Thus, histochemical findings can easily be correlated with familiar staining patterns. Calcium deposits in Carnoy- and alcohol-fixed sections from the same organs are stained equally intensely by alizarin red S and by von Kossa's procedure. This may seem surprising; however, calcium salts are practically insoluble in absolute alcohol-chloroform mixtures, and acetic acid exists in this solvent largely in the undissociated form.

References

1. Bell, E.T., and Clawson, B.J. Primary (essential) hypertension. A study of 420 cases. Arch. Path., 5:939, 1928.
2. Belzer, F.O., Ashby, B.S., and Dunphy, J.E. 24-hour and 72-hour preservation of canine kidneys. Lancet, 2:536, 1967.
3. Biava, C.G., Dyrda, I., Genest, J., and Bencosme, S.A. Renal hyaline arteriolosclerosis: An electronmicroscope study. Amer. J. Path., 44:349, 1964.
4. Bright, R. Reports of Medical Cases. Cited in Major, R.H. Classic Descriptions of Disease, 3d ed. Springfield, Charles C Thomas, Publisher, 1945, pp. 534-540.
5. ——— Reports of Medical Cases. Cited in Major, R.H. A History of Medicine, Springfield, Charles C Thomas, Publisher, 1954, pp. 688 (illustration) and 699.
6. Burkholder, P.M. Malignant nephrosclerosis: An immunohistopathologic study of localized γ-globulin and fixation of guinea pig complement in human kidneys. Arch. Path., 80:583, 1965.

7. Chandler, A.B. Thrombosis in the pathogenesis of atherosclerosis. J. Med. Ass. Georgia, 56:319, 1967.
8. Conn, J.W. Hypertension, the potassium ion and impaired carbohydrate tolerance. New Eng. J. Med., 273:1135, 1965.
9. ——— Cohen, E.L., Rovner, D.R., and Nesbit, R.M. Normokalemic primary aldosteronism: Detectable cause of curable "essential" hypertension. J.A.M.A., 193:200, 1965.
10. Cornil, and Brault. Études sur la Pathologie du Rein. Paris, Germer, Baillière et Cie., 1884.
11. Dickinson, C.J. The heart in hypertension. Lancet, 1:855, 1968.
12. Editorial. A new look at pressor mechanisms. New Eng. J. Med., 278:1399, 1968.
13. Evans, G. A contribution to the study of arterio-sclerosis with special reference to its relation to chronic renal disease. Quart. J. Med., 14:216, 1920-21.
14. Fennell, R.H., Jr., Reddy, C.R.R.M., and Vazquez, J.J. Progressive systemic sclerosis and malignant hypertension. Arch. Path., 72:209, 1961.
15. Fishberg, A.M. Anatomic findings in essential hypertension. Arch. Intern. Med., 35:650, 1925.
16. Fisher, E.R., Perez-Stable, E., and Pardo, V. Ultrastructural studies in hypertension. I. Comparison of renal vascular and juxtaglomerular cell alterations in essential and renal hypertension in man. Lab. Invest., 15:1409, 1966.
17. ——— and Rodnon, G.P. Pathologic observations concerning the kidney in progressive systemic sclerosis. Arch. Path., 65:29, 1958.
18. Goldblatt, H. The Renal Origin of Hypertension. Springfield, Charles C Thomas, Publisher, 1948.
19. ——— Hypertension due to renal ischemia. Bull. N. Y. Acad. Med., 40:745, 1964.
20. ——— In Moyer, J.H. Hypertension. The First Hahnemann Symposium on Hypertensive Disease. Philadelphia, W.B. Saunders Company, 1959, p. 171.
21. Gull, W., and Sutton, H.G. (B) On the arterio-capillary system in connection with kidney disease. 1. On changes in the spinal cord and its vessels in arterio-capillary fibrosis. Trans. Path. Soc. London, 28:361, 1877.
22. ——— and Sutton, H.G. On the pathology of the morbid state commonly called chronic Bright's disease with contracted kidney ("arterio-capillary fibrosis"). Med.-Chir. Trans., London, 55:273, 1872.
23. Humphries, A., and Stoddard, L.D. Unpublished observations.
24. Jackson, J.G., Puchtler, H., and Sweat F. Investigation of staining, polarization and fluorescence microscopic properties of pseudoelastic fibers in the renal arterial system. J. Royal Micr. Soc., 88:473, 1968.
25. Johnson, G. (B) On the arterio-capillary system in connection with kidney disease. 2. On the changes in the blood vessels and in the kidney, in connection with the small red granular kidney. Trans. Path. Soc. London, 28:381, 1877.
26. Joiner, D.W., Puchtler, H., and Gropp S. Lesions resembling hyperplastic arteriosclerosis in infants: Staining, polarization and fluorescence microscopic studies. Lab. Invest., 16:651, 1967 (abstract).
27. ——— Puchtler, H., and Sweat, F. Staining of immature collagen by resorcinfuchsin in infant kidneys. J. Royal Micr. Soc., 88:461, 1968.
28. Jores, L. Über die Arteriosklerose der kleinen Organarterien und ihre Beziehungen zur Nephritis. Virchow. Arch. Path. Anat. 17:367, 1904.
29. Kimmelstiel, P., Kim, O.J., Beres, J.A., and Wellmann, K. Chronic pyelonephritis. Amer. J. Med., 30:589, 1961.
30. ——— and Wilson, C. Benign and malignant hypertension and nephrosclerosis: A clinical and pathological study. Amer. J. Path., 12:45, 1936.
31. ——— and Wilson, C. Intercapillary lesions in the glomeruli of the kidney. Amer. J. Path., 12:83, 1936.
32. Klemperer, P., and Otani, S. Malignant nephrosclerosis (Fahr). Arch. Path., 11:60, 1931.

33. Kuhns, J.G., Puchtler, H., and Sweat, F. Histochemical evidence for plasma proteins in arteriolosclerosis. Lab. Invest., 11:681, 1962.
34. Lillie, R.D. The allochrome procedure: A differential method segregating the connective tissues: Collagen, reticulum and basement membranes into two groups. Amer. J. Clin. Path., 21:484, 1951.
35. MacCallum, W.G. A Textbook of Pathology, 7th ed. Philadelphia, W.B. Saunders Company, 1941, pp. 286-297.
36. MacMahon, H.E. Malignant nephrosclerosis—a reappraisal. In Pathology Annual 1968, Sommers, S.C., ed. New York, Appleton-Century-Crofts, 1968, Vol. 3, pp. 297-334.
37. Mahomed, F.A. (B) On the arterio-capillary system in connection with kidney disease. 3. On the sphygmographic evidence of arterio-capillary fibrosis. Trans. Path. Soc. London, 23:394, 1877.
38. McGee, W.G., and Ashworth, C.T. Fine structure of chronic hypertensive arteriopathy in the human kidney. Amer. J. Path., 43:273, 1963.
39. Moritz, A.R., and Oldt, M.R. Arteriolar sclerosis in hypertensive and nonhypertensive individuals. Amer. J. Path., 13:679, 1937.
40. Osler, W. Principles and Practice of Medicine, 1st ed. New York, D. Appleton and Company, 1892, pp. 628, 664, 749.
41. Paronetto, F. Immunocytochemical observations on the vascular necrosis and renal glomerular lesions of malignant nephrosclerosis. Amer. J. Path., 46:901, 1965.
42. Puchtler, H. Unpublished observations.
43. ——— and Sweat, F. Histochemical specificity of staining methods for connective tissue fibers: Resorcin-fuchsin and Van Gieson's picro-fuchsin. Histochemie, 4:24, 1964.
44. Riva-Rocci. Cited in Bard, P. MacLeod's Physiology in Modern Medicine, 9th ed. St. Louis, The C. V. Mosby Company, 1941, pp. 414-415.
45. Rodgers, J.C., Puchtler, H., and Gropp, S. Staining, polarization, and fluorescence microscopic studies of medial sclerosis in the renal arterial system. Lab. Invest., 16:651, 1967 (abstract).
46. ——— Puchtler, H., and Gropp, S. Transition from elastin to collagen in internal elastic membranes. Arch. Path., 83:557, 1967.
47. Ryle, J.A. The Natural History of Disease, 2nd ed. London, Oxford University Press, 1948, pp. 305-314.
48. Skelton, F.R. Experimental hypertensive vascular disease accompanying adrenal regeneration in the rat. Amer. J. Path., 32:1037, 1956.
49. Sweat, F., Puchtler, H., and Terry, M.S. Staining isolated proteins and polysaccharides on slides: Phosphotungstic acid-hematoxylin versus the rosindole reaction. Stain Technol., 43:283, 1968.
50. ——— Puchtler, H., and Woo, P. Periodic acid-Schiff-picro-Sirius supra blue GL: A light fast modification of Lillie's allochrome stain. Arch. Path., 78:73, 1964.
51. Volhard, F., and Fahr, T. Die Brightsche Nierenkrankheit. Berlin, Julius Springer, 1914. Cited by MacMahon, H.E.[36] and Kimmelstiel, P., personal communication, as the discoverers of malignant hypertension.

References on Methods

A. Stains Suitable for Carnoy-, Formalin- and Zenker-Fixed Tissues:
52. Puchtler, H., and Sweat, F. Commercial resorcin-fuchsin as a stain for elastic fibers. Stain Technol., 35:347, 1960. Eliminates the cumbersome preparation of resorcin-fuchsin with its fire hazard; the dry commercial dye keeps indefinitely.
53. Puchtler, H., Sweat, F., and Doss, N.O. A one-hour phosphotungstic acid-hematoxylin stain. Amer. J. Clin. Path., 40:334, 1963. Eliminates mordanting, reduces staining time from 24-48 hours to one hour.

54. Sweat, F., Puchtler, H., and Rosenthal, S.I. Sirius red F3BA as a stain for connective tissue. Arch. Path., 78:69, 1964. *A modification of Van Gieson's picro-fuchsin which stains collagen, reticulum fibers, and basement membranes intensely and selectively. Permits demonstration of fine collagen fibers in the intima.*

55. See reference 50. *No fading has been observed in sections stored for more than five years; Lillie's original stain fades in less than a year. Excellent for demonstration of hyaline arteriolosclerosis.*

56. Sweat, F., and Puchtler, H. Demonstration of amyloid with direct cotton dyes. Arch. Path., 80:613, 1965. *Stains amyloid selectively without differentiation.*

57. Sweat, F., Meloan, S.N., and Puchtler, H. A modified one-step trichrome stain for demonstration of fine connective tissue fibers. Stain Technol., 43:227, 1968. *Does not require differentiation; staining time: 1 minute.*

B. Methods Suitable Only for Carnoy-Fixed Tissues:

58. Puchtler, H., Chandler, A.B., and Sweat, F. Demonstration of fibrin in tissue sections by the rosindole method. J. Histochem. Cytochem., 9:340, 1961. *Method of choice for demonstrating plasma proteins in hyaline deposits.*

59. Puchtler, H., and Sweat, F. A Selective stain for renal basement membranes. Stain Technol., 39:163, 1964.

60. See reference 27.

61. Puchtler, H., Sweat, F., Terry, M.S., and Conner, H.M. Investigation of staining, polarization, and fluorescence microscopic properties of myoendothelial cells. J. Royal Micr. Soc. in press.

C. Papers Dealing with Specificity of Methods:

62. See reference 43.

63. See reference 24.

64. See reference 49.

65. Puchtler, H., Waldrop, F.S., Conner, H.M., and Terry, M.S. Carnoy Fixation: Practical and theoretical considerations. Histochemie, 16:361, 1968.

Two recent reviews not cited contain numerous references:

    Adams, C.W.M. Vascular Histochemistry in Relation to the Chemical and Structural Pathology of Cardiovascular Disease. Chicago, Year Book Medical Publishers, Inc., 1967.

    Page, I.H., and McCubbin, J.W., eds. Renal Hypertension. Chicago, Year Book Medical Publishers, Inc., 1968, Ch. 16. Relationship of hypertension to vascular changes, pp. 372-396 and bibliography ff.

MYELOPROLIFERATIVE DISORDERS
AND DISSEMINATED INTRAVASCULAR COAGULATION

DONALD G. McKAY

The occurrence of bleeding of varying degrees of severity in myeloproliferative disorders has long attracted the attention of students of these diseases. A variety of explanations has been offered. Perhaps the most time-honored is the concept, particularly in leukemias, that the replacement of the bone marrow by leukemic cells has resulted in a destruction of megakaryocytes with the production of thrombocytopenia and consequent hemorrhage. In some cases this may be an adequate explanation. Another theory suggests that in certain leukemias there is activation of the fibrinolytic enzyme system with a resultant degradation of fibrinogen in the circulating blood, leading to hemorrhage because of a diminished circulating fibrinogen level or abnormal aggregation of fibrinogen into fibrin at sites of vascular trauma. There is clear evidence that plasminogen is activated in some patients with leukemia,[1] but it is doubtful that this is more than a secondary response or that it could explain the bleeding tendency in all of these patients.

We have recently encountered several patients, with different types of myeloproliferative disorders, who demonstrate clearly that the bleeding tendency, in some patients, is triggered by disseminated intravascular coagulation. These cases shed new light on the problem and also raise important questions of a fundamental nature concerning the influence of leukocytes, platelets, tumor cells, and damaged endothelium on the blood coagulation mechanism in vivo.

Eosinophilic Leukemia

CASE. This 57-year-old businessman had a chief complaint of pleuritic pain for 12 days and numbness and weakness of the left arm with blurred vision for one day. His present illness began with the chest pain. One week later his physician found a blood pressure of 130/86, decreased resonance and fremitus at the left base without rales, and a left upper quadrant mass extending to the iliac crest. Chest X-rays showed a normal

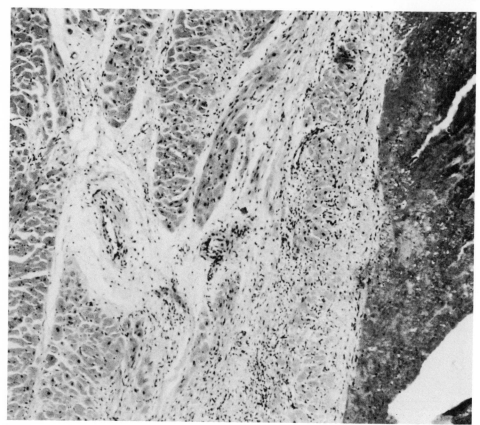

Fig. 1.   Eosinophilic leukemia: mural thrombus, heart. The dark material at the right is the mural fibrin deposit. The endocardium and subendocardium are replaced by a layer of connective tissue. H&E. X165.

heart, minor areas of bilateral pleural thickening, and splenomegaly. The initial laboratory examination showed a hemoglobin of 12.2 grams, hematocrit 37 percent, and a white blood cell count of 35,000 (33 percent were polymorphonuclears, 9 percent myelocytes, 11 percent lymphocytes, 10 percent monocytes, and 37 percent eosinophils). The erythrocyte sedimentation rate was 59 mm/hr. The blurred vision and numbness of his left arm brought him to the Presbyterian Hospital.

Physical examination on entry revealed a well-nourished, well-oriented man with a good memory but strangely unconcerned about his illness. There was no papilledema and no abnormal reflexes. Sensory examination was normal, as was position sense except in the left arm. The liver was one fingerbreadth below the costal margin and the spleen was enlarged.

A repeat laboratory examination revealed a white blood cell count of 43,050 (54 percent polymorphonuclears, 15 percent lymphocytes, 10 percent monocytes, and 24 percent eosinophils). The reticulocyte count was 2.3 percent. Urinalysis showed a specific gravity of 1.026, 1+ albumin, and 6 to 8 white cells per high power field.

During his hospital stay, his neurologic signs progressed rapidly. By the following day, he was obtunded, and the paralysis of his left arm was complete. Lumbar puncture revealed a clear fluid with an initial pressure of 250, sugar 82, protein 29 mg percent, 18 red cells, 1 white cell, and cultures were negative. An electroencephalogram showed several areas of slowing, and a right carotid arteriogram was normal. Five days after admis-

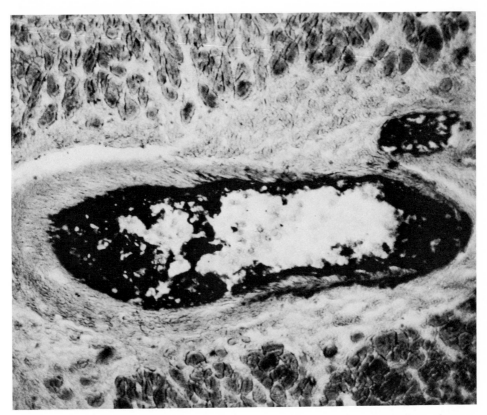

Fig. 2. Eosinophilic leukemia: myocardium. An arteriole in the myocardium shows a mural deposit of fibrin. H&E. X400.

sion, he had a flaccid quadriplegia, and on the ninth day he lapsed into a coma from which he never recovered even though he lived for another month.

A bone marrow aspiration showed 49 percent eosinophils and hypoplasia of the erythrocyte series. He was treated with prednisolone and Achromycin initially. The Achromycin was replaced by penicillin, Chloromycetin, Streptomycin, and INH. A repeat lumbar puncture yielded an initial pressure of 90, sugar 95, protein 43, and 38 red blood cells.

During the first two weeks, his temperature ranged from 101 to 103°, but in the third week he became afebrile. During the fourth week, a comparison of sera of 7/30 and 8/16 showed no rise in titre of antibodies to influenza, polio, herpes, lymphocytic choriomeningitis, Eastern or Western equine encephalitis, St. Louis encephalitis, mycoplasma pneumoniae, or leptospira. Tests for trichinosis, toxoplasmosis, histoplasmosis, and blastomycosis were negative.

In his final week, his temperature rose to 104°, and he developed respiratory distress which increased until his death 39 days after admission.

Autopsy

1. Eosinophilic leukemia
   a) Leukemic infiltration of
     (1) bone marrow

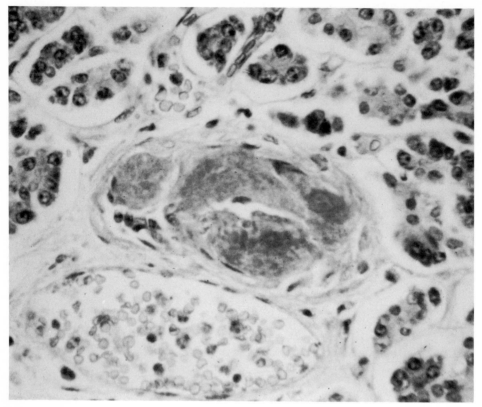

Fig. 3.   Eosinophilic leukemia: pancreas. Fibrin thrombus in venule. H&E. X400.

(2) spleen
(3) striated muscle
(4) adrenal
(5) kidney
(6) urinary bladder
(7) testis

2. Disseminated intravascular coagulation with thrombosis of
   a) Mural endocardium, right ventricle (Fig. 1)
   b) Arterioles of myocardium, with multiple foci of necrosis of cardiac muscle (Fig. 2)
   c) Spleen, with multiple small infarcts
   d) Capillaries of pancreas (Fig. 3)
   e) Cerebral capillaries: encephalomalacia, recent, multiple in frontal, parietal, and occipital lobes bilaterally; right inferior temporal gyrus; left caudate nucleus and right cerebellar hemisphere (Fig. 4)

In this patient, the cerebral, splenic, and myocardial infarcts were caused by thrombi in the capillaries of these organs. The mural endocardial thrombus was another manifestation of an increased coagulability of the blood.

Patients with eosinophilic leukemia present many clinical manifestations common to other forms of leukemia.[2] Chronic fatigue, weakness, weight loss, anorexia,

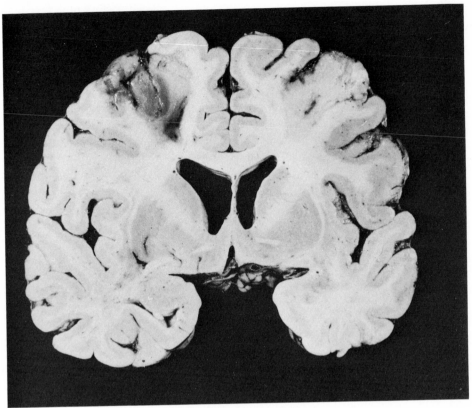

Fig. 4.   Eosinophilic leukemia: brain. Multiple small infarcts of the cortex.

lassitude, bone and joint pains, fever, sore throat, bleeding, and purpura are among these symptoms and signs. Splenomegaly, hepatomegaly, lymphadenopathy, bone tenderness, retinitis, and skin lesions also occur.

A few findings, however, seem peculiar to eosinophilic leukemia. There is a high incidence of chronic cough, transient pulmonary infiltrates seen by chest film, rales, and cyanosis. These are apparently related to the eosinophilia. Also, there is a high incidence of myocardial damage, and mural thrombi in both ventricles and the left auricle are more frequent. There is also a predilection for involvement of the central nervous system. Drowsiness, coma, convulsions, delirium, or hemiplegia are frequent. The clinical occurrence of bleeding and purpura, respiratory distress with cyanosis, myocardial damage, coma, convulsions, and hemiplegia, in association with the pathologic findings of cerebral, splenic, pulmonary, and myocardial infarcts, are due to platelet and fibrin thrombi in the microcirculation. These were clearly demonstrated in the case reported above.

In our studies of disseminated intravascular coagulation, we have found that the localization of thrombi in the microcirculation is extremely variable from one disease process to the next. This is due to the variations in the mechanism by which and the rate at which the clotting mechanism is triggered. In eosinophilic leukemias, there is a strong suggestion that the clotting is somehow related to the eosinophil itself. Archer[3] studied the effect of eosinophils on the plasma prothrombin time with the following results:

	CLOTTING TIME
Brain thromboplastin; plasma: 0.024 M $CaCl_2$	18 seconds
Eosinophils in saline; plasma: 0.025 M $CaCl_2$	344 seconds
Saline; plasma: 0.025 M $CaCl_2$	480 seconds

Although the eosinophils appeared to shorten the prothrombin time when compared to simple recalcification of plasma, the effect was minor when compared to tissue (brain) thromboplastin. These studies indicate that the eosinophil does not contain a substance equivalent to tissue (complete) thromboplastin but does have a slight procoagulant activity comparable to the phospholipid of normal platelets, leukocytes, and red blood cells. It is possible that this "partial thromboplastin" effect may be enough to induce blood coagulation in vivo.

Another possibility is that the eosinophilic granule may play a role in triggering clotting. The granules contain crystals which, when released from cytoplasm of the eosinophil upon death of the cell, might act as particulate matter and cause not only agglutination of platelets but activation of Hageman factor. It has long been known that particulate matter is capable of triggering blood coagulation in vivo and in vitro.[4]

Promyelocytic Leukemia

CASE. The patient was a 20-year-old female with a chief complaint of excessive bleeding during the last menstrual period and bruises on her legs for the past five days. Past history revealed that she had had psychomotor seizures consisting of dizziness, shaking of the right arm, and occasional falls without loss of consciousness since 1957. She was treated with Dilantin and Mysoline and had not had a seizure for the past two years. Prior to the present illness, she had not noticed any bleeding tendency. She felt weak and tired but had had no weight loss.

Physical examination on admission on 5/11/66 revealed a well-developed, well-nourished female in no acute distress. Temperature was 99.8°, pulse 120, blood pressure 120/70, and respirations 16. Over the skin of both legs were 10 ecchymotic areas and a large firm one (4 × 4 cm) over the left hip. There were petechial hemorrhages on the uvula and palate, ecchymosis of the lower lip, and blood was oozing from the gums, without any gingival hypertrophy. Lymph nodes, spleen, and liver were not palpable.

Laboratory examination revealed a hematocrit of 38 percent; hemoglobin of 12.8 grams; a white blood cell count of 22,800 with 36 percent polymorphonuclear leukocytes, 24 percent immature granulocytes, 38 percent blasts, 1 percent lymphocytes, and 1 percent basophils. No platelets were found on the blood film. Urinalysis was within normal limits. The blood urea nitrogen (BUN) was 15 mg percent, and uric acid was 4.5 mg percent. Bacterial culture of the urine and bone marrow yielded no growth.

Initial coagulation studies included a bleeding time of 12 minutes and a venous clotting time in which the first tube showed a small clot after 5 minutes, which gradually became smaller with continued tilting. There was poor clot retraction at the end of 10 hours. The prothrombin time was 20.4 seconds and a Rumpel-Leede test produced 40 petechiae in a 2.5 square centimeter area.

Bone marrow aspiration showed a hypercellular marrow with numerous immature cells of the myeloid series, many with abundant nonspecific granules characteristic of promyelocytes.

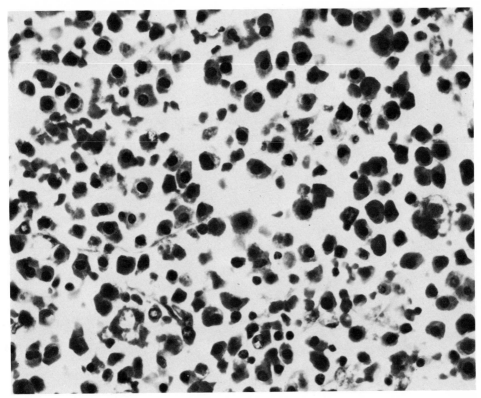

Fig. 5.   Promyelocytic leukemia: bone marrow. The marrow is completely replaced by leukemic cells. H&E. X300.

On 5/12/66, the prothrombin time was 28 seconds; Factor V was 35 percent of normal; platelets 29,000; prothrombin consumption time was 12 seconds (normal: >20 sec); a partial thromboplastin was 75 seconds (normal: 60 to 85 sec); and a fibrinogen was 26 mg percent. At this point heparin was started as a continuous intravenous infusion amounting to 7,200 units every four hours.

On 5/13/66, the fibrinogen level was 62 mg percent (12 hours after heparin was started) and 80 mg percent within 24 hours. Bleeding from the gums stopped within four hours after heparin was started, and vaginal bleeding ceased within 24 hours. On 5/15/66, the fibrinogen was 151 mg percent. The platelet count remained low (19,000), and there was a drop in hematocrit from 34 to 20 percent. This was not accompanied by any obvious bleeding, but later that day the patient developed fever. Blood cultures were negative.

On 5/16/66, a platelet transfusion was started, and the patient's white blood count rose to 92,600 with 64 percent blasts. A course of Prednisone, Vincristine and 6-mercaptopurine was started. Following transfusion of 6 platelet units, the platelet count was 72,000, and the fibrinogen was 243 mg percent.

On 5/17/66, she complained of a severe headache and became progressively lethargic. At 4:00 P.M. her platelet count was 36,000, white blood cell count 91,000, and fibrinogen 229 mg percent. The headache became more severe, and she complained of diplopia. By 11:00 P.M. she had a dilated right pupil (poorly reactive) and a fully dilated left pupil which was completely unreactive. She responded only to painful stimuli. Respirations and pulse ceased at noon on 5/18/66. Unfortunately, autopsy permission could not be obtained.

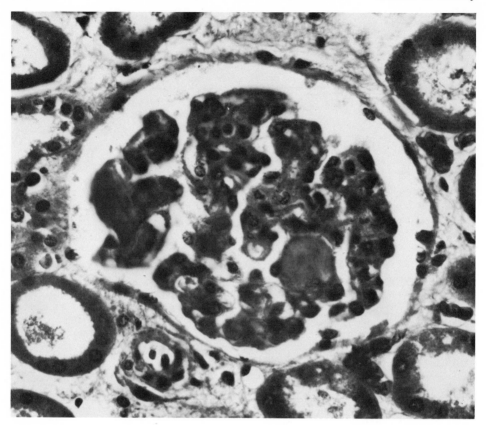

Fig. 6.   Promyelocytic leukemia: kidney. Two capillary loops are distended and obstructed by recent fibrin deposits. H&E. X400.

We have observed several cases of disseminated intravascular clotting in pro-myelocytic leukemia at autopsy. One such case is illustrated in Figures 5, 6, and 7. There were thrombi in the glomerular capillaries and in the adrenal sinusoids, with hemorrhagic necrosis of the adrenal. The bone marrow was replaced by leukemic cells. Pittman, et al.[5] have described three cases of acute promyelocytic leukemia with disseminated thrombi at autopsy and clear evidence of intravascular coagulation from studies of the hemostatic mechanism.

In an attempt to determine the cause of intravascular coagulation in promyelo-cytic leukemia, we investigated the thromboplastic properties of the leukemic cells. Suspensions of white cells (WBC) and red cells from the patient were prepared by differential centrifugation from EDTA plasma.[6] Washed cells were sonicated and lyophilized. Optimal concentrations of the sonicates and other substances in a partial thromboplastin test system formed clots in the following times:

1. Calcium   117 seconds
2. Red blood cell stroma   112 seconds
3. Partial thromboplastin (platelet factor 3 substitute,
   Thrombofax)   58 seconds

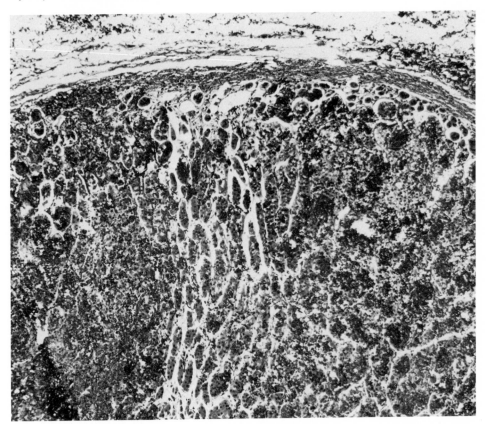

Fig. 7. Promyelocytic leukemia: adrenal. The foci of hemorrhage and necrosis in the cortex are due to deposition of fibrin thrombi in the sinusoids. H&E. X165.

4. Complete (tissue) thromboplastin (Simplastin)	18 seconds
5. White cell (leukemic) sonicates	20 seconds

One milligram of Simplastin had the thromboplastic activity of 8.5 mg of leukemic cell extract. Promyelocytic WBC preparations yielded short clotting times with Factor VIII and IX-deficient plasma, but not with fibrinogen or prothrombin-deficient plasma.

The fact that extracts of the leukemic cells shortened the partial thromboplastin times to this extent indicates that these cells contain "tissue thromboplastin." A similar examination of normal human leukocyte extracts resulted in a shortening of the partial thromboplastin time to approximately 80 seconds. Normal rabbit leukocytes from the peritoneal cavity behaved the same.[7] This indicates that normal leukocytes contain little or no "tissue thromboplastin." Hjort and Rappaport[8] arrived at a similar conclusion.

In addition, we studied the leukocytes from one or two cases of acute and chronic lymphocytic leukemia and chronic granulocytic leukemia, and all of these shortened the clotting time to the same extent as normal leukocytes.

Acute Leukemia

The major causes of death in acute leukemia are infection and hemorrhage. Hersh, et al.[9] attributed death to infection in 70 percent of patients and to hemorrhage in 52 percent in a series of 414 patients. The majority of these patients had acute lymphocytic and acute myelogenous leukemias. Evidence that disseminated intravascular coagulation is a major complication of acute leukemias comes eventually from three sources: 1) pathology; 2) alterations of the hemostatic mechanism; and 3) response of the hemostatic mechanism to heparin.

Pathologic Changes

The best described and correctly interpreted case was studied by Baker, et al.[10] The patient died of acute myelogenous leukemia and at autopsy showed capillary and arteriolar thrombi in renal glomerular capillaries, hepatic arterioles, pulmonary vessels, and right middle cerebral artery. These thrombotic occlusions had produced ischemic necrosis or hemorrhage in the respective tissues. This demonstration by pathologic means constitutes certain evidence of disseminated intravascular coagulation.

Another case of disseminated intravascular coagulation demonstrated at autopsy in a patient with acute leukemia was described by Rosenzweig and Kendall.[11] Pathologic examination revealed thrombosis of the microcirculation in the intermediate lobe of the pituitary, paraventricular nuclei, gastric mucosa, colonic mucosa, adrenals, and spleen. Hemorrhagic infarction due to the thrombi was present in all of these tissues. The major feature of this patient's disease was the presence of acquired diabetes insipidus which was due to the damage to the paraventricular and supraoptic nuclei and possibly the posterior lobe of the pituitary. We have previously shown that thrombosis of the microcirculation of the posterior pituitary, supraoptic, and supraventricular nuclei is a cause of diabetes insipidus in patients with disseminated intravascular coagulation[12] due to other causes. Rosenzweig and Kendall[11] found in the literature eleven cases of leukemia and diabetes insipidus.

Bone and bone marrow infarcts are fairly common in acute leukemia. Nies, et al.[13] found at autopsy bone necrosis in 15 percent of patients with acute lymphocytic leukemia and in three percent of those with acute myelogenous leukemia. The infarcts were of varying ages and some could be demonstrated by X-ray as radiolucent defects, osteoporosis, subepiphyseal radiolucencies, periosteal lesions, and, in one case, aseptic necrosis of the femoral head. Bone infarct (aseptic necrosis of bone) is a complication of disseminated intravascular coagulation in sickle cell anemia, cases of spontaneous fibrinolysis inhibition, and in patients with rheumatoid arthritis and prolonged administration of cortisone. Although the leukemic infiltration of the bone may play a major role in the localization, occlusion of capillary beds by thrombi is the most likely explanation of bone infarcts in leukemia and these other disorders.

The gastrointestinal tract is frequently involved in acute leukemia. Massive hemorrhage from the gastrointestinal tract may be a cause of death. More frequently, the hemorrhage is not lethal but is high in incidence. Pathologic involvement of the

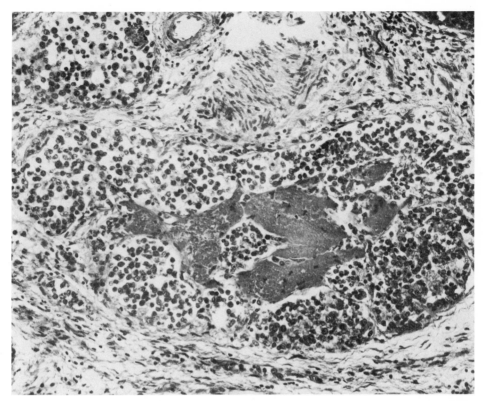

Fig. 11.   Leukemic spread of reticulum cell sarcoma: ovary. The tumor cells line the vessel and the lumen is obliterated by thrombus. H&E. X300.

several years which was treated with Reserpine, and recurrent epistaxes for many years requiring cauterization in 1963 and 1964. He also complained of dysphagia for the past 10 years. A report from his local physician indicated a red blood cell count of 6 million, six months prior to admission.

His present illness began on 11/28/64 with the sudden onset of a headache with a profound sense of fatigue and malaise. After transient improvement, symptoms recurred on 12/2 when his wife noted that he was jaundiced. This was followed by recurrent daily vomiting and a 12-hour period of hiccoughs. On 12/6, he developed pain and cyanosis of his toes and was admitted to a local hospital.

On admission, although the toes were cyanotic, there were strong pulses in the arteries of the leg. His blood pressure was 150/80; the erythrocyte sedimentation rate 6; hemoglobin 15.8 grams; hematocrit 50 percent; white blood cell count was 17,750 with 79 percent polymorphonuclears, 21 percent lymphocytes and 5 nucleated red blood cells per 100 white cells. The urine contained 2+ albumin, 4 to 5 white cells and 2 to 3 red cells per high power field. Serum bilirubin was 3.8 mg percent; serum albumin 2.9 g and serum globulin 3.1 g. The SGOT rose from 220 to 2,000 units in a short period of time. A reticulocyte count was 1.2 percent, and a bone marrow aspiration revealed erythroid hyperplasia with some myelocytic hyperplasia. A phlebotomy of 300 ml led to a drop in blood pressure to 90/50. He was then transferred to the Presbyterian Hospital on 12/9/64.

On admission, his blood pressure was 108/68, pulse 100, respirations 20, and temperature 98.8°. He was lethargic, with slow mentation, and plethoric, with acrocyanosis. His sclerae were icteric, and there was some dried blood in the left naris. Auscultation

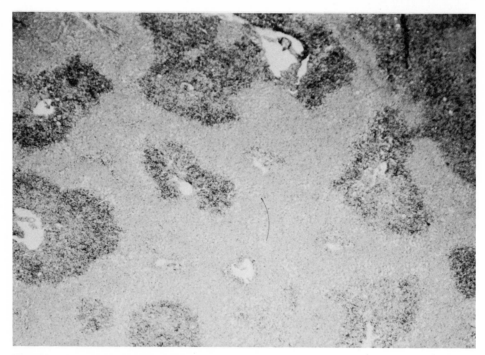

Fig. 12.   Polycythemia vera: liver. The dark patches around central veins are deposits of fibrin in the sinusoids with areas of central hemorrhagic necrosis. PTAH. X60.

revealed scattered rales at both lung bases extending one-third of the way up on the left. There was a protodiastolic rhythm and a systolic murmur at the apex and base, the latter transmitted faintly to the neck. A loud "to and fro" abdominal bruit was heard, but the liver and spleen were not enlarged. The fingers were clubbed, and there was a livid reticulum of both legs to the knees, with a deep cyanosis of all toes. The feet were cool in spite of bounding bilateral arterial pulses.

At this point, laboratory studies revealed a hemoglobin of 13.5 grams; hematocrit 41 percent; reticulocyte count of 4.6 percent; an erythrocyte sedimentation rate of 4; and 50 nucleated red blood cells per 100 white cells. The platelet count was 85,000, pro-thrombin time 21 seconds (normal: 13 sec), and fibrinogen 176 mg percent. The urinalysis exhibited a trace of albumin with a rare white cell. The blood urea nitrogen (BUN) was 86 mg; serum calcium 8.1 mg percent; phosphorus 4.4 mg percent; bilirubin 3.8 mg percent; alkaline phosphatase 22 units; SGOT 740 units; serum glutamic-pyruvic transaminase (SGPT) 800 units; cephalin flocculation and thymol turbidity negative; and uric acid 16 mg percent.

During his hospital stay, the patient had a temperature ranging from 100 to 101°, and he remained confused. He was given penicillin, Streptomycin, and Hydrocortisone. Three days after admission, he became suddenly more cyanotic about the head, his respirations slowed, and shortly thereafter he died.

Autopsy

1. Polycythemia vera
    a) Hyperplasia of bone marrow, all elements
    b) Extramedullary hematopoiesis, spleen
2. Disseminated intravascular coagulation
    a) Thrombosis of hepatic veins and sinusoids of liver, with extensive central necrosis of liver (Budd-Chiari syndrome) (Figs. 12 and 13)

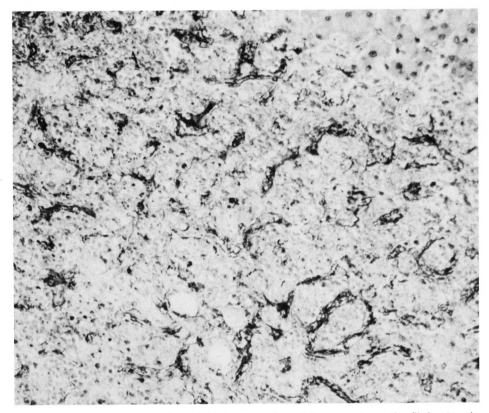

Fig. 13.   Polycythemia vera: liver. A high power view of the liver shows the fibrin strands in the sinusoids of the central lobular zones. PTAH. X300.

     b) Thrombosis of arterioles, capillaries, and venules of
        (1) skin of feet
        (2) kidney
        (3) testis (Fig. 14)
        (4) prostate (Fig. 15)
  3. Hypertensive arteriosclerotic heart disease
     a) Cardiomegaly (640 grams)
     b) Severe coronary artery atherosclerosis, with complete occlusion of the right
     c) Benign nephrosclerosis
     d) Abdominal aneurysm (fusiform), 10 cm long, below renal arteries
     e) Cerebral arteriosclerosis: encephalomalacia, old, microscopic, right middle
        frontal gyrus and right putamen
  4. Congenital hypoplasia
     a) Left cerebellar hemisphere
     b) Inferior and middle cerebellar peduncles

    Intravascular thrombosis is a well-known complication of polycythemia vera. The paradoxical occurrence of thrombosis and hemorrhage provides the major complications of the disease. Thromboses occur in one-fourth of the patients and account for one-fourth of the deaths.[17] Cerebral, coronary, and mesenteric arteries are frequently involved, as are peripheral arteries and veins. Gastrointestinal tract lesions, such as peptic ulcer, are secondary to thrombosis of the small vessels of the mucosa.

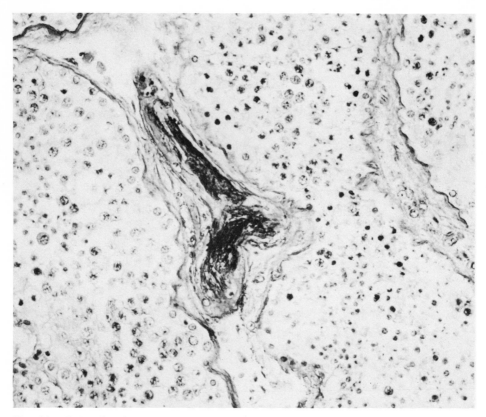

Fig. 14.   Polycythemia vera: testis. An intertubular capillary is obstructed by a fibrin thrombus. PTAH. X300.

Massive subcutaneous bleeding with hematomas containing 3 to 4 liters of blood were described by Whitelaw and Thomas,[18] and massive adrenal hemorrhage has been reported.[19]

Studies of the blood coagulation components have not been systematic but have shown that blood clots formed in vitro are unstable, dissolve easily, and show poor retraction. In a study of 19 cases, Björkman, et al.[20] found that the fibrinogen levels were within normal limits but that increased fibrinolytic activity was present in all cases. No increased fibrinolysis was found in three patients with secondary polycythemia.

The occurrence of thrombotic episodes explains the hemorrhagic diathesis. The bleeding is due to a depletion of coagulation factors which are used up in the clotting process and also to the activation of fibrinolysin which further depletes the clotting factors.

Hemorrhagic Thrombocythemia

Hemorrhagic thrombocythemia is a clinical syndrome with the presenting symptom of recurrent spontaneous hemorrhages, either external or into the tissues, and often preceded or accompanied by thromboses in the superficial or deep veins.

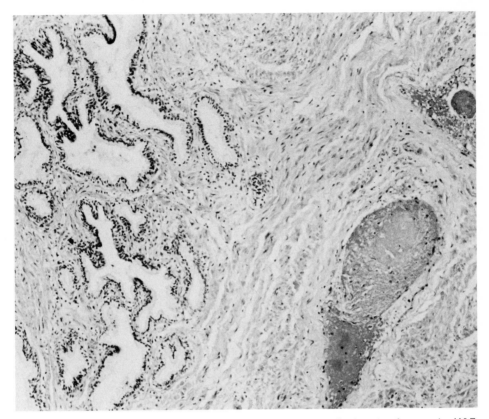

Fig. 15.   Polycythemia vera: prostate. A thrombus obstructs the lumen of a venule. H&E.
X165.

An extremely high platelet count, leukocytosis, splenomegaly, and a hypochromic
anemia with a tendency to slightly polycythemic red cell counts in intervals between
hemorrhages are common. Gunz[21] reviewed 50 cases and found that there is approximately an equal sex ratio and that the mean age of the patients is 51 years.
Bleeding occurs in all cases and is spontaneous, repeated, and of varying severity.
The duration of the bleeding tendency is often from one to five years, but in one instance it extended over a 27-year period.[22] The most common site of bleeding is the
gastrointestinal tract, but hemoptysis, menorrhagia, hematuria, and excessive bleeding after minor trauma, dental procedures, or operations may occur. Although spontaneous bruising with the formation of large hematomata after insignificant trauma
is frequent, purpura does not occur. The hemorrhagic tendency may manifest itself
initially within a few months after splenectomy. Splenectomy is usually followed by
progression of the disease with exacerbation of the bleeding tendency and sometimes
a rapid demise. Splenic enlargement is the most consistent finding at physical examination. The most common site of thrombosis is the splenic vein, although the veins
of the leg and penis may also be involved. A patient rarely dies of pulmonary
embolus or portal vein thrombosis. The liver may be enlarged and peptic ulcer will
be found in about 20 percent of the cases.

Platelet counts are invariably high. The mean platelet count is approximately

3.2 million per cu ml but may even reach 14 million. The structure of the platelets is often abnormal with the appearance of chains, irregular shapes, and giant forms. Very large clusters of platelets are seen in the blood or bone marrow smears. Leukocytosis with a predominant rise in polymorphonuclear leukocytes is usually present. Myelocytes or myeloblasts account for 1 to 3 percent of the total count. Hypochromic anemia of variable severity is usually observed. Abnormally high red cell counts are found in one-third of the cases, but polycythemia is transient and always alternates with anemia.

The platelet survival time in in vivo clinical experiments is either normal[21] or prolonged.[23] Platelet function, as determined by the thromboplastin generation time, is either increased, normal, or decreased and varies from patient to patient and from time to time in the same individual. Some evidence exists that an anticoagulant activity is present in the blood of some of the patients. This anticoagulant activity may be derived from the platelets themselves.[24, 25] The bleeding time is normal in half the cases and prolonged in the remainder. It may become prolonged but revert to normal in any one patient. Capillary resistance is usually within normal limits, as is the coagulation time, prothrombin consumption, and clot retraction. Decreases in prothrombin activity, fibrinogen, and Factors V, VII, and VIII may be encountered.

Treatment with P[32] is as effective in this syndrome as it is in polycythemia vera.[26] With the resultant decrease in platelets, there is a concomitant diminution in the hemorrhages which may cease altogether.

Although hemorrhagic thrombocythemia is a rather distinct clinical entity, it is best regarded as a variant of the myeloproliferative disorders, such as myelogenous leukemia and polycythemia vera. These two processes show the same age and sex incidence, splenomegaly, hyperplasia of all the cells of the bone marrow, and extramedullary hematopoiesis. They are frequently associated with peptic ulcer and occasionally, with gout. The chief difference lies in the higher incidence of hemorrhage. Because of this, the clotting mechanism in hemorrhagic thrombocythemia has received closer scrutiny.

The increased tendency to thrombosis in these diseases is due to the increased number of platelets in the circulating blood. Even though the rate of destruction is the same, an increased amount of thromboplastin is released into the circulating blood as the platelets die. When this increased amount of thromboplastin can no longer be removed by the reticuloendothelial system, it reaches a level which induces thrombus formation. Stasis, eddies, and endothelial damage are the vascular factors determining the location of the thrombi.

When enough thrombosis occurs, certain of the coagulation factors are consumed in the process. These include fibrinogen, prothrombin, and Factors V, VII, and VIII. Associated with the thrombosis is an activation of the fibrinolytic enzyme, which in turn tends to further deplete the components of the hemostatic mechanism. Eventually, a severe bleeding tendency appears, which may be augmented by the anticoagulant effect of the abnormally large numbers of platelets. The idea that multiple capillary thrombi, causing an excessive consumption of coagulation factors, are responsible for the bleeding tendency was first proposed by Arlotti and Ballerini.[27]

Summary

The cases cited illustrate the fact that disseminated intravascular coagulation is a complication of myeloproliferative disorders. The clotting episode seems to occur predominantly as a terminal event. In many instances, it is the major cause of death. The evidence for its occurrence comes from three sources: 1) pathologic demonstration of fibrin and platelet thrombi or emboli in vessels of the microcirculation; 2) depletion of the factors of the hemostatic mechanism of the circulating blood; and 3) the restoration of the clotting factors toward normal upon administration of heparin. Sometimes the latter is accompanied by a cessation of a hemorrhagic diathesis.

Unfortunately, although the response to heparin is an important pharmacologic tool in demonstrating the presence of disseminated intravascular coagulation, it has not prevented death in some patients. It should be emphasized that disseminated intravascular coagulation is an intermediary mechanism of disease behind which there is always a fundamental etiologic agent. Ideally, the best treatment is that directed toward the etiologic agent or the prevention of the underlying disease process.

In the case of neoplastic processes, it is likely that the inexorable lethal effects will not be greatly affected by therapy directed against disseminated intravascular coagulation. The most that can be hoped for is a slight prolongation of life.

From the practical as well as the theoretical standpoint, the pathogenesis of the clotting episode in these diseases is of great interest. The evidence so far suggests that there are multiple mechanisms which trigger the clotting. These mechanisms are mentioned below.

BACTEREMIA.   Endotoxemia is a frequent cause of intravascular coagulation in terminal disease. In myelogenous leukemias, the immature granulocytes are incapable of phagocytizing either bacteria or endotoxin, and this allows proliferation of bacterial cells in tissues such as the lungs and in the blood stream. Infections in various local sites are frequent in these cases. In patients with other forms of leukemias (lymphocytic or monocytic), there is also a high incidence of bacteremia. In these cases, the increased susceptibility is due to the crowding of the marrow by leukemic cells with a granulocytopenia due to myelophthisis. Endotoxemia can be a major cause of disseminated intravascular coagulation in leukemias and, in the analysis of any single case, must be ruled out before any other mechanism can be adduced.

TISSUE THROMBOPLASTIN.   Most tissues of the body contain complete (tissue) thromboplastin, and there are several conditions in man in which the exposure of the bloodstream to tissue thromboplastin results in intravascular coagulation. Invasion of the bloodstream by cancer is the most frequent situation.[4] When the cancer cells die within the bloodstream they release tissue thromboplastin into the plasma.

Since leukemia is a neoplastic disease, one might expect that leukemic cells might similarly be the source of a clot-promoting agent when they die within the circulation. Although the studies are far from complete, we have found evidence of tissue thromboplastin only in the leukemic cells of one case of promyelocytic leukemia. It seems quite likely that these cells are responsible for the intravascular coagulation in this type of leukemia. However, examination of cells in one or two cases of acute and chronic lymphocytic and myelogenous leukemia have failed to show evidence of tissue thromboplastin by use of the partial thromboplastin time.

PARTIAL THROMBOPLASTIN.   Extracts of normal leukocytes of rabbits and man shorten the partial thromboplastin time to about the same extent as platelet factor 3 or substitutes for platelet factor 3 such as inosithin and Thrombofax. For want of a better name, this is called partial thromboplastin. We have observed such a material in the cells of one or two cases of lymphocytic and chronic myelogenous leukemia. A similar activity has been reported for extracts of horse eosinophils.

The role of partial thromboplastin in triggering intravascular coagulation is problematic. When substances such as platelet factor 3 or other phospholipid substitutes are infused into experimental animals, there is a slight reduction in the levels of circulating platelets and fibrinogen. This suggests the induction of a minor degree of intravascular clotting. However, we have never observed capillary thrombi in these experiments.[28] Therefore, it seems unlikely that such a material derived from the breakdown of normal leukocytes or of certain leukemic cells could be the sole cause of the observed intravascular clotting in these cases, although it might be contributory.

PARTICULATE MATTER.   Particulate matter and certain foreign colloidal substances are capable of triggering the clotting mechanism. These agents act by causing platelet agglutination *pari passu* with activation of Hageman Factor.

Eosinophils contain large granules which, under the electron microscope, have a dense central shaft. It has been demonstrated[29] that when eosinophils are destroyed they release Charcot-Leyden crystals. These granules and/or crystals, released in relatively large amounts in eosinophilic leukemia, may be responsible for the clotting in these patients.

ENDOTHELIAL DAMAGE.   There are several diseases in which endothelial damage in the microcirculation seems to be the trigger mechanism of disseminated intravascular coagulation. Among the leukemias we have studied, the case of reticulum cell sarcoma or histiocytic leukemia presents good evidence that this was the mechanism. The neoplastic cells were found closely adherent to and beneath the endothelium of these vessels that were thrombosed. This phenomenon was not observed in any other type of leukemia.

THROMBOCYTHEMIA.   Increase in the number of circulating platelets occurs in polycythemia vera, hemorrhagic thrombocythemia, and in rare cases of myelogenous leukemia. With the increase of platelets in the circulating blood, an increased number of platelets is being destroyed in the circulation. The consequence is a release of an increased amount of platelet phospholipid (partial thromboplastin) into the circulation. Although partial thromboplastin is not considered a substance that can trigger blood coagulation by itself, we have observed in animal experiments that infusion of platelet factor 3 and artificial substitutes for platelet factor 3 are capable of reducing the levels of circulating fibrinogen. Even though thrombi were not formed in these experiments, the decreased fibrinogen level indicates a mild stimulus to clotting in vivo.

Stasis may occur due to the increased viscosity of the blood in these diseases and may be the vascular factor determining the localization of the thrombi.

Results

Although several types of cells were seen within the tumor, the dominant type was a relatively mature smooth muscle cell. Sections from these tumors in multiple locations repeatedly demonstrated a large branched smooth muscle cell in which the nucleus appeared to occupy approximately 50 percent of the total volume. The cytoplasm was electron dense, limited by a basement membrane and contained myofilaments, fusiform bodies, and many micropinocytotic vesicles (Figs. 2, 3, 4). Few strands of granular endoplasmic reticulum and a few mitochondria also were present. There were other cells whose morphology suggested a smooth muscle histogenesis, but they appeared less mature. These cells were characterized by variable numbers of the above characteristic internal organelles, an increased amount of rough endoplasmic reticulum, and increased numbers of mitochondria.

Another group of cells, believed to be fibrocytes (Fig. 5) were characterized by abundant granular endoplasmic reticulum with saccular and tubular outlines, increased numbers of oval mitochondria, and prominent Golgi apparatuses.

A third group of cells, believed to be endothelial (Figs. 6, 7, 8), were characterized by a partial basement membrane, microvilli, numerous pinocytotic vesicles, clusters of fine fibrils including rod-shaped bodies,[4] and varying numbers of lipid droplets.

In many micrographs, clear definition and classification of individual cells could not be made. Small numbers of primitive cells had so few internal organelles that they could not be classified. In other cells, there were cytoplasmic organelles which indicated lines of differentiation other than the dominant pattern within the cell. These immature or abortive structural characteristics support the multipotentiality of the reserve cell. However, it was clear that we were documenting at least three lines of differentiation that included smooth muscle cells, fibrocytes, and endothelial cells. Each of these was associated with its characteristic location or end product. The muscle cells were related to electron microscopically acellular stroma associated with mucopolysaccharides; the fibrocytes were associated with collagen or elastic fibrils; the endothelial cells were associated with lipid accumulation, necrosis, and the linings of small vessels that contained red blood cells.

Discussion

Matsuyama and Ooneda[5] have discussed the histogenesis of primary myxoma of the heart based on electron microscopic examination. They noted a preponderance of electron-dense spindle cells with surrounding basement membranes and central oval large nuclei. Abundant rough endoplasmic reticulum and filamentous elements, in addition to other common organelles, were present in the sarcoplasm. The matrix contained a small amount of collagen, elastic fibers, and diffusely distributed fine electron-dense granules. We have observed the same tumor cells electron microscopically.

In 9 of 11 autopsies on infants under four months of age, islands of myxomatous or myxofibromatous tissue were found in the endocardium near the foramen ovalis with the use of light microscopy.

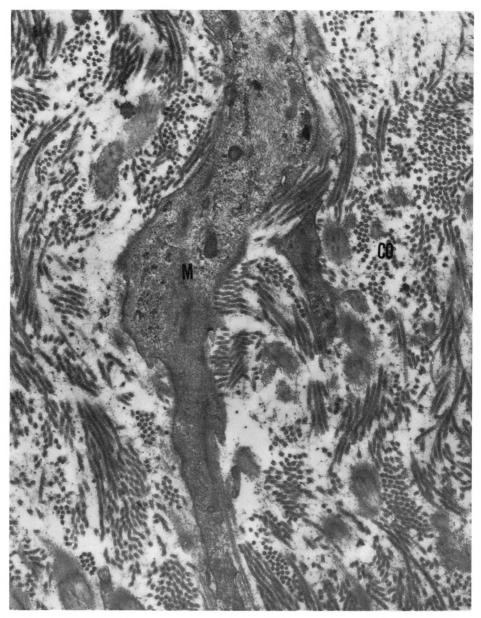

Fig. 2.   Cardiac myxoma. A mature smooth muscle cell is surrounded by collagen fibrils
in mucopolysaccharide-rich stroma. M = smooth muscle cell; CO = collagen. X28,000.

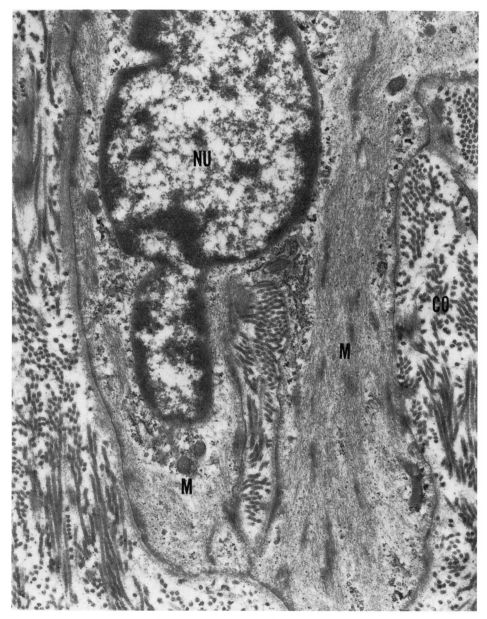

Fig. 3.   Cardiac myxoma. NU = nucleus. X28,000.

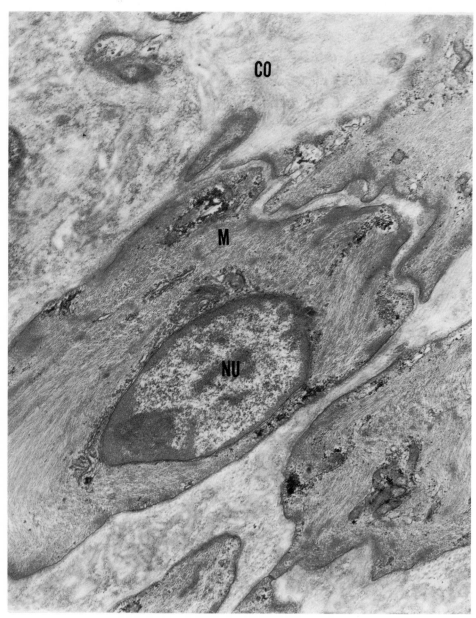

Fig. 4. Cardiac myxoma. The characteristic internal organelles, including myofilaments, fusiform bodies, and micropinocytic vesicles, are demonstrated. X28,000.

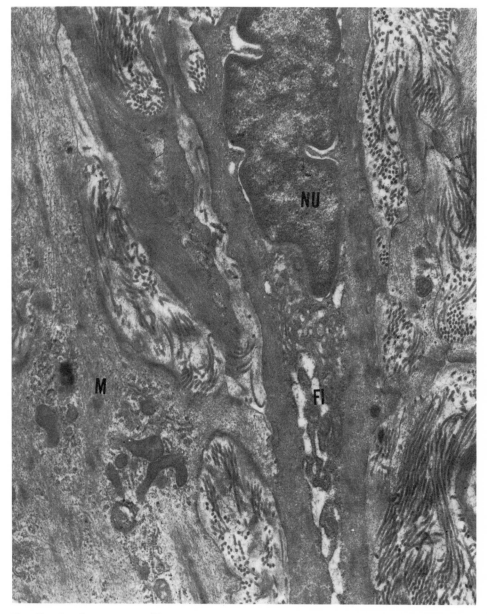

Fig. 5.   Cardiac myxoma. The central elongate cell has the structural characteristics of a fibrocyte embedded in collagen. Nearby a portion of a smooth muscle cell is seen. Fl = fibrocyte. X28,000.

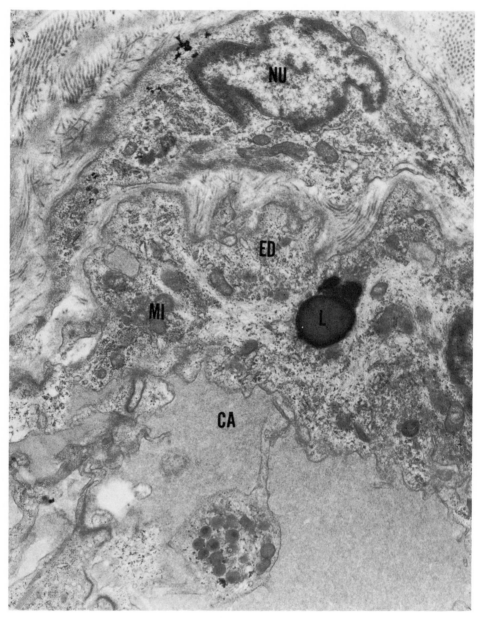

Fig. 6.   Cardiac myxoma. ED = endothelial cell; MI = mitochondria; CA = capillary
lumen; L = lipid. X28,000.

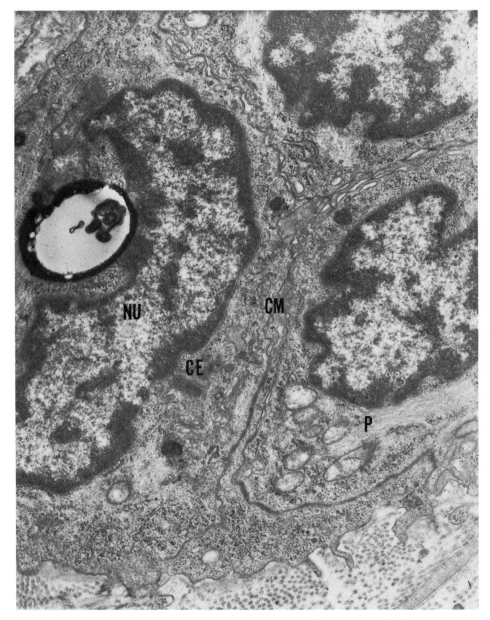

Fig. 7.   Cardiac myxoma. An endothelial cell lining a capillary is seen. In the sarcoplasm there are large lipid droplets. CE = centriole; P = primitive cell; CM = cell membrane. X28,000.

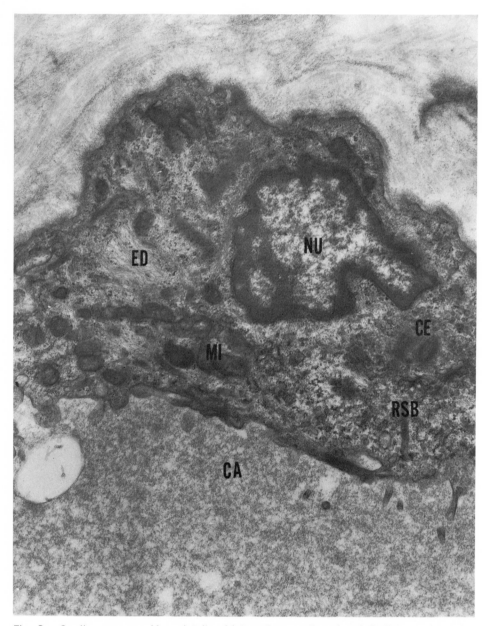

Fig. 8.   Cardiac myxoma. More details of internal organelles of endothelial cells including pinocytic vesicles and rod-shaped bodies. RSB = rod-shaped bodies. X28,000.

Matsuyama and Ooneda[5] concluded that the myxoma was derived from residual islands of embryonal undifferentiated residual tissue in the endocardium, believed to be closely related to embryonal botryoid rhabdomyosarcoma. However, we believe that myxomas represent a benign tumor of the ubiquitous subendothelial vasoformative reserve cell. The residual islands of myxomatous tissue in the endocardium near the fossa ovalis may represent foci of vasoformative reserve cell hyperplasia related to intrauterine flow patterns through the foramen ovale.

Relation to Other Prospective Diseases of the Subendothelial Vasoformative Reserve Cell

To further the concept, we reviewed other vascular lesions characterized electron microscopically by proliferation of these subendothelial reserve cells. In the proliferative phase of the intimal atherosclerotic lesion, the predominant cell electron microscopically is the smooth muscle cell. It has been described in experimental atherosclerosis in the rat,[6, 7] rabbit,[8, 9] dog,[10] and monkey.[11, 12] The smooth muscle cells in the human intimal proliferative lesion have been described by Geer, et al.,[13, 15] Haust, et al.,[14] and Scott, et al.[16]

Electron microscopic studies of the proliferative lesions induced by diet in the rhesus monkey indicated several morphologic type of cells which have been interpreted as being interrelated histogenetically.[11] Clearly evident were mature smooth muscle cells with surrounding basement membrane and electron dense sarcoplasm in which marginal pinocytic vesicles and myofilaments were readily demonstrated. In less mature cells, there were still abundant myofilaments, the hallmark of the smooth muscle cell. Also noted were large lipid-laden cells whose histogenesis could not be definitely related to the smooth muscle cell or to macrophages. In addition, fibroblast-like cells and primitive cells were described. This group of cells closely resembled the cell types seen electron microscopically in the myxomas of the heart.

We collected tissue in the operating room from the thickened whitish endocardium overlying hypertrophied infundibular muscle beneath the pulmonary stenosis of two children with tetralogy of Fallot. Electron microscopic study of this thickened endocardium again demonstrated abundant proliferation of subendothelial cells including numerous smooth muscle cells and fibrocytes (Figs. 9, 10, 11, 12, 13).

We studied a thickened aortic cusp from a 52-year-old patient with rheumatic aortic stenosis. Again, different cells, including smooth muscle cells and fibrocytes, were found within abundant collagen electron microscopically. We also obtained portions of congenitally abnormal stenosed pulmonary valve leaflet from a child with tetralogy of Fallot (Fig. 14). Again, there was abundant proliferative response with different cells, including smooth muscle cells.

Comments on Comparative Histogenesis

Sabin[17, 18] has described embryogenesis of blood vessel walls from the area vasculosa of the yolk sac in chicks. She concluded that angioblasts differentiated from mesenchyme and produced blood vessels, primitive plasma, and red blood cells. Within angioblastic cell masses, the formation of vessels was initiated by marked cytoplasmic vacuolization, death, and liquefaction of central cells, with resultant

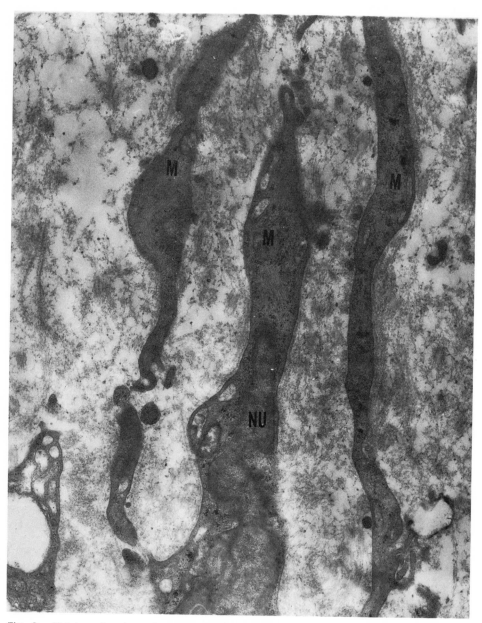

Fig. 9.   Thickened endocardium over hypertrophied infundibular muscle, from tetralogy of Fallot. X28,000.

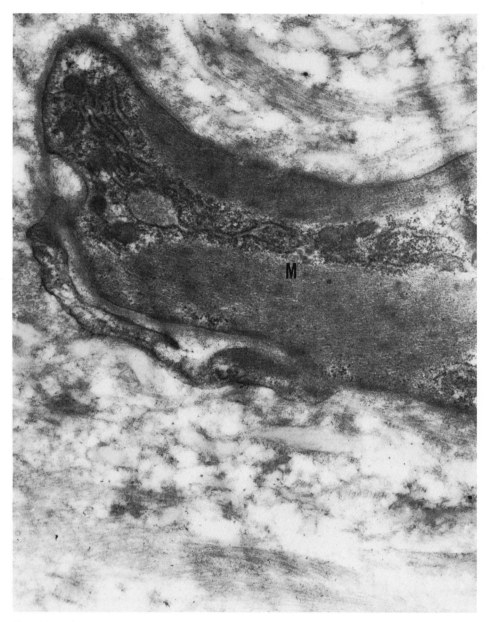

Fig. 10.   Thickened endocardium over hypertrophied infundibular muscle from tetralogy of Fallot. Smooth muscle cells are surrounded by collagen fibrils in mucopolysaccharide-rich stroma. X40,000.

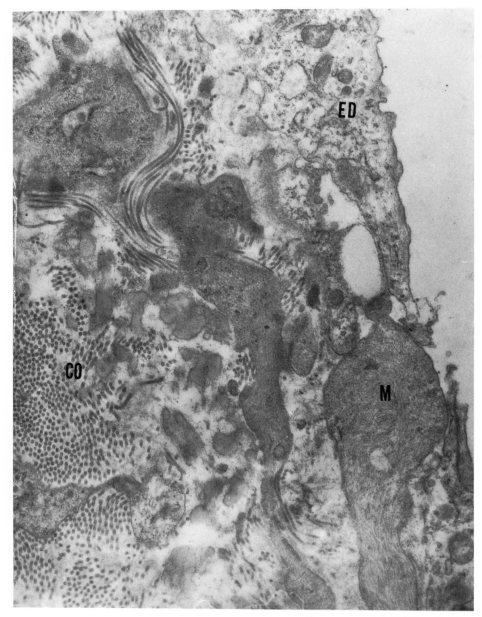

Fig. 11.   Thickened endocardium over hypertrophied infundibular muscle from tetralogy of Fallot. X28,000.

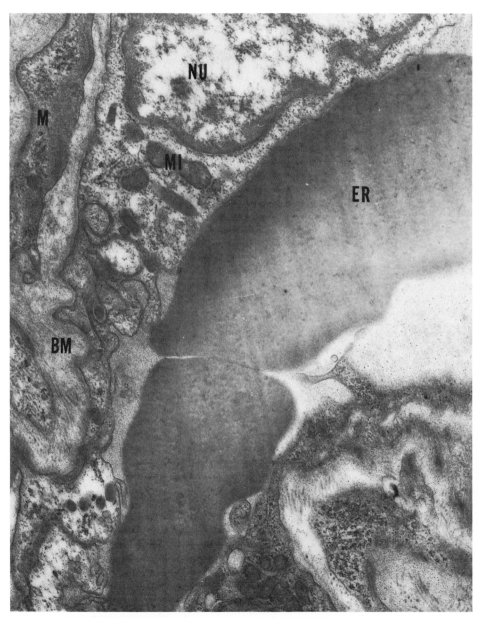

Fig. 12.   Thickened endocardium over hypertrophied infundibular muscle from tetralogy of Fallot. ER = erythrocyte, X28,000.

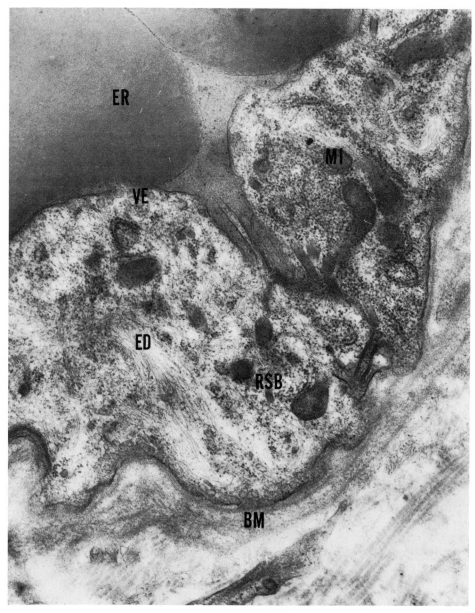

Fig. 13.   Thickened endocardium over hypertrophied infundibular muscle from tetralogy of Fallot. Endothelial cell differentiation can be seen. Foci of varying degrees of maturation are present. BM = basement membrane; VE = pinocytic vesicles. X40,000.

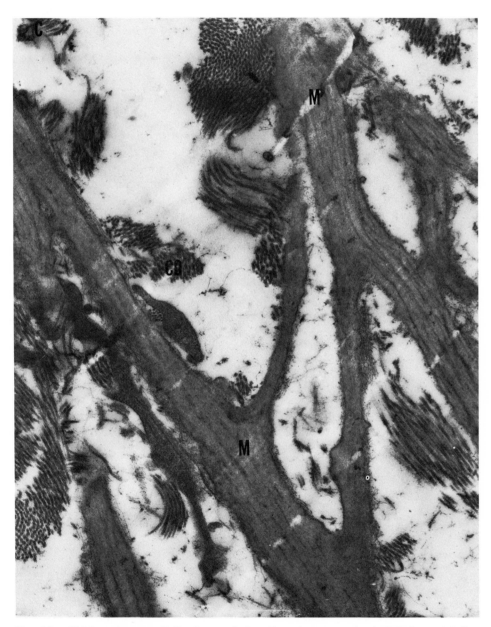

Fig. 14. Thickened congenitally abnormal stenotic pulmonary valve in tetralogy of Fallot. Branching smooth muscle cells are found in abundant mucopolysaccharide stroma. X28,000.

production of primitive plasma. The future lining cells of the vascular channels also developed large eccentric cytoplasmic vacuoles and liquefied until only a rim of granular cytoplasm surrounded an elongated nucleus. Primitive red blood cells were formed from angioblasts and endothelial cells, but this differentiation did not occur before the formation of primitive plasma.

Utilizing these observations, the histogenetic origin of multiple gross variants of hemangioblastoma of the brain have been considered.[19]

Comments on Kinetics of Cell Replacement

In many hollow organs such as the bronchus, cervix, urinary bladder, esophagus, and others, the lining cell is continuously replaced by a sublining multipotent reserve cell. In these different situations, we recognize the concept of reserve cell hyperplasia. In some locations, the foci of reserve cell hyperplasia may persist for years without apparent differentiation or maturation. However, they may undergo spontaneous regression or may show different lines of differentiation with varying degrees of maturation. On the other hand, functional stimulation of the reserve cells with or without cellular hyperplasia may produce a local increase in secretory products.

Generally, at the light microscope level, we recognize differentiation through morphologic structural characteristics and intra- or extra-cellular elements identified by specific or nonspecific histochemical techniques.

There is a multipotent vasoformative reserve cell in the subendothelial layer of vascular channels. This cell appears to be a normal reserve cell required for continuous replacement of the overlying endothelial cells. Numerous studies indicate that, in the early proliferative vasoformative reserve cell intimal response to injury, the subendothelial smooth cells are characterized by the production of mucopolysaccharides.[20, 21, 22] In other areas, or later, there may appear focal deposits of lipid, focal necrosis, and strands of collagen and elastic fibrils. These products, readily demonstrated by light microscopy, are manifestations of different lines of differentiation in the proliferative vasoformative reserve cell response. The interrelation of these variants is schematically represented in Table 2.

Table 2.   Lines of Differentiation of Vasoformative Reserve Cells

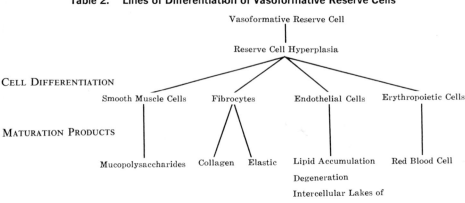

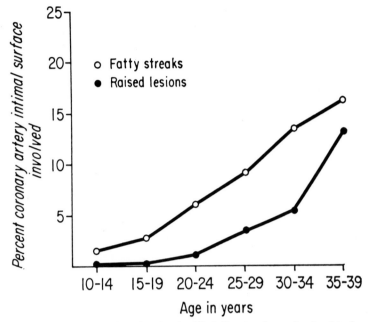

Fig. 2. Percent of intimal surface involved with fatty streaks and raised lesions in Negro males from New Orleans. (From McGill. *Lab. Invest.*, 18:560, 1968. Courtesy of The Williams & Wilkins Co.)

A borderline suggestive association of cancer of the lung with increased severity of atherosclerosis was revealed in this study. No correlation was found between body weight, body height or trunk length, and severity of atherosclerosis.[9] The authors concluded that if obesity by itself is a risk factor in coronary artery disease, then it would seem to act by a mechanism other than by aggravating mural atherogenesis.

Correlation of Severity of Atherosclerosis with Mortality

The severity of atherosclerosis and its correlation with environmental agents revealed a change in the severity of the disease in the populations several years before morbidity and mortality statistics from coronary heart disease reveal any such association.

An especially important contribution of the study was the finding that with few exceptions the ranking of autopsy groups according to the severity of raised atherosclerotic plaques correlated closely with the ranking of the same population by mortality from coronary heart disease.[10] Furthermore, the ranking was similar among the various autopsy groups regardless of sex, arteries evaluated, or the decade being considered.[11] These observations strongly support the prevailing view that environmental factors exert predominant control over the pathogenesis of this disease and that the severity of the disease in the artery wall is closely correlated with the incidence of clinical manifestations.

Reversal of Lesions?

This study also contributed tantalizing facts regarding reversal of atherosclerotic lesions, since in some of the populations aortic fatty lesions tended to diminish
in extent over those seen in earlier decades.[6] This observation could, of course, be a
reflection of changing social and economic patterns of living rather than true reversal of lesions. Since the autopsies were performed in a relatively small span of
years, one could assume that the younger representatives of the postmortem populations had been exposed more heavily early in life to changing mores which cause
acceleration of the atherosclerotic process, such as the consumption of richer diets,
decreasing exercise, increasing use of cigarettes, etc.

Histogenesis and Progression

In one of the most challenging parts of the study, the histologic characteristics
of the atherosclerotic lesions were determined from a standard site in the left
anterior descending coronary artery of 315 males between 10 and 39 years of age
from seven different populations.[12] These seven location-race groups were ranked
according to the mean extent of atherosclerotic lesions in the coronary artery and
aorta as a measure of the tendency of each group to develop atherosclerosis. It was
found that the amount of deposited intimal lipid and the degree of cellular infiltration and of intimal proliferation all helped to predict the disposition toward the
development of severe raised atherosclerotic plaques with fibrous caps later in life.
As will be summarized in the following section of this paper, a similar conclusion
can be made from the study of experimentally induced lesions in animals such as
Rhesus monkeys[13] and swine.[14] In general, the essential features of the histogenesis
of progressive atherosclerosis in the artery wall were proliferation or immigration of
medial cells into the intima and evidence of injury or "irritation" of the artery as
indicated by signs of cell damage and/or inflammation.

Report of First International Symposium

Signs of reaction of the arterial wall to injury, particularly when certain food
fats are fed to experimental animals, were reported in a second monograph on
atherosclerosis published within the last few months. This monograph entitled *Recent Advances in Atherosclerosis* contains the complete proceedings, including the
discussions, of the First International Symposium on Atherosclerosis held in Athens
in June of 1966.[2] Although publication was delayed, it is the only recently available
volume which presents a comprehensive review of recent progress in the study of
this disease. It, too, reflects substantial progress in the understanding of the pathogenesis of this disease.

Epidemiology and Atherosclerosis Control

Two of the epidemiologic studies which are reported in the first section of this
monograph have important implications in terms of pathogenesis, prevention, and

reversal of atherosclerosis. J. J. Groen[15] of Israel reported recent studies indicating that members of the Bedouin population as well as Jewish portworkers and Arab villagers with serum cholesterol levels below 150 mg percent demonstrated a virtual absence of myocardial infarction or coronary heart disease; whereas patients with serum cholesterol in the 200 to 300 mg percent range demonstrated a substantial attack rate from this disease. Groen and his co-workers further interpreted some of the very low attack rates, particularly those in the Bedouin and in the Jewish portworkers, as reflecting the protective effects of habitual vigorous physical exercise combined with diets conducive to low serum lipid levels.[16] They emphasized the predominance of cereals in these diets.

In a most stimulating report, Dr. Jeremiah Stamler[17] presented early results of his long-term study of "high risk" male participants in the Coronary Prevention Evaluation Program of the Board of Health of the City of Chicago which is supported by the Chicago Heart Association and the National Heart Institute. The 6-year mortality rate of the 82 very high-risk participants, who were included in the study and who had followed the multiple recommendations designed to reduce their risk factors, was approximately one-tenth of that of a control group composed of dropouts from the program who had had similar but no more severe risk factor abnormalities. The two death rate figures available at the time of this report were 21.7 per thousand for the treated group and 228.7 for the dropout group (Table 1).

Table 1. Six Year Mortality Rates from Coronary Heart Disease in Very High Risk Participants in the Coronary Prevention Evaluation Program*

GROUP	NUMBER OF MEN	NUMBER OF DEATHS	DEATH RATE	S.E.
All	117	6	108.9	45.3
Non-drop-outs	82	1	21.7	19.8
Drop-outs	35	5	228.7	90.0

* From Stamler, et al. *Progr. Biochem. Pharmacol.*, 4:30, 1968. Courtesy of S. Karger, Basel.

Of the 35 dropouts, five died, all of coronary heart disease. These results must be considered as preliminary, but they are encouraging and certainly demonstrate the ability to maintain free-living, high-risk, middle-aged men in a coronary disease prevention program designed to counteract multiple risk factors on a long-term basis.

Control of Cholesterol Synthesis

In the section on lipid metabolism of intact animals, two contributions—one by C. Bruce Taylor's group of Chicago[18] and one by Professor Börgstrom of Lund which was quoted by Ahrens in his presentation[19]—indicate that two of the long-held opinions regarding the lack of danger in consuming large amounts of dietary cholesterol are probably incorrect. Dr. Taylor reported a virtual absence of depression of hepatic cholesterol synthesis when large amounts of dietary cholesterol are given to man. Dr. Börgstrom's report suggested that there is no effective ceiling for cholesterol absorption in man. He reported that with intakes varying from 150 mg to 2 g of dietary cholesterol per day the same percent of the daily intake was absorbed. This means that at least 600 mg per day can be absorbed from dietary sources. Each of these reports have important implications in terms of pathogenesis, prevention, and the reversal of atherosclerosis in man.

Lipoprotein Deposition in the Artery

Many of the intact artery and tissue culture studies reported in this volume[2] helped reinforce the emerging view that intact lipoproteins, particularly the low-density varieties, make their way into the artery wall[20, 21] and into the pre-existing medial (smooth muscle) mesenchymal cells where a number of important biochemical events take place. These include splitting off the protein moiety of the lipoprotein,[22] further synthesis or at least a change in the fatty acids of the cholesterol ester molecules,[23] and stimulation of synthesis of phospholipid by these arterial wall cells.[23, 24, 25] Furthermore, increasing evidence indicates that the cells of the artery wall, far from being inert and static, have a remarkable capacity for proliferation in response to various kinds of stimuli.[26, 27, 28] This appears to be true of the subintimal smooth muscle cells, the endothelial cells, and the stellate cells of the actual atheromatous lesions. In contrast, endothelial and smooth muscle cells located away from the plaque are rarely labelled by tritiated thymidine and probably divide relatively rarely. Of particular interest was the report by Hollander, Kramsch, and Inoue,[29] whose more recent work will be reviewed later in this report. They have obtained substantial evidence that extractable low-density lipoproteins but not high-density lipoproteins accumulate in the human and experimental atherosclerotic plaque (Table 2).[30] Much of the accumulated cholesterol is deposited

Table 2. Extractable Lipoprotein Content of the Human Aortic Intima with Atherosclerosis*

Content	Low-density fractions			High-density fractions
	$d < 1.063$ mg/g.d.t.	%		d 1.063–1.210 mg/g.d.t.
		$d < 1.019$	d 1.019–1.063	
Lipoprotein content	101	44%	56%	8.6
Total lipid	91	40%	47%	4.3
Total protein	10	4%	9%	4.3

* From Hollander. *Exp. Molec. Path.,* 7:248, 1967. Courtesy of Academic Press, Inc.

intracellularly and still retains its linkage to low-density lipoproteins. The reduced cholesterol specific activity in the plaque, together with radioautographic findings, suggest that there is an impaired transport of arterial cholesterol in the plaques. This metabolic deficiency may play an important role in the accumulation of cholesterol in the arterial intima (Table 3).

Anoxia and Other Factors in Pathogenesis of Atherosclerosis

Studies reported by Abel Robertson[22] indicate that reduced oxygen availability at the cellular level may play an important part in accelerating human atherogenesis

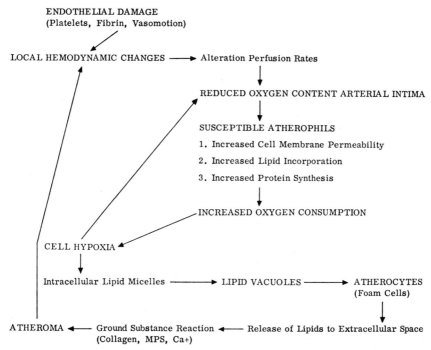

Fig. 3. Reduced oxygen availability at the cellular level and its part in accelerating human atherogenesis by initiating a chain-reaction of self-sustaining metabolic abnormalities. (Lazzarini-Robertson. *Progr. Biochem. Pharmacol.*, 4:305, 1968. Courtesy of S. Karger, Basel.)

by initiating a chain reaction of sustained metabolic abnormalities (Fig. 3). He concludes that many of the theories of pathogenesis of atherosclerosis may be explained by a common denominator of reduced oxygen transport.

There appears to be emerging evidence that enzyme activity in the intact smooth muscle cell is important in determining the overall metabolic activity in the artery wall. The smooth muscle cell appears to be vulnerable to anoxia, and its metabolic activity declines rapidly after various injuries. In fact, Adams et al.[31] have reported that respiratory function is decreased in the senescent aorta. This is correlated with depression of lipolytic and triglyceride degrading enzyme activity.

Table 3. Subcellular Distribution of Intravenously Administered ³H Cholesterol in Aortic Intima of Man Suggests Accumulation in the Arterial Intima*

FRACTION	UNINVOLVED INTIMA			ATHEROSCLEROTIC PLAQUE		
	CHOLESTEROL MG/G.D.T.	³H-CHOLESTEROL CPM/G.D.T.	CHOLESTEROL SP. ACTIVITY	CHOLESTEROL MG/G.D.T.	³H-CHOLESTEROL CPM/G.D.T.	CHOLESTEROL SP. ACTIVITY
Nuclear debris	15.6	8946	573	71.3	7653	107
Mitochondria	2.4	574	239	7.6	1436	189
Microsome	1.5	416	277	13.8	1894	137
Supernatant	3.7	1686	455	50.4	4328	86

A.C. ♀, 34.

* From Hollander, et al. *Progr. Biochem. Pharmacol.*, 4:270, 1968. Courtesy of S. Karger, Basel.

Progressive intimal thickening also impairs the diffusion of oxygen into the inner and middle parts of the media, leading to hypoxic damage of this region.[32]

The thickness of the avascular inner arterial wall in man (0.84 mm to 1.00 mm) borders on a limiting diffusion distance for oxygen. Therefore, this part of the artery is constantly on the verge of anoxia. Furthermore, cholesterol feeding alters respiratory kinetics of the arterial cell. It lowers the efficiency of phosphorylation and depresses the mitochondrion's machinery for fatty acid synthesis. Anaerobic glycolysis then makes the largest contribution to this cell's energy requirement due to inadequate supply of oxygen and deficient "Pasteur effect" in the artery wall.[33]

When middle arterial zones are poorly supplied with oxygen, the activity of many enzymes decline, but lactate dehydrogenase rises.[34] This is compatible with the view that the hypoxic middle layers of the artery wall utilize partial glycolysis for their energy needs. This is also true in the atherosclerotic lesion according to the results of lactate dehydrogenase isoenzyme studies by Lojda and Fric.[35] In a recent article, Zemplenyi[36] explains the relationship between enzymatic disturbances and some events of genesis in atherosclerosis as follows: In arteries susceptible to atherosclerosis, the activity of Krebs cycle enzymes decreases, respiration and oxidative phosphorylation are impaired, so that there is a decreased production of energy rich phosphate bonds and reduced vascular synthetic activity. The result of the above biochemical abnormalities might be expected to be reduced protein and phospholipid synthesis which in turn could result in decreased solubilization of hydrophobic lipids (especially cholesterol) and the decreased removal of "sclerogenic" lipids from the arterial wall. Therefore, Zemplenyi reasons, it appears that the defensive mechanism in the arterial medial cells of the artery wall is reduced, resulting in an unfavorable balance between lipid transportation from plasma and the artery's metabolism.

Other new and informative data which may have a bearing on the pathogenesis of atherosclerosis in man and which were presented for the first time at the Athens Symposium are reported by Beaumont[37] who studied patients who have produced antibodies to their own low-density (beta) lipoproteins. The report by K. W. Walton[38] implicated and also demonstrated connection of the low-density lipoproteins to the pathogenesis of human atherosclerosis both in the male and in the female. Furman, et al.,[39] taking into consideration the importance of the serum lipids, particularly their physical state, in atherogenesis, indicated that androgen-induced reduction in apoliprotein A synthesis (α-lipoproteins) will result in diminution of serum lipoprotein stability and will thus augment atherogenesis.

Effects of Drugs on Reversal of Atherosclerosis

New data on the effects of some of the most promising therapeutic agents were recorded for the first time. Among these was the report by Lars Karlson[40] of Stockholm who reviewed the most recent advances in the understanding of the blood lipid lowering effects of nicotinic acid. It now appears that it lowers lipoprotein concentration by inhibiting the usual free fatty acid supply to the liver from adipose stores, thus resulting in a decrease of lipoprotein synthesis in the liver, which in turn results in decreasing concentrations of lipoproteins in the blood. Gould and

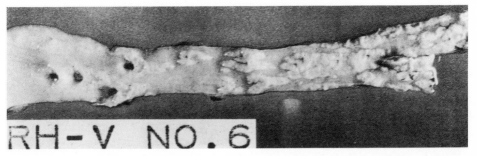

Fig. 4. Severe atherosclerotic lesion in the abdominal aorta of the Rhesus monkey fed a mixture of butterfat and coconut oil. (From Wissler. *Progr. Biochem. Pharmacol.*, 4:378, 1968. Courtesy of S. Karger, Basel.)

Swyryd[41] presented extensive evidence indicating that CPIB (Atromid S) inhibits cholesterol synthesis in the liver at a very early biochemical stage in the conversion of acetate to mevolonate, with no resulting accumulation of any identifiable intermediate in the cholesterol biosynthesis chain. They concluded that the CPIB acts in a manner similar to exogenous cholesterol in inhibiting cholesterol synthesis and thus should be considered as having a physiologic mechanism of action.

Experimental Atherogenesis

Among the reports most pertinent to an understanding of the pathogenesis of atherosclerosis were those which dealt with the development of this disease in primates and nonprimates, both experimentally manipulated and studied in the normal situation. The accelerated development of severe, far advanced atherosclerosis in the Rhesus monkey by pure dietary means involving the use of a mixture of butterfat and coconut oil was documented (Figs. 4, 5).[28] In addition, the importance of certain food fats such as coconut oil and peanut oil in the stimulation

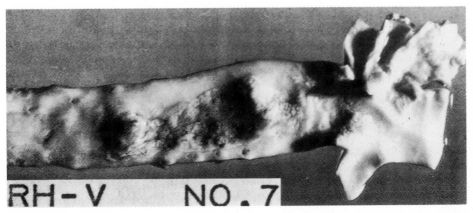

Fig. 5. Severe atherosclerotic lesion in the thoracic aorta of a Rhesus monkey fed a mixture of butterfat and coconut oil. (From Wissler. *Progr. Biochem. Pharmacol.*, 4:378, 1968. Courtesy of S. Karger, Basel.)

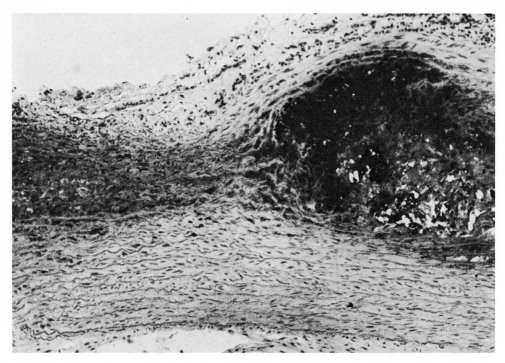

Fig. 6. Photomicrograph of a severe atherosclerotic lesion produced by a diet containing butterfat and coconut oil in the aorta of a Rhesus monkey. Oil Red 0. X 100. (From Wissler. *Progr. Biochem. Pharmacol.*, 4:378, 1968. Courtesy of S. Karger, Basel.)

of arterial medial cells proliferation was reported in several species. These included studies in the squirrel monkey, rabbit, and dog.[42, 43, 44] The ensuing discussion suggested that myristic acid or perhaps lauric acid may be particularly potent in producing this substantial arterial cell reaction. This phenomenon is of considerable practical importance since some populations, notably Scandinavians, are recorded to consume very large amounts of coconut oil. Furthermore, the experimental disease produced by rather simple manipulation of the monkey so closely resembles the complicated and far advanced lesions in man (Figs. 6, 7) that this model may present a promising approach to further studies of methods to additional documentation of the important factors influencing pathogenesis, prevention, and reversal of atherosclerosis.

Platelets, Fibrin and Atherogenesis

There were numerous reports in this monograph which indicates the growing recognition of the substantial role played by platelets and fibrin in the development of the atherosclerotic lesion in man and experimental animals. Although the precise mechanisms are not yet clear, it is becoming more and more evident that platelets or platelet products not only enter the arterial wall, but they may have an important role in unlocking the arterial endothelium so that larger quantities of low-density lipoproteins can be deposited in focal areas. Of particular interest were the results

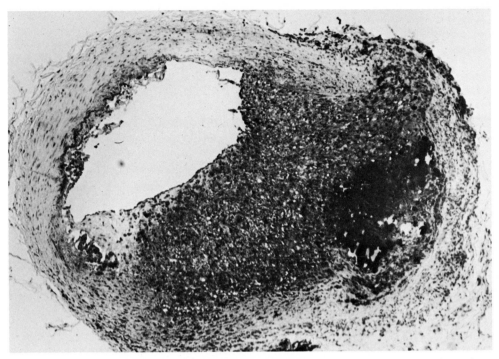

Fig. 7 Photomicrograph of a severe atherosclerotic lesion in the cross section of a major coronary artery of a Rhesus monkey fed a mixture of butterfat and coconut oil. Oil Red 0. X 100. (From Wissler. *Prog. Biochem. Pharmacol.*, 4:378, 1968. Courtesy of S. Karger, Basel.)

summarized by Frazier Mustard[45] which indicate that adenosine diphosphate causes platelet aggregation and appears to be a final common pathway for many stimuli which induce platelet aggregation. He suggests that surfaces such as collagen and particulate matter such as antigen-antibody complexes, viruses and bacteria all induce platelet aggregation (Fig. 8). Further, the interaction of platelets with these stimuli can be inhibited by several "anti-inflammatory" compounds. The electron-microscopic and immunohistochemical studies of "fatty streaks" of the human aorta by M. Daria Haust[46] also implicate fibrin in the early atherosclerotic lesion in man and further support the concept that several blood elements as well as the smooth muscle cell are involved in the development and progression of the fatty lesion.

In general, these studies further emphasize the combined roles of lipoprotein and fibrin (with or without platelet products) in the development of atherosclerosis in man. They also indicate the importance of further studies of the interactions among these substances if we are to understand completely the early pathogenesis of this important disease.

Arterial Localization and Metabolism of Lipid

The importance of lipoprotein inhibition in the development of atherosclerosis has been given a further impetus from the recent work on the composition of the

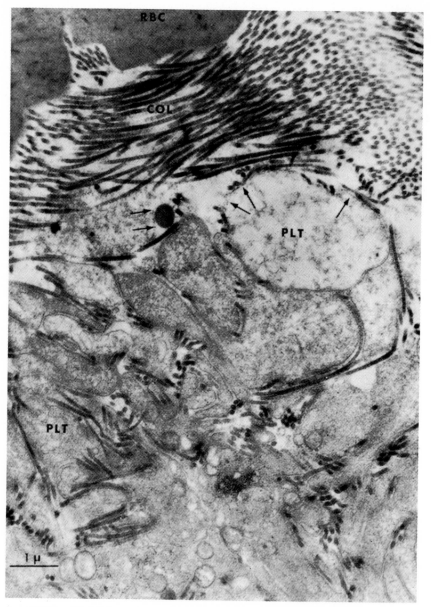

Fig. 8.   Electronmicrograph of the platelets in contact with collagen on an injured vessel wall. X14,500. (From Mustard, et al. *Progr. Biochem. Pharmacol.*, 4:508, 1968. Courtesy of S. Karger, Basel.)

atherosclerotic plaque as compared to normal intima.[30] Hollander[29] and his co-workers have found that the plaque area in both man and dog is much more likely to take up labelled cholesterol than is the normal-looking area (Table 3). Furthermore, they report that the concentration of low-density lipoproteins is about four times as high in atherosclerotic plaques as compared to normal intima, while high density lipoprotein content is comparable in diseased and normal intima. By means of other calculations, it is apparent that low-density to high-density lipoprotein ratios are about 14 to 1 in diseased intima and about 2.5 to 1 in "normal" intima.[30] In contrast, nonprotein bound cholesterol is not readily transportable or metabolizable by the artery; in addition, it is capable of producing substantial inflammation. Studies on the subcellular distribution of intravenously administered tritium-labelled cholesterol in dog and monkey indicated that the uptake is greatest in the microsomal fraction with decreasing amounts in "nuclear debris," mitochondria, and in supernatant fluid.

More recent studies by Hollander[47] indicate the ^{131}I-labelled low-density lipoprotein are also taken up by both the aortic intima and media of the dog. In the intima, much of this appears in the nuclear debris fraction and in the supernatant fluid which may contain some of the "plasma membrane." In the aortic media, the largest proportion of the label appears in the supernatant fluid and lesser quantities are associated with the microsomes, mitochondria, and with the "nuclear debris." Similar results are obtained with samples of femoral artery.

Of equal interest is the fact that over 80 percent of ^{14}C-labelled acetate was incorporated with both the lipid and protein components of the low-density lipoprotein fractions when intimal segments are incubated for eight hours. About three times more ^{14}C acetate was converted into the protein associated with the low-density fraction than in the proteins bound with the high-density fractions. Additional incubation studies with ^{14}C leucine revealed a similar distribution of radioactive protein moieties. In general, the results of these studies by Hollander and his collaborators suggest that lipid and protein components of the low-density lipoprotein fractions are being incorporated into and kept by the artery wall to a much greater extent than those of the high-density fraction.[30, 47, 48]

The studies of Hollander and co-workers also help to increase the evidence that the medial mesenchymal cell of the artery is of critical importance in trapping low-density lipoproteins. In fact, the accumulation of these lipid moieties appears to be of paramount importance in the development of the typical atherosclerotic lesion in man.[48] The importance of localization of low-density lipoprotein in this cell has also been recently supported by new evidence which indicates that the cells in which low-density lipoprotein (and lipid droplets) can be identified by immunohistochemical means are also the same cells which contain myosin.[49, 50] Furthermore, there is increasing evidence that most, if not all, of the cells which proliferate in a number of types of experimentally induced atherosclerosis are modified, lipid-containing, and smooth muscle-containing cells when studied by electronmicroscopy.[51, 52, 53, 54] This concept of a single cell type which responds to injury by means of proliferation and migration, and in some instances by altered synthesis of collagen, elastin, and ground substance, offers an unitarian (Fig. 9) hypothesis for the understanding of the pathogenesis of atherosclerosis.[54, 55] Assuming that this medial cell is more easily injured by accumulating lipid or lipid products than is a histocyte or a fibroblast, this helps one to understand the severe necrosis that is observed in human and non-human primate atherosclerosis, as compared to a relative absence of necrosis in the typical acute foam-cell lesions which have been studied as a part

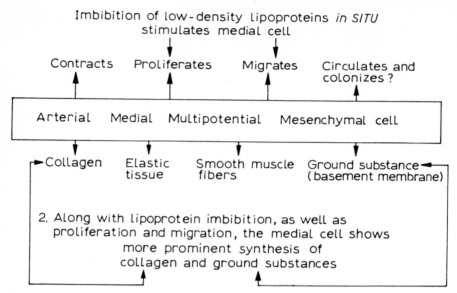

Fig. 9.   Unitarian cellular hypothesis for atherogenesis. (From Wissler. *J. Atheroscler. Res.*, 8:201, 1968. Courtesy of Elsevier Publishing Co., Amsterdam.)

of cholesterol induced generalized xanthomatosis in rabbits and fowl, and to a lesser extent in the cholate-thiouracil-treated, cholesterol-fed rat.[56]

Recently, the major questions which need to be answered about the reaction of the medial cell to this disease have been listed.[49] These include further study of the factors which control the entrance of a number of serum constituents into the arterial medial cell, the factors which stimulate the proliferation and migration of this cell type, identification of the constituents of lipoprotein molecules which are injurious to this cell especially when certain food fats are fed, and the constituents of the lipoprotein molecules which are difficult or impossible for the cells to metabolize. Furthermore, it appears that the mechanisms which can divert the cell from elastin formation to a more abundant collagen or acid mucopolysaccharide formation should be identified.

Thomas and his co-workers[56] have recently reported studies of the pre-proliferative phase of the atherosclerosis in swine fed cholesterol in combination with peanut oil and butter. Observations were made on the abdominal aorta before proliferative lesions became evident. They observed that an increased rate of DNA synthesis in both the intima and media began three days after the experimental dietary regimen was started. At the same time, they observed ultrastructural changes in small clusters of cells in the intima and inner media suggestive of cell damage or even death. Although they did not imply that this pre-proliferative phase always develops into proliferative lesions, it is highly probable that progression by cell multiplication occurs in many cases (Figs. 10, 11).

Imai and Thomas[51] examined and described middle cerebral arteries of young swine fed either a stock or an "atherogenic" diet for 160 days. They observed a transitional state of lesions in the artery between the proliferative and atheromatous

Tamayo, R., Restrepo, C., Robertson, W.P., Salas, Y., Solberg, L.A., Strong, J.P., Tejada, C. and Wainwright, J. General findings of the international atherosclerosis project. Lab. Invest., 18:498, 1968.

6. McGill, H.C., Jr. Fatty streaks in the coronary arteries and aorta. Lab. Invest., 18:560, 1968.

7. Robertson, W.B. and Strong, J.P. Atherosclerosis in persons with hypertension and diabetes mellitus. Lab. Invest., 18:538, 1968.

8. Restrepo, C., Montenegro, M.R., and Solberg, L.A. Atherosclerosis in persons with selected disease. Lab. Invest., 18:552, 1968.

9. Montenegro, M.R., and Solberg, L.A. Obesity, body weight, body length and atherosclerosis. Lab. Invest. 18:594, 1968.

10. Strong, J.P., Solberg, L.A., and Restrepo, C. Atherosclerotic lesions in persons with coronary heart disease. Lab. Invest., 18:537, 1968.

11. Montenegro, M.R., and Strong, J.P. Comparison in four broad causes of death groups. Lab. Invest., 18:503, 1968.

12. Geer, J.C., McGill, H.C., Jr., Robertson, W.B., and Strong, J.P. Histologic characteristics of coronary artery fatty streaks. Lab. Invest., 18:565, 1968.

13. Wissler, R.W., Vesselinovitch, D., Getz, G.A., and Hughes, R.H. Aortic lesions and blood lipids in rhesus monkeys fed three food fats. Fed. Proc., 26:2, 1967.

14. Thomas, W.A., Jones, R.M., and Lee, K.T. Electron microscopy study of pre-atherosclerotic aortas of cholesterol-fed swine. Fed. Proc., 27:575, 1968.

15. Groen, J.J. Recent advances in the epidemiology of atherosclerosis. *In* Progress in Biochemical Pharmacology: Recent Advances in Atherosclerosis, Miras, C.J., Howard, A.N., and Paoletti, R., eds. S. Karger, New York, 1968, Vol. 4, p. 1.

16. Groen, J.J., Dreyfuss, F., and Gutmann, L. Epidemiological, nutritional and sociological studies of atherosclerotic (coronary) heart disease among different ethnic groups in Israel. *In* Progress in Biochemical Pharmacology: Recent Advances in Atherosclerosis, Miras, C.J., Howard, A.N., and Paoletti, R., eds. S. Karger, New York, 1968, Vol. 4, p. 20.

17. Stamler, J., Berkson, D.M., Majonner, L., Lindberg, H.A., Hall, Y., Levinson, M., Burkey, F., Miller, W., Epstein, M.B., and Andelman, S.L. Epidemiological studies on atherosclerotic coronary heart disease: Causative factors and consequent prevention approaches. *In* Progress in Biochemical Pharmacology: Recent Advances in Atherosclerosis, Miras, C.J., Howard, A.N., and Paoletti, R., eds. S. Karger, New York, 1968, Vol. 4, p. 30.

18. Taylor, C.B., Mikkelson, B., Anderson, J.A., and Forman, D.T. Human serum cholesterol synthesis. *In* Progress in Biochemical Pharmacology: Recent Advances in Atherosclerosis, Miras, C.J., Howard, A.N., and Paoletti, R., eds. S. Karger, New York, 1968, Vol. 4, p. 71.

19. Ahrens, E.H., Jr. Studies of cholesterol metabolism in intact organism. *In* Progress in Biochemical Pharmacology: Recent Advances in Atherosclerosis, Miras, C.J., Howard, A.N., and Paoletti, R., eds. S. Karger, New York, 1968, Vol. 4, p. 54.

20. Krut, L.H., and Wilkens, J.H. The filtration of plasma constituents into the wall of the aorta. *In* Progress in Biochemical Pharmacology: Recent Advances in Atherosclerosis, Miras, C.J., Howard, A.N., and Paoletti, R., eds. S. Karger, New York, 1968, Vol. 4, p. 249.

21. Hollander, W., Kramsch, D.M., and Inoue, G. The metabolism of cholesterol, lipoproteins and acid mucopolysaccharides in normal and atherosclerotic vessels. *In* Progress in Biochemical Pharmacology: Recent Advances in Atherosclerosis, Miras, C.J., Howard, A.N., and Paoletti, R., eds. S. Karger, New York, 1968, Vol. 4, p. 270.

22. Robertson, L.A., Jr. Oxygen requirements of the human arterial intima in atherogenesis. *In* Progress in Biochemical Pharmacology: Recent Advances in Atherosclerosis, Miras, C.J., Howard, A.N., and Paoletti, R., eds. S. Karger, New York, 1968, Vol. 4, p. 305.

23. Bowyer, D.E., Howard, A.N., Gresham, G.A., Bates, D., and Palmer, B.V. Aortic perfusion in experimental animals. A system for the study of lipid synthesis and accumulation. *In* Progress in Biochemical Pharmacology: Recent Advances in Atherosclerosis, Miras, C.J., Howard, A.N., and Paoletti, R., eds. S. Karger, New York, 1968, Vol. 4, p. 235.

24. Christensen, S. Intimal uptake of plasma lipoprotein and atherosclerosis. *In* Progress in Biochemical Pharmacology: Recent Advances in Atherosclerosis, Miras, C.J., Howard, A.N., and Paoletti, R., eds. S. Karger, New York, 1968, Vol. 4, p. 244.

25. Billimoria, J.D., and Rothwell, T.J. Factors affecting the synthesis of individual phospholipids in the rat aorta. *In* Progress in Biochemical Pharmacology: Recent Advances in Atherosclerosis, Miras, C.J., Howard, A.N., and Paoletti, R., eds. S. Karger, New York, Vol. 4, 1968, p. 225.

26. Thomas, W.A., Lee, K.T., and Kim, D.N. Metabolic studies of protein synthesis in aortas of monkeys fed atherogenic diet. *In* Progress in Biochemical Pharmacology: Recent Advances in Atherosclerosis, Miras, C.J., Howard, A.N., and Paoletti, R., eds., S. Karger, New York, 1968, Vol. 4, p. 445.

27. McMillan, G.C., and Story, H.C. Radioautographic observations on DNA synthesis in the cells of atherosclerotic lesions of cholesterol-fed rabbits. *In* Progress in Biochemical Pharmacology: Recent Advances in Atherosclerosis, Miras, C.J., Howard, A.N., and Paoletti, R., eds. S. Karger, New York, 1968, Vol. 4, p. 280.

28. Wissler, R.W. Recent progress in studies of experimental primate atherosclerosis. *In* Progress in Biochemical Pharmacology: Recent Advances in Atherosclerosis, Miras, C.J., Howard, A.N., and Paoletti, R., eds. S. Karger, New York, 1968, Vol. 4, p. 378.

29. Hollander, W., Kramsch, D.M., and Inoue, G. The metabolism of cholesterol lipoproteins and acid mucopolysaccharides in normal and atherosclerotic vessels. *In* Progress in Biochemical Pharmacology: Recent Advances in Atherosclerosis, Miras, C.J., Howard, A.N., and Paoletti, R., eds. S. Karger, New York, 1968, Vol. 4, p. 270.

30. Hollander, W. Recent advances in experimental and molecular pathology influx synthesis and transport of arterial lipoproteins in atherosclerosis. Exp. Molec. Path., 7:248, 1967.

31. Adams, C.W.M., Abdulla, Y.H., Bayliss, O.B., Mahler, R.F., and Root, M.A. Quantitative histochemical observations on certain oxidative and lipolytic enzymes in human aortic wall. *In* Progress in Biochemical Pharmacology: Recent Advances in Atherosclerosis, Miras, C.J., Howard, A.N., and Paoletti, R., eds. S. Karger, New York, 1968, Vol. 4, p. 248.

32. Zemplenyi, T., Urhova, O., Urbonova, D., and Kohout, N. Study of factors affecting arterial enzymic activities in man and some animals. *In* Progress in Biochemical Pharmacology: Recent Advances in Atherosclerosis, Miras, C.J., Howard, A.N., and Paoletti, R., eds. S. Karger, New York, 1968, Vol. 4, p. 325.

33. Whereat, A.F. Recent advances in experimental and molecular pathology. Atherosclerosis and metabolic disorders in the arterial wall. Exp. Molec. Path., 7:233, 1967.

34. Adams, C.W.M. Vascular histochemistry. Lloyd-Lecke, London, 1967.

35. Lojda, L., and Fric, P. Lactic dehydrogenase isoenzymes in the aortic wall. J. Atheroscler. Res., 6:264, 1966.

36. Zemplenyi, T. Vascular enzymes and atherosclerosis. J. Atheroscler. Res., 7:725, 1967.

37. Beaumont, J.L. Hyperlipidemia with circulating anti-β-lipoprotein autoantibody in man. Autoimmune hyperlipidemia, its possible role in atherosclerosis. *In* Progress in Biochemical Pharmacology: Recent Advances in Atherosclerosis, Miras, C.J., Howard, A.N., and Paoletti, R., eds. S. Karger, New York, 1968, Vol. 4, p. 110.

38. Walton, K.W. The role of low density lipoproteins in the pathogenesis of human atherosclerosis. *In* Progress in Biochemical Pharmacology: Recent Advances in

Atherosclerosis, Miras, C.J., Howard, A.N., and Paoletti, R., eds. S. Karger, New York, 1968, Vol. 4, p. 159.

39. Furman, R.H., Alaupovic, P., Bradford, R.H., and Howard, R.P. Gonadal hormones, blood lipids and ischemic heart disease. *In* Progress in Biochemical Pharmacology: Recent Advances in Atherosclerosis, Miras, C.J., Howard, A.N., and Paoletti, R., eds. S. Karger, New York, 1968, Vol. 4, p. 334.

40. Carlson, L.A. Recent advances in the metabolism of plasma lipids. *In* Progress in Biochemical Pharmacology: Recent Advances in Atherosclerosis, Miras, C.J., Howard, A.N., and Paoletti, R., eds. S. Karger, New York, 1968, Vol. 4, p. 170.

41. Gould, R.G., and Swyryd, E.A. Metabolism of plasma lipids. *In* Progress in Biochemical Pharmacology: Recent Advances in Atherosclerosis, Miras, C.J., Howard, A.N., and Paoletti, R., eds. S. Karger, New York, 1968, Vol. 4, p. 191.

42. Clarkson, T.B., Bullock, B.C., and Lehner, N.D.M. Pathologic characteristics of atherosclerosis in New World monkeys. *In* Progress in Biochemical Pharmacology: Recent Advances in Atherosclerosis, Miras, C.J., Howard, A.N., and Paoletti, R., eds. S. Karger, New York, 1968, Vol. 4, p. 420.

43. Malmros, H., and Sternby, N.H. Induction of atherosclerosis in dogs by a thiouracil free semisynthetic diet, containing cholesterol and hydrogenated coconut oil. *In* Progress in Biochemical Pharmacology: Recent Advances in Atherosclerosis, Miras, C.J., Howard, A.N., and Paoletti, R., eds. S. Karger, New York, 1968, Vol. 4, p. 182.

44. Kritchevsky, D., and Tepper, S.A. Influence of special fats on experimental atherosclerosis in rabbits. *In* Progress in Biochemical Pharmacology: Recent Advances in Atherosclerosis, Miras, C.J., Howard, A.N., and Paoletti, R., eds. S. Karger, New York, 1968, Vol. 4, p. 474.

45. Mustard, J.F., Glynn, M.F., Jorgensen, L., Nishizawa, E.E., Packham, M.A., and Rowsell, H.C. Recent advances in platelets, blood coagulation factors and thrombosis. *In* Progress in Biochemical Pharmacology: Recent Advances in Atherosclerosis, Miras, C.J., Howard, A.N., and Paoletti, R., eds. S. Karger, New York, 1968, Vol. 4, p. 508.

46. Haust, M.D. Electron microscopic and immunohistochemical studies of fatty streaks in human aorta. *In* Progress in Biochemical Pharmacology: Recent Advances in Atherosclerosis, Miras, C.J., Howard, A.N., and Paoletti, R., eds. S. Karger, New York, 1968, Vol. 4, p. 429.

47. Hollander, W., and Kramsch, D.M. The distribution of intravenously administered (^{3}H) cholesterol in the arteries and other tissues. J. Atheroscler. Res., 7:491, 1967.

48. Kramsch, D.M., Gore, I., and Hollander, W. The distribution of intravenously administered (^{3}H) cholesterol in the arteries and other tissues. J. Atheroscler. Res., 7:501, 1967.

49. Knieriem, H.J., Kao, V.C.Y., and Wissler, R.W. Actomyosin and myosin in the deposition of lipids and serum lipoproteins. AMA Arch. Path., 84:118, 1967.

50. ——— Kao, V.C.Y., and Wissler, R.W. Immunohistochemical administration of smooth muscle cells in human and bovine arteriosclerosis. Amer. J. Path., 50:58, 1967.

51. Imai, H., and Thomas, W.A. Cerebral atherosclerosis in swine: Role of necrosis in progression of diet induced lesions from proliferative to atheromatous. Exp. Molec. Path., 8:330, 1968.

52. Florentin, R.A., and Nam, S.C. Dietary-induced atherosclerosis in miniature swine. I. Gross and light microscopy observations: Time of development and morphologic characteristics of lesions. Exp. Molec. Path., 8:3, 1968.
    Daoud, A.S., Jones, R., and Scott, R.F. I. Electron microscopy observations: characteristics of endothelial and smooth muscle cells in the proliferative lesions and elsewhere in the aorta. Exp. Molec. Path., 8:3, 1968.
    Scott, R.F., and Morrison, E.S. III. Lipid values: Cholesterol, triglyceride and phos-

pholipid and esterified fatty acid values in serum and in aortic intima-media tissue. Exp. Molec. Path., 8:3, 1968.

Kim, D.N., Lee, K.T., and Thomas, W.A. IV. Metabolic studies: *In vitro* protein synthesis by aortic strips from swine fed atherogenic diets. Exp. Molec. Path., 8:3, 1968.

Dodds, W.J., and Miller, K.D. V. Hematologic studies: Clotting factors and related hematologic values. Exp. Molec. Path., 8:3, 1968.

53. Geer, J.C., Catsults, C., McGill, H.C., Jr., Strong, J.P. Fine structure of the baboon fatty streak. Amer. J. Path., 52:265, 1968.

54. Wissler, R.W. The arterial medial cell, smooth muscle or multifunctional mesenchyme. J. Atheroscler. Res., 8:201, 1968.

55. ──── and Vesselinovitch, D. Experimental models of human atherosclerosis. *In* Atherosclerosis: Recent Advances, 1966. New York, New York Academy of Science (in press).

56. Thomas, W.A., Florentin, R.A., Nam, S.C., Kim, D.N., Jones, R.N., and Lee, K.T. "Pre-proliferative phase" of atherosclerosis in swine fed cholesterol. Arch. Path., 1968 (in press).

57. Scott, R.F., Morrison, E.S., Jarmolysch, J., Nam, S.C., Kroms, M., and Coulston, F. Experimental atherosclerosis in rhesus monkeys. I. Gross and light microscopy feature and lipid values in serum and aorta. Exp. Molec. Path., 7:11, 1967.

58. Frederickson, D.S., Levy, R.G., and Lees, R.S. Fat transport in lipoproteins—An integrated approach to mechanisms and disorders. New Eng. J. Med., 276:34, 1967.

59. ──── Levy, R.I., and Lees, R.S. Fat transport in lipoproteins—An integrated approach to mechanisms and disorders (continued). New Eng. J. Med., 276:148, 1967.

60. ──── Levy, R.I., and Lees, R.S. Fat transport in lipoproteins—An integrated approach to mechanisms and disorders (continued). New Eng. J. Med., 276:215, 1967.

61. ──── Levy, R.I., and Lees, R.S. Fat transport in lipoproteins—An integrated approach to mechanisms and disorders (concluded). New Eng. J. Med., 276:273, 1967.

62. Lewes, L.A. Broadening perspectives of electrophoresis as seen from twenty-five years of use at the Cleveland Clinic. Cleveland Clin. Quart., 34:141, 1967.

63. Smithies, O. Zone electrophoresis in starch gels; group variations in the serum proteins of normal human adults. Biochem. J., 61:629, 1955.

64. Raymond, S., Miles, J.L., and Lee, J.C.J. Lipoprotein patterns in acrylamide gel electrophoresis. Science, 151:346, 1966.

65. Margolis, S. Separation and size determination of human serum lipoproteins by agarose gel filtration. J. Lipid Res., 8:501, 1967.

66. International Workshop on Lipoproteins, Chicago. Nature, 219:10, 1968.

67. Sones, F.M. Cine coronary arteriography. Anesth. Analg., 46:499, 1967.

68. Kemp, H.G., Evans, H., Elliott, W.C., and Gorlin, R. Diagnostic accuracy of selective coronary cinearteriography. Circulation, 361:526, 1967.

69. Hermon, M.V., Elliott, W.C., and Gorlin, R. An electrocardiographic, anatomic and metabolic study of zonal myocardial ischemia in coronary heart disease. Circulation, 35:834, 1967.

70. McGill, H.C., Brown, B.W., Gore, I., McMillan, G.C., Pollak, O.J., Robbins, S., Roberts, J.C., and Wissler, R.W. Grading stenosis in the right coronary artery. Circulation, 37:460, 1968.

71. ──── Brown, B.W., Gore, I., McMillan, G., Paterson, J.C., Pollak, O.J., Roberts, J.C., and Wissler, R.W. Grading human atherosclerotic lesions using a panel of photographs. Circulation, 37:455, 1968.

INDEX